ADVANCES IN SURGERY

VOLUME 11

ADVANCES IN SURGERY

ADVANCES *in* SURGERY

EDITOR

CHARLES ROB
Rochester, New York

ASSOCIATE EDITORS

JAMES D. HARDY
Jackson, Mississippi

GEORGE L. JORDAN, JR.
Houston, Texas

WILLIAM P. LONGMIRE, JR.
Los Angeles, California

LLOYD D. MACLEAN
Montreal, Canada

G. THOMAS SHIRES
New York, New York

CLAUDE E. WELCH
Boston, Massachusetts

VOLUME 11 • 1977

YEAR BOOK MEDICAL PUBLISHERS • INC.
CHICAGO • LONDON

Library of Congress Catalog Card Number: 65-29931

International Standard Serial Number: 0065-3411

International Standard Book Number: 0-8151-7365-2

Editor's Preface

THIS 11TH VOLUME OF ADVANCES IN SURGERY contains 10 chapters; 7 by surgeons and one each by an anesthesiologist, a radiologist, and an internist who specializes in chemotherapy and medical oncology. Our policy of selecting as contributors people who are acknowledged authorities has been continued. The general plan has been to provide practical and useful advice for active surgeons and for residents at all levels of training. The 10 subjects chosen for this volume were selected because the Editor and Associate Editors felt that they represented important material at the advancing or changing edge of surgery.

Microsurgery is not new, but it is rapidly expanding into new fields. Doctor R. Daniel of Montreal has dealt with this subject in an instructive and practical way. The Editors believe that as techniques of microsurgery improve and as more experience is gained, surgeons will use microsurgery in other regions of the body and that eventually members of every specialty and division of surgery will be using microsurgical techniques in one form or another.

Four chapters deal with postoperative problems. Doctor J. Carrico in his chapter "Monitoring of the Critically Ill Surgical Patient" provides invaluable advice for all of us who are responsible for the care of a patient in a modern intensive unit. Doctor J. A. Collins, the new Chairman of the Department of Surgery at Stanford University Medical School, presents a splendid review of the acute respiratory distress syndrome. The problems of postoperative drug therapy are reviewed by Doctor F. Colgan who writes from the vantage point of an anesthesiologist specially interested in postoperative care and patient management. Hyperalimentation has always been a difficult field and Doctor J. E. Fischer in an excellent chapter provides sound advice and a review of the current status of this therapeutic modality.

Ultrasound is a diagnostic tool which is safe to use and which is providing more and more information as experience increases. Doctor R. Gramiak describes the theory, technique and value of ultrasound in the diagnosis of abdominal disease. Adjuvant therapy for cancer is at a point in development where general guidelines exist but it is often difficult and sometimes impossible to establish the true place of adjuvant therapy in the management of an individual patient. Doctor John Bennett has done well to state the present place of adjuvant therapy in several forms of cancer. Injuries of the hand have interested surgeons for decades and major advances have been made. Doctor R. Smith in this chapter concentrates upon injuries of the metacarpal bones and their articulations.

Ulcerative colitis and granulomatous disease of the colon have caused more confusion than appears to have been justified. Professor John Goligher of Leeds University in England clarifies this problem. He has been a pioneer in this field and he has written an important chapter.

The management of peripheral arterial embolism improved in a most dramatic manner when Doctor John Cranley and his associates introduced the Fogarty balloon embolectomy catheter. Doctor Cranley, in this chapter "Arterial Embolism," writes not only about conventional arterial embolism but also about microemboli and the prevention and treatment of the problems they cause such as the "Blue Toe Syndrome."

We thank the contributors and believe that they have produced a fine book.

CHARLES ROB

Table of Contents

Hyperalimentation

JOSEF E. FISCHER

Department of Surgery, Massachusetts General Hospital, Boston, Massachusetts

We are at the end of a decade of progress in an area that has seen some of the most significant advances in patient care of this century. It is approximately 10 years since Dudrick, working in Rhoads's laboratory, showed that it was possible to maintain young animals and ultimately patients in reasonable health with parenterally administered nutrition and even to have normal growth under these circumstances.[36] What is surprising, however, is that with the exception of a few workers, nutrition was neglected for as long as it was. Perhaps this was because taking nutrition was so natural that when it stopped no one noticed. In any event, patients have starved and probably succumbed to starvation at a time when perhaps they most required protein and caloric intake.

The casual attitude toward nutrition in hospitals throughout the world is not merely evidenced by unappetizing food delivered cold. The diet kitchen is looked upon as a place where financial savings can easily be achieved. Instead of tempting patients who often are mildly anorectic, the food, if anything, adds to anorexia. Patients are kept on NPO status for the most trivial of tests, tests in which it has not been demonstrated that eating interferes even to the slightest extent. Liquids are given in the form of water with no caloric value, although Wilmore and his co-workers have recently demonstrated that up to 1,000 calories in liquid supplements alone can be administered while achieving adequate fluid intake.[110] For all of these reasons our

1

thoughts about nutrition need to be radically revised as evidence gradually emerges that the maintenance of an adequate nutritional state in patients may not only result in earlier return to function in society, but perhaps contribute significantly to survival as well.

History of Parenteral Nutrition

The first experiments in parenteral administration of nutritious material date back to the 17th century. The first materials that were administered intravenously, besides blood, were milk, oil, wine and other materials of nutritional value. These, however, were administered as the result of occasional insights that cannot even vaguely be considered as part of an overall attack on the problem of malnutrition. Not until the 1930s did the first systematic investigation of protein requirement in illness begin. Abbott, Elman and their co-workers began to experiment with the peripheral administration of casein hydrolysates and 5% dextrose.[30] Others used 10% dextrose in an attempt to increase caloric intake.

The first apparently successful case of parenteral nutrition in an infant was reported in 1944 from the Johns Hopkins University, Department of Pediatrics, when an infant with intractable diarrhea who had been abandoned as unsalvageable was supported for a period of time by means of peripheral protein administration and a homemade concoction of intravenous fat. Over the next decade, with the availability of intravenous fat in Europe, interest in nutrition gradually increased, so that by the early 1960s there emerged a group of workers interested in parenteral nutrition. In the United States, however, the mechanism by which positive caloric and nitrogen balance could be steadily achieved had not emerged.

In 1952 Aubaniac, a French surgeon working in Vietnam, perfected subclavian venipuncture to achieve rapid transfusion in Vietnamese battle casualties. In 1966 Dudrick, working in Rhoads's laboratory, realized that positive nitrogen balance could not be achieved unless 150 calories/gm of nitrogen, a figure suggested by Moore but largely overlooked, could be achieved. He adapted the subclavian administration technique, first to beagle puppies and then, in the first case so managed, to a young baby. Parenteral nutrition was on its way.[25]

Since that time progress has been rapid. After an initial period of claims and counterclaims, it is now realized that both peripheral and central techniques are efficacious and both have their indications. With the realization that the average patient can easily be supported, the next decade will presumably see (as has already begun) a differentiation of parenteral nutrition for patients with different needs. We now realize that patients with renal disease and those with hepatic disease have different requirements. The same may be said for pediatric patients and perhaps for the regrowing patient—the adult who is terribly depleted and must grow his entire lean body mass again. Cardiac failure, burns and massive trauma also may constitute special cases. The next decade may also see the emergence of an actual subspecialty of parenteral nutrition, with increased understanding of the metabolic derangements and nutritional needs of injured patients.

Nutritional Requirements in Disease

It is beyond the scope of this review to go into great detail about the enteral approach to nutritional support in disease. Most of our knowledge of patient requirements is, however, derived from oral intake. In the United States dietary intake is excessive. The adult male, when not doing heavy labor, needs only 2,000 calories. We take in approximately 15% of our calories as protein, approximately 50% as carbohydrate and 35% as fat. These figures obviously vary. For individuals doing heavy manual labor, requirements are increased by 300–600 calories/24 hours. In disease, however, caloric requirements increase. Thus, each degree of fever (Fahrenheit) apparently increases oxygen consumption and presumably energy consumption approximately 7%. While herniorrhaphy changes energy requirements not at all[59] (and may in fact decrease them because the patient is put to bed), operations of slightly greater magnitude, such as cholecystectomy, pyloroplasty and vagotomy, all increase energy requirements by 20–30%. Sepsis, when present, increases energy requirements out of proportion to the fever, and increases of 40–50% above normal in infected patients are not uncommon. These pale by comparison with those of patients with major burns, in whom nitrogen excretions of up to 30 gm are common,[110] reflecting massive catabolism.

RELATIONSHIP BETWEEN ROUTE OF ADMINISTRATION AND REQUIREMENTS.—The enteral route is much more efficacious than the intravenous route in providing calories and nitrogen in the most economical form.[16c] The reasons for this are not entirely clear. Certain metabolic processes are more efficiently carried out when the nutrient enters the portal circulation rather than the systemic circulation. Examples include transamination of certain amino acids, which normally takes place in the wall of the gut, and the metabolic processes engaged in by the liver. It is not surprising, then, that administration of certain amino acids is associated with a 15–20% increase in splanchnic blood flow, much of which is required by the liver for its metabolic processes. The exact amount of "caloric wastage" brought about by intravenous administration is not entirely clear but is estimated to be as high as 50%.[60] This should be taken into account when calculating metabolic requirements for patients. Translated into practice, intravenous calories should exceed estimated oral requirements by 50%.[60]

PROTEIN

The requirement for protein is critical in all considerations of parenteral nutrition. In traumatized, especially septic, patients caloric needs are met by the breakdown of lean body mass. It is said, although supporting data are difficult to find, that when patients lose 40% of their lean body, mass death ensues, generally from pneumonia secondary to catabolism of the muscles of respiration so that the patients cannot clear their own secretions or breathe effectively. Much of the work in calculating protein requirements has been carried out in normal individuals. Whether this information can be applied to patients who are depleted, sick or septic is not clear.

In a series of investigations stretched over 2 decades, Rose and his co-workers defined a group of amino acids they termed essential, i.e., the carbon skeleton could not be synthesized and these amino acids were therefore not synthesized by transamination as the other, "nonessential," amino acids were.[85, 86] These essential amino acids include phenylalanine, methionine, lysine, threonine, tryptophan and the 3 branched chain amino acids, valine, leucine and isoleucine. All of these are critical in the number of metabolic steps. Other amino acids such as arginine and histidine may be required in infants, as histidine almost certainly is,[111] and in renal failure, although plasma amino acid concentrations in patients with short-term renal failure are normal.[6, 15]

The essential amino acids, however, may be synthesized by transamination if the carbon skeleton is provided, as recently demonstrated by Walser et al.[106, 108] The utilization of excess nitrogen, in the form of ammonia or glutamine, or as urea, may thus be accomplished provided the proper metabolic background is present. This will be subsequently discussed in the sections on renal failure and the administration of the alpha-keto acids.

The requirement for protein, however, cannot be viewed as separate from the requirement for calories. Nitrogen retention and equilibrium can be achieved by the use of protein alone in amounts of up to 2 gm of synthetic L-amino acids/kg without the provision of adequate carbohydrate calories.[9, 47] When glucose in the amount of 55 calories/kg is provided, only 0.5 gm of crystalline amino acids is required for nitrogen equilibrium.[9] The fate of the ingested or administered protein is also dependent on the type and number of calories provided. With carbohydrate alone most of the administered protein is incorporated into lean body mass under the influence of insulin. With fat and carbohydrate, however, amino acids are distributed both to the periphery and to the liver, and liver weight and nitrogen increase.[74]

ENDOGENOUS AMINO ACIDS. — Administered or ingested protein does not form the greater part of available amino acids, however, as there is rapid turnover of body protein. Up to 160 gm of free amino acids may be available within the total body pool. It is estimated that only 2% is present within the circulation as free amino acids at any given time. Much of this free amino acid is resynthesized to protein, provided adequate amounts of energy are available. When adequate amounts of energy are not administered, catabolism apparently proceeds unchanged, but synthesis of protein apparently decreases, as after trauma or in the presence of infection. This is not surprising, as protein synthesis is an energy-requiring reaction. Thus, administration of adequate calories is important, not only for the maintenance of lean body mass by the prevention of catabolism, i.e., by the carbohydrate protein-sparing effect, but also to maximize the efficiency of utilization of the administered protein and the reincorporation of endogenously available amino acids into protein.

PLASMA FREE AMINO ACIDS VS MUSCLE FREE AMINO ACIDS. — As just stated, approximately 160 gm of amino acids is available in the rapidly turning over pool of body protein per day. Only 2% of this is present in the circulation as free amino acids. Because of ease of access, plasma amino acid patterns have been widely studied as being indicative of the metabolic state of the patient. It now appears that absolute plasma amino acid patterns do not reflect the static conditions within the muscle pool of free amino acids as estimated by muscle biopsy, nor do changes in plasma amino acid patterns accurately reflect changes either within muscle or, it appears, within the brain.[39, 104] Because of the ease of access, however, plasma amino acids will continue to be widely studied, with the proviso that extrapolation should be cautious with respect to tissue amino acid content.

THE BRANCHED CHAIN AMINO ACIDS. — The branched chain amino acids, valine, leucine and isoleucine, are unique in that they represent a source of energy for muscle capable of providing energy without going through glucose. This becomes of increasing importance when glycogen stores are depleted or, for example, when an intracellular block to the utilization of glucose exists in the presence of sepsis or massive trauma. It is also clear that the branched chain amino acids represent one aspect of critical control of muscle breakdown,[75] a factor that has just begun to be exploited in the treatment of patients. It may be possible, for example, to exert maximal protein sparing with small amounts of amino acids if these are given entirely in the form of the branched chain amino acids.[40a] An application of this principle has recently been applied in the treatment of patients in hepatic failure in whom muscle catabolism may contribute to hepatic encephalopathy. It has been possible in both animals[38] and man[39] to demonstrate a decreased release of endogenous amino acids by providing a solution high in calories and especially high in branched chain amino acids. One would expect that similar benefits will accrue in patients with renal failure, in whom increased survival with better nutrition has been demonstrated,[5] and in patients with sepsis, whose increased requirement for branched chain amino acids has recently been stressed.

CARBOHYDRATE

Glucose is the coin of the realm. Six carbon fragments broken down into 3 carbon fragments, which then enter the Cori cycle, provide a major portion of energy requirements. While other carbohydrates, such as fructose, xylitol and sorbitol, have been utilized as carbohydrate energy sources, especially in Europe, it is reasonable to point out that up to 80% of these administered carbohydrates are converted to glucose prior to utilization. Thus, the argument that other carbohydrates may be more suitable in posttraumatic glucose intolerance rings rather hollow. It makes little sense to administer other carbohydrates, which require energy for transformation into glucose prior to utilization, as opposed to glucose itself with adequate insulin to promote utilization. Thus, while the practice of administering other carbohydrates is widespread in Europe, there appears to be little advantage to introducing this practice into the United States. There are other disadvantages:

1. Fructose, the most widely mentioned of these substrates, is largely converted into glucose. Production of lactate and pyruvate is increased, and fructose, especially in the severely ill and septic patient, has a tendency to provoke lactic acidosis, which, once established, may be fatal.

2. Xylitol, another widely regarded substitute for glucose, is hepatotoxic. The patient with trauma and sepsis is already at risk for hepatic decompensation and does not need the added insult of xylitol.

3. Glucose is relatively easy to measure in all hospitals. This is not the case for other carbohydrates. Fructose and other substances may be detected as reducing substances in the urine, provided glucose oxidase methods for determining urine glucose are not utilized. Glucose oxidase techniques (Dextrostix) will not detect fructose, xylitol and sorbitol. Thus, excessive blood concentrations of these substances are not as easily detected as excessive concentrations of glucose.

Sorbitol and xylitol are not available for intravenous administration in this country, whereas fructose is. Fructose is approximately 3 times as expensive as glucose.

FAT

With the exception of the essential fatty acids, linoleic, linolenic and some of the polyunsaturated fatty acids that the body apparently cannot synthesize except from other unsaturated fatty acids, the presence of fat in the diet may not be essential.

Excessive carbohydrate and protein may ultimately end up as adipose tissue. There are, however, several theoretical advantages for utilizing fat in any intravenous regimen:

1. Fat is part of the normal diet, and there may be beneficial effects of dietary fat of which we are unaware.

2. In its anhydrous form, fat yields 9 calories/gm when totally oxidized as opposed to 3.3 – 4 calories/gm of glucose when totally oxidized.

3. As stated earlier, protein is distributed both to the liver and to the periphery in the presence of fat and carbohydrate, while it is not clear that protein is distributed as much to the liver in the absence of fat.[74]

A number of fat emulsions have been available in the past, but until recently the incidence of anaphylactic reactions, fever, thrombocytopenia, bleeding tendency and other toxic manifestations of administration have by far outweighed any theoretical advantage. More recently, however, what appears to be an excellent fat emulsion, a soybean-egg-phosphatide emulsion, has become available in this country as 10% Intralipid, which may require us to rethink this position.[72, 114] With 10% glucose and amino acids, fat may be administered peripherally for patient support.

It should be made clear at the outset, however, that all lipid systems use glucose for a substantial portion of the calories, and this in part is responsible for some of the confusion concerning the effects of fat. In addition, a certain amount of glycerol is present as a stabilizing agent in the emulsion, and this is easily available as 3 carbon fragments to be rapidly synthesized to glucose. A certain amount of carbohydrate (although small) is therefore available within the lipid emulsion itself. One should also make clear that, whereas in Europe Intralipid is available as a 10% or 20% emulsion (more concentrated in terms of calories), the 20% emulsion is not available in the United States. Thus, all discussions of fat administration must be limited to the 10% solution, with which the advantage of a more concentrated form of calories is lost.

Nor is it clear that fat is protein sparing under all circumstances. Gamble's classic work established the protein-sparing effect of small amounts of glucose.[41] Fat may not spare protein when administered without amino acids.[16] In sick and septic patients, free fatty acid mobilization may be maximal and rates of fat utilization suboptimal. Thus, administration of additional fat when endogenous fat cannot be utilized does not appear to have any salutory effect. This may explain, at least in part, recent publications suggesting that in the presence of a given amount of carbohydrates the added administration of 1,500 calories of fat did not result in decreased urea nitrogen excretion.[65, 66] When equivalent amounts of glucose alone vs glucose plus fat are administered with amino acids, nitrogen excretion is, if anything, greater with fat, although perhaps not significantly.[57a] After 5–7 days adaptation to the use of fat occurs, and the advantage of glucose disappears.

PREVENTION OF ESSENTIAL FATTY ACID DEFICIENCY.—Despite our lack of ability to define indications for use of fat in routine intravenous nutrition, essential fatty acid deficiency may be prevented by the administration of 4–10% of the caloric requirement as Intralipid.[72] Essential fatty acid deficiency has become increasingly recognized both biochemically and clinically in chronically depleted patients on total parenteral nutrition, as in regional enteritis. While it has not been clearly established that essential fatty acid deficiency is injurious, except perhaps to red cell membranes and (to a questionable extent) to wound healing, it seems best to avoid it, as a 500-ml bottle of 10% Intralipid every other day or twice weekly will essentially remove concern about this complication. Equally efficacious prevention of essential fatty acid deficiency will be accomplished by the oral ingestion of any unsaturated oil such as corn, sunflower or safflower oil, in approximately 25–50 ml/day into any orifice in the gastrointestinal tract. Corn oil margarine, which some patients prefer, may be ingested as well. This also has the advantage of being less expensive. In severe cases, intravenous lipid may be required.[16a]

Hormonal Background

As investigations into the area of parenteral nutrition become more sophisticated, inevitably the role of the various hormones becomes an integral part of such investigations. Most agree that in adults insulin is the major known storage hormone. The synthesis of amino acids into muscle is clearly affected by insulin, especially in the presence of adequate carbohydrate calories and protein. The effect of insulin on the liver is not clear, although recent isolated hepatocyte studies[57] as well as studies on liver regeneration following portacaval shunt have indicated that insulin is essential in maintenance of both hepatic morphology and hepatic function.[97] Glucagon has recently been suggested as a catabolic stimulus, or at least a hormone whose elevation is coincident with the catabolic state.[102] Indeed, it has been suggested that insulin-glucagon ratio is a reasonable indication of whether an animal is anabolic or catabolic.[102] This assumption has been recently challenged.[47]

While steroids exert a permissive action for hepatic protein synthesis overall, steroids, especially in excess, contribute to muscle catabolism. Epinephrine and norepinephrine certainly are catabolic stimuli, and their concomitant release with steroids as well as glucagon may have resulted, in part, in the confusion surrounding glucagon as a catabolic agent,[109] although some disagree.[102]

Although glucagon clearly contributes to the glucose resistance in hyperglycemia following trauma, sepsis and perhaps hepatic failure,[93, 94] it is diffucult to ascribe an actual catabolic action to it. The contributions from Jeejeebhoy's group[47] therefore are most welcome, as they appear to have clearly shown that the insulin-glucagon ratio is determined in part by the substrate provided but does not really in itself influence whether the patient goes into nitrogen retention (anabolism) or not. Thus, while glucagon is generally elevated in circumstances when patients are catabolic, Brennan[15] infused glucagon without observing any catabolic effect. A direct effect of glucagon on muscle has not been observed, and it cannot therefore be said that glucagon is a catabolic stimulus. Thus, the insulin-glucagon ratio, while in general reflecting anabolism or catabolism, is not an absolute indicator of these 2 states.

Other Dietary Components

VITAMINS. — Vitamins are an essential part of our diet, performing as cofactors in metabolism. There is comparatively little information concerning the need for vitamins in health and disease, and much of what is available is dated. Estimates of vitamin requirements are periodically published; these are generally based on a revision of preceding estimates. The safest view is that with respect to the relatively nontoxic B and C vita-

TABLE 1.—SUGGESTED DOSAGE OF
VITAMINS DURING SEVERE ILLNESS

	MG/DAY	IV/DAY
Water-soluble		
Thiamine	25	
Riboflavin	25	
Niacin	200	
Pantothenic acid	50	
Pyridoxine	50	
Folic acid*	2.5	
B_{12}†	5	
Ascorbic acid	500–2,000	
Fat-soluble		
A†		5,800
D†		400
E†		
K*	10	

*Inactivated (oxidized) by addition to hypertonic glucose amino acid solutions.
†Sufficient states of these vitamins exist so that deficiency states are unlikely during short-term (2–4 weeks) parenteral nutrition. In practice, however, it is wise to provide them.

mins, increased requirements are present in disease and large excesses may be given with impunity.

With respect to the fat-soluble vitamins, some authorities doubt that they need be given at all. Diseases of excess of vitamins A, D and E do exist and have been observed in patients receiving parenteral nutrition. Thus it seems wise to limit these vitamins, which in general are stored in adequate amounts, to barely above minimal requirements until further data are forthcoming. A table of vitamin dosage is included (Table 1).

TRACE METALS. — Trace metals are another dietary component we take for granted. Here even less is known. Whereas there has been a significant amount of work concerning zinc and its possible importance,[58, 100] we know very little about copper, chromium, selenium, iodine, etc. Most of our knowledge concerning trace metals comes from the development of deficiency states, especially in long-term patients. Thus, requirements for trace metals that have been suggested derive from the study of patients on long-term parenteral nutrition in whom deficiency states have developed (Table 2). This is further discussed under "Complications of Parenteral Nutrition."

TABLE 2.—SUGGESTED INTAKE OF
TRACE METALS*

TRACE ELEMENT†	SALT	INPUT MG	μG	COMMENTS
Zinc	$ZnCl_2$	3		
Copper	$CuSO_4$	1.6		
Manganese	$MnCl_2$	2		
Chromium	$CrCl_3$		2	Trivalent
Selenium			120	
Iodine			120	

*Modified after Jeejeebhoy et al.[55]
†Fe is given intramuscularly once every week or every other week (25 mg).

Present Practice in Parenteral Nutrition

In defining objectives for parenteral nutrition, it seems wiser to accept the more limited goal of maintaining lean body mass rather than the actual repletion of such lean body mass. Non-fluid weight gain has been extensively documented now, but it is not clear, at least to this author, that in routine practice this weight gain represents anything but, in the majority of cases, fat. The fatigue that persists in salvaged, severely depleted patients for as long as 1–2 years suggests that the weight gain initially represents fat and some small amount of lean body mass and that subsequently, with normal nutrition and the passage of time, body composition is extensively reworked to replete lean body mass completely at the expense of the fat that has been laid down. This is a process that takes months, not days, for complete full vigor, stamina and usefulness in society to return.

Even while accepting this more limited goal, present practice consists of administering a protein source, now increasingly the crystalline amino acids instead of the earlier hydrolysates[9] with up to 47% dextrose as a caloric source. The ready availability of crystalline amino acids has made possible the modification of certain solutions for special disease requirements, as in patients with nitrogen intolerance, i.e., renal failure[5, 26] or hepatic failure,[38, 39] or perhaps the altered requirements of pediatric patients[14, 111] and the "regrowing" patient.[98]

The use of Intralipid in significant amounts as part of a regimen depends on location, indications, age of the patient and the individual investigator's feeling about the usefulness of fat.

Indications for Parenteral Nutrition

LIMITATIONS IN USE. — It is a truism that the frequency of the use of total parenteral nutrition (TPN) will depend largely on the safety with which it is used. Thus, indications in different institutions will vary, the most liberal being in institutions where TPN is safe for those "who cannot or will not eat," as originally espoused by Dudrick.[25] A very limited use — in patients in whom it is obvious that some nutrition must be provided to avoid a fatal outcome — will be indicated in institutions whose familiarity with the technique is limited or whose complication rate, especially that of sepsis, is so high as to cast doubt on the value of this therapy. Were it not for the complications of the technique, all patients would "eat" with TPN for the duration of their hospitalization.

An additional consideration, and one that becomes more important with the increased intervention of third-party payers in the practice of American medicine, is cost effectiveness. Crystalline amino acid solutions in glucose are expensive, as is Intralipid. Proper quality control and the prevention of complications require a highly trained parenteral nutrition team, which is also expensive. These potential objections might be more easily overcome if randomized prospective studies[18] had been carried out suggesting that parenteral nutrition increases survival, decreases incapacitation or decreases hospital time. Unfortunately, only a few such studies[5, 51] have been forthcoming in the 1st decade of parenteral nutrition. We apparently are so impressed with the technique that anecdotal experiences are deemed sufficient. The increasing cost of the technique, as well as its potential complications and the objections of third-party payers to paying for costly sophisticated methods of treatment whose efficacy remains unproved, will make the performance of randomized prospective studies imperative in the years to come.

INDICATIONS. — Despite these objections, an order is emerging out of the chaos, and certain things can be stated about the indications for parenteral nutrition. Initially, one must consider not only the patient and his disease, but also his prior nutritional state. All would agree that the aged patient without adequate fat stores, with rampant sepsis and the inability to take anything orally should be treated with TPN. The well-nourished

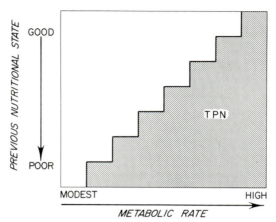

Fig 1.— A concept originally proposed by Dudrick and Winters by which a given patient may be judged as requiring or not requiring total parenteral nutrition *(TPN)*. Note that in the patient who is in previously good nutritional state, a modestly elevated metabolic rate may be tolerated. In contrast, the patient with a previously poor nutritional state should be considered for parenteral nutrition even with relatively modest metabolic demands.

patient, however, with limited deprivation of oral intake and with only moderate catabolism, for example after injury or fracture, may not be one in whom the indications are clear. Taking these factors — the previous nutritional state of the patient and the degree of catabolism — into account, one can arrive at a concept pictured in Figure 1. Another important factor is the age of the patient. With only a moderate degree of catabolism a well-nourished young patient can probably withstand 14 days of peripheral administration of amino acids (with or without dextrose) or dextrose alone without entering a phase of illness from which he could not be retrieved. Above age 60 time becomes more limited, however, and above age 70 it is rare that a patient, unless moderately obese and especially spry, can withstand deprivation of oral intake for longer than 10 days without showing the effects. Lean body mass can be lost to about 35%, after which it is said that death, usually from pneumonia and inability to clear secretions, often results.

It is useful to order indications in respect to what one is trying to achieve and whether parenteral nutrition has any effect on the disease process itself other than nutritional support.

I. Primary therapy
    A. Value appears established
       1. Fistulas
       2. Short bowel syndrome
       3. Renal failure
    B. Value not totally established, but suggestive
       1. Inflammatory bowel disease
         a) Crohn's disease with small bowel involvement
       2. Anorexia nervosa
II. Supportive therapy
    A. Value established
       1. Burns
       2. Radiation enteritis and enteritis secondary to chemo-
         therapy
    B. Value not totally established
       1. Prior to major surgery
       2. Cardiac surgery
       3. Pancreatitis
       4. Major nitrogen loss
       5. Prolonged ileus or stomal dysfunction
       6. Prolonged respiratory failure
    C. Experimental indications
       1. Neoplastic disease
       2. Hepatic failure

Solutions Available

Within the past 5 years the original protein hydrolysate (casein or fibrin) has given way to a profusion of solutions, which seems to increase with each passing year. These solutions include:

1. *Protein hydrolysate.* — According to law, protein need only be hydrolyzed 50% to component amino acids; thus hydrolysates are only 55% hydrolyzed. Since peptides are not utilized when administered directly into the circulation, approximately 45% of the protein administered is wasted and generally excreted in the urine. This has given rise to

2. *Synthetic amino acid solutions.* — These solutions are generally compounded in a composition similar to that of some naturally occurring protein of high biologic value, such as casein,

fibrin or egg albumin. There is less wastage, as there are no peptides and nitrogen equilibrium can be achieved at a much lower infusion rate of L-synthetic amino acids as compared with protein hydrolysates.[9]

3. *Essential amino acids.* — This solution has been extensively used (also in randomized trials) for the treatment of acute renal tubular necrosis, and is apparently associated with an increased survival rate.[1, 4-6, 26] This solution will be commercially available in 1977. It is further discussed under "Renal Failure."

4. *Hepatic formulation.* — This is available only as an experimental solution in several centers. It is a completely different amino acid composition,[38, 39] which seems to be well tolerated without encephalopathy in patients with cirrhosis and hepatic decompensation. This solution requires much study before proof of efficacy and general acceptance.

All 4 of these solutions are generally administered with hypertonic dextrose, in concentrations between 23% and 47%, varying with the disease conditions in which they are given.

5. *Intralipid.* — This is available as a peripheral solution. It has been discussed earlier under "Fat."

Magic Numbers and Limitations in Amount Used

Although one may theoretically consider that any number of calories and any amount of protein may be infused in parenteral nutrition, the amount administered is limited in practice by several considerations, among which are the calorie-nitrogen ratio and the inability of patients to metabolize more than a theoretical limit of glucose and amino acids without toxic consequences.

CALORIE-NITROGEN RATIO. — Synthesis of protein in lean body mass is an energy-consuming process. As stated earlier, this synthesis occurs not only with exogenously administered protein and amino acids, but from the endogenously, internally generated pool of free amino acids. Synthesis in the absence of an external energy supply is decreased; this is probably the site of interaction of parenteral nutrition with the catabolic organism. The calorie-nitrogen ratio required for positive energy balance is generally estimated as between 150 and 250 nonprotein calories/gm of administered nitrogen. It appears, however, that this ratio is not constant but varies at different times of the disease. In renal failure, for example, the value may be much higher, as optimal figures for the decrease in blood urea nitrogen may require calorie-nitrogen ratios as high as 300:1 or even higher. In the moderate catabolic state, a ratio of approximately 200:1 has been adopted by most institutions for their infusions, although 150:1 is probably adequate for most situations. It also seems that later in a patient's course, when catabolism has decreased, a ratio of 100–125:1 is probably adequate and that excessive amounts of glucose may contribute to the deposition of fat in the liver and to the accumulation of fat as opposed to lean body mass.

PROTEIN. – We have previously spoken of an optimal requirement of 0.2–0.24 gm nitrogen/kg in most situations. In severely catabolic patients this figure may be higher. Excessive administration of nitrogen, even in patients with adequate hepatic and renal function, leads to an accumulation of 1 of the 2 nitrogen waste products, urea or ammonia. In neither of these cases do most patients become symptomatic at modest levels of elevation of blood urea nitrogen and ammonia. An occasional elderly patient may manifest disorientation as a consequence of inability to utilize many amino acids, which then accumulate in the circulation and presumably affect the brain. The limit on nitrogen administration is imposed by another factor, the calorie-nitrogen ratio and limitations on the utilization of glucose. This has been variously estimated as 0.8–1.2 gm glucose/minute in most adults. This again depends on the age and the state of the patient, glucose and insulin resistance, the presence or absence of sepsis, state of the pancreas and the ability of the patient to increase secretion of insulin. As there are 1,440 minutes within a 24-hour period, taking the lowest figure, 0.8 gm glucose/minute, 1,100 gm of glucose seems to be the lower limit of the theoretical maximum that can be achieved. This is equivalent to approximately 4.5 L of 23% dextrose solution, which in widespread experience is what most patients can tolerate without hyperglycemia, excessive fatty deposition in the liver and other metabolic complications. Although the theoretical limit for the intravenous administration of glucose has been reached, oral administration of carbohydrate simultaneously with intravenous administration may be associated with a salutory effect, increased weight gain and nitrogen deposition. Apparently the theoretical threshold for glucose applies to intravenous glucose only, and the oral route enables one to achieve levels of 10,000 calories by the combined routes, as for example in burns.[110]

Primary Therapy: Value Established

FISTULAS

Fistulas remain the classic indication for parenteral nutrition, as eating is contraindicated in these patients. Hyperalimentation, as compared with the administration of an elemental diet or normal food, is associated with a marked decrease in intestinal secretion in animals with established fistulas.[112] There is little doubt that complete gut rest may actively aid the spontaneous closure of fistulas. Small bowel fistulas, particularly those of the high-output type, have in the past been associated with an extraordinarily high mortality. In the classic review, published from our institution in 1960, mortality of patients with high-output fistulas ranged between 47 and 62%.[29] Mortality seemed directly related to output and was due to 3 factors: sepsis, malnutrition and electrolyte imbalance. These factors seemed to be interrelated. Sepsis contributed to malnutrition, and output was directly related, with high-output fistulas having the highest incidence of electrolyte imbalance, malnutrition and sepsis. The authors noted that no patient judged to have severe malnutrition (the criteria were a total protein level of less than 4.8 and loss of greater than 25% of the body weight), survived. Sheldon et al.[92a] further recognized the importance of nutrition in these patients and noted that when more than 3,000 calories were provided, mortality fell to 14%. Over the past several years (the "hyperalimentation era"), a number of papers dealing with fistulas and parenteral nutrition have appeared, in which we see that:

1. The spontaneous closure rate appears to have gone up, varying from 31%[8] in our institution to 70% in other reports.[67]

2. Mortality varies widely, from 6% to 21%, depending on the institution and the type of patient.[8, 37, 67, 92a] The differences among these series are easily explained on the basis of:

a) The etiology of the fistulas. Those series with the higher mortality appear to have a higher percentage of postoperative fistulas. In the series with the lowest mortality, 6%, postoperative fistulas constituted approximately 50% of the total.[67]

b) Mortality varied depending on whether each individual fistula was considered as a separate fistula, or whether each patient with a fistula was considered separately.[8, 37, 67, 83, 92a]

c) Mature fistulas are either included or excluded.

Despite this, genuine differences appear in the management of fistulas. In our institution, where spontaneous closure has gone from 10 to 31% with the introduction of hyperalimentation, a review of 119 patients with fistulas treated in the prehyperalimentation era reveals that the mortality was only 15% in 1960–70.[93a]

Thus, much of the decrease in mortality can correctly, at least in our institution, be attributed to better perioperative and intensive care. Sepsis remains the major killer in fistula patients.

In summary, there seems to be little question that spontaneous closure of fistulas has increased with the use of parenteral nutrition. There are certain fistulas that will not close, and criteria have been established suggesting when operative closure should be undertaken.[8, 37] Certain high-output fistulas, particularly those of the ileum, appear less likely to close than those in other areas, such as gastroduodenal fistulas. All in all, parenteral nutrition remains a valuable addition to the armamentarium of fistula therapy but clearly, at least in our experience, is not the entire answer.

THE SHORT BOWEL SYNDROME

The short bowel syndrome may arise in a number of ways, particularly following massive resection for mesenteric thrombosis due to malrotation and volvulus and in patients with regional enteritis who have undergone multiple resective procedures. The advent of parenteral nutrition has been a significant advance in the treatment of these patients. Most of these patients are totally incapable of taking any nourishment by mouth in the early period after operation; even water taken by mouth will provoke profuse diarrhea. Standard management for this group of patients involves no attempt to feed them by mouth for the first 2 months. In patients with minimal amounts of gut remaining, i.e., 6–12 in. of jejunum and only the left colon, it is probably reasonable to assume that "permanent" hyperalimentation on an outpatient basis will be required for a period of at least 1 or 2 years until hypertrophy takes place. Some have

likely to have much effect in renal failure, as previously noted in an early study.[63]

What solution is used when parenteral nutrition is indicated depends on tactics and goals. If it is not clear that routine dialysis is not necessary, essential amino acids and hypertonic dextrose should be started early in an attempt either to delay or to avoid dialysis. In patients with a violated retroperitoneum, such as patients with acute tubular necrosis following resection of a ruptured abdominal aortic aneurysm, amino acids with 47% dextrose may delay the necessity for dialysis until the patient is stable and the retroperitoneum is sealed.[1]

An outstanding problem in the treatment of renal failure is to determine which amino acids are considered essential. Some advocate the addition of arginine and histidine as essential amino acids which, in the presence of renal failure, cannot be synthesized by the body.[11] However, in acute renal failure, amino acid patterns done at this institution suggest that there is no deficiency in plasma histidine and arginine.[6] Once renal failure becomes established and the need for dialysis becomes chronic, both essential and nonessential amino acids will be lost. A rough estimate for hemodialysis is 2.5 gm amino acids/hour of hemodialysis. Once a schedule has been established, both essential and nonessential amino acids should be administered, as this will help prevent protein depletion. The use of a balanced mixture of essential and nonessential amino acids to approximately 35 gm of protein equivalent, as advocated by Lee,[64] presumably will require more frequent dialysis, but there is no evidence that this is a superior program or that increased survival will occur, as has been demonstrated.[5] A slower rate of rise of blood urea nitrogen will be achieved on the basis of administration of only L-essential amino acids, 26 gm protein equivalent/24 hours, as suggested by studies at our institution. It is not clear from various studies how long it will take for nonessential amino acids to be depleted, but studies by Giordano and Giovanetti[43, 44] suggest that protein depletion does not take place even with chronic diets that would generally be considered protein-deficient, i.e., 0.5 gm protein/kg in patients with chronic renal failure.

The mechanisms of these changes remain a somewhat disputed point. Whereas Walser and his colleagues[107] have suggested that urea recycling (the mechanism suggested by Abel and his co-workers[4, 5]) is responsible for only 6% of the effect in patients with chronic renal failure, it is likely that in acute renal failure this mechanism is more important, as with increased catabolism in the setting of acute tubular necrosis it would appear that the amount of broken-down amino acids present in the free amino acid pool is somewhat larger than in the comparatively protein-depleted patient with chronic renal failure. Thus, it is likely that the Giordano principle is more important in the presence of adequate calories in the hypercatabolic state of acute tubular necrosis. Additional work remains to be done, and the place of alpha-keto acids in the therapy of this condition is as yet unclear.[108]

Primary Therapy: Value Not Totally Established

INFLAMMATORY BOWEL DISEASE

The concept of bowel rest in inflammatory bowel disease is a natural one; its purpose is to allow inflammation, bleeding and edema to subside. Options are limited, however, with peripheral, conventional hypocaloric glucose infusions, as protein and calories are required for the healing of bowel lesions as well as to prevent body wasting in prolonged starvation. The use, therefore, of parenteral nutrition in the therapy of inflammatory bowel disease is natural. A number of studies, prospective but not randomized, have now been carried out in inflammatory bowel disease, and it is now possible to make several generalizations.[34, 80, 81]

1. The best results in inflammatory bowel disease are in those patients with regional enteritis confined to the small bowel. A remission rate of as high as 75% has been reported, and this has lasted for approximately 5 years in the longest-studied patient we are aware of.[80]

2. Under the cover of parenteral nutrition, steroids may be tapered to approximately 5–10 mg prednisone/24 hours. With low-dose steroids, remission, even in patients who are admitted with acute obstruction, may last for as long as 5 years. In those few patients in whom a flaring up of disease has occurred, steroids have been tapered completely and omitted, which might well lead to early recurrence of symptoms.[39a]

In granulomatous disease involving the colon a lower remission rate has occurred, whereas in ulcerative colitis the value of parenteral nutrition, especially in hypercatabolic patients, appears to be supportive only. Under such circumstances, earlier discharge, fewer complications and less ileostomy malfunction appear to be the result of parenteral nutrition carried out in patients with ulcerative colitis who subsequently undergo total proctocolectomy.[81] One advantage in the latter situation might be to convert a 2-stage operation, i.e., subtotal colectomy with subsequent proctectomy, into a 1-stage procedure. Although this is a matter of some controversy, a 1-stage operation is desirable. I personally have seen patients whose rectums urgently required removal 1 week following initial subtotal colectomy; these patients failed to respond to the colectomy and continued to bleed or to manifest perirectal sepsis.

ANOREXIA NERVOSA

No one individual interested in parenteral nutrition has an extensive experience with these difficult patients. It seems, however, that what starts as a "voluntary" anorexia develops into a complex pathophysiologic situation and a vicious cycle once the pattern of weakness and anorexia is established. We have had the opportunity to treat several of these patients with parenteral nutrition. It appears that reversal of the cachexia may be part of the process in which the patient's improvement and greater well-being make psychiatric therapy easier and make the patient more tractable. Future studies will be required to verify or negate this hypothesis.

Supportive Therapy: Value Established

BURNS

Large burns represent the epitome of trauma. It is in these patients that the hypercatabolic state reaches its maximum. Basal metabolic requirements 200% of normal are common in patients with major burns, although rarely seen elsewhere. The demands on lean body mass are extraordinary, and urinary excretion of nitrogen may reach 30 gm/24 hours. Indeed, even when 9,000–10,000 calories a day by a combined enteral and parenteral route are achieved, it is not possible to avert the weight loss seen in these massive injuries completely but merely to lessen it.[110]

Numerous energy-linked metabolic derangements have been documented in this group of patients. Thus, Curreri and his co-workers[22] documented increased red cell sodium levels in a group of malnourished burn patients. They interpreted this data as showing an energy deficit of the sodium:potassium adenosine triphosphate (ATP)-dependent sodium pump. When the nutritional deficit was corrected by parenteral nutrition, red cell sodium levels returned to normal, suggesting that the primary defect in allowing sodium to accumulate in the red cell (and presumably in the cells elsewhere) was energy dependent. Similar defects in neutrophil function have also been observed. Since sepsis remains the major killer in burns, any defect in host resistance to infection may be lethal.

Other defects are not quite as apparent, but as costly. With the tremendous catabolic stimulus, these patients may catabolize their lean body mass to the extent that respiratory muscles may be utilized for gluconeogenesis and weaning from a respirator may be impossible. In view of these facts, it is not surprising that there is increased survival in a group of patients with major burns treated with nutritional supplementation as opposed to those treated with standard therapy.[110]

A few words of caution appear appropriate. First, although generally hematogenous seeding of catheters is unusual in the unburned patient and most catheter sepsis appears related to breaks in technique and catheter care,[19, 28, 89, 90] bacteremias in burn patients are so regular and of such virulence that catheter contamination by hematogenous spread is common. Thus, the protocol that is used so successfully in "normal" patients on parenteral nutrition must be radically altered for burn patients.

1. Catheters must be kept in place no longer than 48–72 hours and sites rotated on a regular basis. Since sites of access in severely burned patients may be limited, in our own institution we alter our protocol so that catheters are used for the administration of all fluids, antibiotics and protein supplements, as well as for parenteral nutrition. Lines are changed scrupulously every 48 to 72 hours, and sites may be rotated between the internal jugulars and subclavians. While it is preferable to have lines

through unburned skin, this may only be possible in some patients by using the femoral route. This is at best a poor second choice as compared with catheters terminating in the superior vena cava, and the risk of thrombophlebitis, sepsis and pulmonary embolism is extraordinarily high.

2. One cannot expect parenteral nutrition alone to be sufficient for these severely catabolic patients. Despite their anorexia and despite early malfunction of the gastrointestinal tract, these patients should be "stuffed" like geese. A daily caloric intake of approximately 9,000–10,000 calories, achievable only with difficulty, is a useful target. Wilmore and co-workers have pioneered the concept of never giving fluids of noncaloric value.[110] Fluids are given as juices, frappes or other nutritional materials.

3. A certain caution in the use of fat appears appropriate here. Long el al. could find no effect of 1,500 calories given as 10% Intralipid on urinary nitrogen excretion in patients receiving either suboptimal or optimal amounts of carbohydrates.[65, 66] This experience is supported by the lack of utilization of exogenously administered fat in severely traumatized patients.[49] The reason for this may be that these patients have maximal mobilization of their own free fatty acids, which they do not appear to utilize. The addition of exogenously administered fat merely adds to overload of a system in which fat accumulates.

RADIATION ENTERITIS AND ENTERITIS SECONDARY TO CHEMOTHERAPY

When the gut is poisoned, either by chemotherapeutic agents that prevent the normal replacement of gastrointestinal cells every 36 hours with resulting decreased absorption or by injury, edema and ulceration as well as malfunction secondary to acute radiation damage, one has no alternative but to utilize the parenteral route. Since after a limited period the gastrointestinal tract will recover, supportive parenteral nutrition in this area is a very useful adjunct. There is, however, as will be discussed subsequently, little evidence at the present time that an increased tumor response rate to radiation or chemotherapy will result when patients are treated with simultaneous nutritional support.

Supportive Therapy: Value Not Totally Established

PRIOR TO MAJOR SURGERY

This is perhaps the area where the largest *potential* indication for parenteral nutrition exists. Patients facing major surgery for a variety of reasons, including neoplasms, often have lost a significant amount of weight. While the body economy functions beautifully in an attempt to give the wound primacy and to enable healing at the expense of other tissues, it is not clear that this functions as well in depleted patients.[51] Certainly colonic anastomoses in protein-depleted rats are stronger when these animals are repleted prior to anastomoses. Whether this is applicable clinically remains controversial. As usual, there is a significant margin of error in bodily functions. It is not clear that even in the protein-depleted state a larger percentage of such anastomoses will leak as compared with anastomoses carried out in normally nourished patients. In view of the potential magnitude of the patient population, there is an urgent need for studies to demonstrate a decreased complication rate attributable to malnutrition in this group of patients.

Toward this end, Holter, working in this institution, has carried out a prospective study in which patients with neoplasms who had lost 10–25% of previous body weight were randomized for either perioperative hyperalimentation, beginning 72 hours before surgery and carried out until 1,500 calories were taken by mouth, or standard therapy. These 2 groups in turn were matched for age and operation with a group of patients whose weight loss was minimal or nonexistent.[51] Although the numbers are comparatively small (only 84 patients thus far entered), the results are suggestive. There appears to be a higher incidence of major complications, conceivably interpreted as being secondary to malnutrition, 18% vs. 8% in the control group in a group of patients operated on by the same surgeons. Parenteral nutrition carried out in perioperative fashion (probably for too short a period but carried out in this fashion for economic reasons) appeared to shift the complication rate from its elevated percentage back toward, but not to, normal. If this trend continues and becomes statistically significant, we may find that a large group of patients who have lost a significant amount of weight and are faced with major surgery may benefit from perioperative parenteral nutrition carried out pre- and perioperatively. Even if this is the case in the slightly malnourished patient, it says almost nothing about a similar practice if carried out in a patient with normal nutrition upon presentation. Much additional work remains to be done in this area.

CARDIAC SURGERY

The patient with end stage chronic rheumatic heart disease often manifests cardiac cachexia, a poorly understood chronic disease state in which low cardiac output, presumably low perfusion and low provision of nutrients to various tissues results in an accumulation of edema and a decrease in lean body mass. Since the operative mortality in this group of patients is high, any improvement secondary to nutritional therapy would be most welcome and appropriate. Toward this end, Abel and his co-workers carried out a prospective randomized study in 64 patients with "cardiac cachexia" undergoing cardiac surgery.[3] These patients constituted approximately 3% of the total group at risk. Parenteral nutrition was begun on the day of operation and carried out until patients had either been weaned from the respirator or were able to take a significant amount of their nutrition by mouth. While the rate of complications in this group of patients was low, as no damage was done even to the patients with prostheses in place, no clear discernible benefit was obtained in this group of patients as reflected either in time respiratory support required or other functions. Another report, in which 3 patients with severe trivalvular disease were parenterally nourished prior to operation and all survived, can be taken as anecdotal.[42a] Larger numbers of patients need to be included in such studies with prospective randomization. The complications of parenteral nutrition must be balanced against any benefit, real or imagined, as reflects either survival or morbidity following such operations. At the present writing no such study exists.

PANCREATITIS

Severe pancreatitis with interruption of gastrointestinal function represents a reasonable indication for parenteral nutrition.

One could further argue that as parenteral nutrition decreases exocrine pancreatic function, such therapy might even ameliorate severe pancreatitis. In a recent report, Goodgame and Fischer retrospectively reviewed 46 patients with severe pancreatitis.[46] These patients constituted 11% of the total population at risk admitted with pancreatitis over the years 1972–74, and represented by far the most severe end of the spectrum of severe pancreatitis. Parenteral nutrition was undertaken generally within 4 or 5 days of admission, and one may argue that this was too late to affect the course of pancreatitis. No effect was discerned on the active process of pancreatitis itself, other than that these patients could be supported nutritionally for up to 3 or 4 months. Disturbingly, catheter sepsis was significantly higher in this group of patients, at least early in their course, as compared with the general patient population at this institution. While it would be attractive to presume that parenteral nutrition would beneficially affect the course in this group of patients, no such data were derived. Again, this might be the subject of a prospective randomized study. Nonetheless, in the patient whose gastrointestinal tract cannot be utilized for prolonged periods of time and in whom no other means of nutrition is available, prolonged parenteral nutrition may be lifesaving. One cannot say, however, that parenteral nutrition directly and beneficially affects the course of pancreatitis.

MAJOR NITROGEN LOSS

This group includes patients with major trauma, large open wounds, large decubiti, etc. The catabolic stimulus is severe. One would presume that parenteral nutrition might have a beneficial effect on the course of such disease states. Again, unfortunately, no studies are available at the present time. While one will argue that these patients must be fed and maintained, it is not clear that absence of all but minimal intake over a period of 2 weeks, for example, in patients suffering trauma, results in greater morbidity/mortality as compared with patients treated by parenteral infusions over this period of time. Here again, common sense is no substitute for data. Were we dealing with a completely innocuous technique, we might feel free to utilize this or similar techniques in all patients. Since this is not the case, here again, despite the fact that logic dictates one should support these patients, who perhaps would recuperate faster with parenteral nutrition following major trauma, caution must be exercised. The author is aware of no studies that demonstrate that this is the case. As is so often the situation in parenteral nutrition, one assumes, since we normally eat, that patients, especially with injuries, should be nourished, especially if oral intake is interfered with for a prolonged period of time. How long that period of time is and *whether this makes any difference in outcome* is not clear at the present time. The same may be said for the next group.

PROLONGED ILEUS OR STOMAL DYSFUNCTION

This is not an uncommon situation. An elderly patient may undergo sigmoid resection and may not have a bowel action for a week, during which time oral intake is omitted. A traumatic operation of moderate magnitude has been added to 3 days of bowel preparation, and thus 10 days of starvation result in a patient who can ill afford it. If ileus persists, one is tempted to begin hyperalimentation. In the best sense this may help prevent pneumonia, immobility thrombophlebitis, decubiti, etc. Although this is logical, again one is utilizing a potentially dangerous technique to make the surgeon, and only secondarily perhaps the patient, feel better. With stomal dysfunction following Billroth II gastrectomy, however, one may have little alternative but to provide the patient with parenteral nutrition during the period, sometimes 3–5 weeks, before the stomal edema subsides and the gastrojejunostomy begins functioning. Under such circumstances, in the absence of sepsis such patients (especially those supplemented with albumin) have survived in the past — however, in a weakened state. Whether they return to function in society sooner or whether their convalescence is more rapid with parenteral nutrition is not clear; more data are necessary.

PROLONGED RESPIRATORY FAILURE

As prolonged respiratory support becomes more common and sophisticated the need for nutritional support becomes mandatory. It is my feeling that many patients who are unable to "wean" from the respirator cannot do so because their muscles of respiration are simply not strong enough to support them following prolonged catabolism and use for gluconeogenesis in starvation. Thus, nutritional support to prevent breakdown of the muscles of respiration is essential. In addition, if we knew a bit more about the metabolism of the lung and its preferred nutritional requirements, possibly we might find that provision of adequate nutrition to the lung will aid its recovery from respiratory insufficiency. In the present state of the art this is not possible, and one can merely say that nutritional support to patients on prolonged respiratory assistance is probably essential but has certainly not been established. Again, more data are needed.

Supportive Therapy: Experimental Indications

Neoplastic Disease

If we define neoplastic disease in its largest sense, that is, a group of cells that has escaped from normal homeostatic control, it follows that in injury the wound no longer has primacy. The necessity for nutritional supplementation in neoplastic disease becomes more understandable. If the wound can no longer command the mobilization of all the amino acids and other beneficial factors it usually has available for healing, perhaps adding nutritional support will circumvent the tumor and allow normal wound healing to take place. But the situation becomes much more complicated. On the one hand, there are certainly many patients with neoplasms who die of starvation, the neoplasm taking needed nutrients from the patient. If this cycle can be broken, patients might well do better with whatever therapy is desired. Secondly, malnutrition certainly appears to contribute to the anergy that occurs in the late stages of cancer.[20, 28] This is not to say, however, that the reversal of such anergy means that such patients will tolerate treatment to a better extent, although this has been suggested.[19, 28] Thirdly, there is the spectre of the fear that providing nutrition to the patient will also nourish the cancer. Some experiments suggest that increased tumor growth accompanied increased body weight when adequate nutrition was provided to animals with cancer.[98]

One can identify several groups of patients with malignancy who might potentially benefit from parenteral nutrition:

1. Those patients who have lost a great deal of weight and are

about to undergo radical surgical procedures. These have been previously discussed, and benefits of parenteral nutrition appear likely here, although not definitely proved.[51]

2. Patients who have lost immunologic competence on the basis of malnutrition and in whom the return of immunologic competence might enable them to withstand their tumors better. This remains entirely theoretical. There is no evidence, to the author's knowledge, at the present time that the return of immunologic competence to such patients will signify anything other than the restoration of reasonable nutrition. It has definitely not been established that the patient will be able to deal better with his tumor.

3. Patients who have been denied chemotherapy and radiation therapy for widespread neoplastic disease because of malnutrition. It is in this group that most of the present work has been done.[19, 20, 28] It has been established that parenteral nutrition can be done safely even in patients with low white cell counts who are at risk for sepsis.[19] It has also been demonstrated that there is at least a small group of patients to whom chemotherapy and radiotherapy would have previously been denied who become candidates for such therapy and, presumably, some have benefited from treatment.[20] However, these patients do not constitute all the patients at risk, and indeed there remains a large group of patients in whom neither parenteral nutrition nor any nutritional supplementation can reverse the course of the disease. Anergy remains; the patients continue to deteriorate despite large amounts of calories and nutrients and succumb to cancer. Whether these patients would benefit from altered nutritional supplementation is not clear. This, however, leaves the 2 major questions unanswered. These are:

a) In patients in whom malnutrition and anergy have been reversed and who are now candidates for chemotherapy and radiation therapy, is the remission obtained justified in view of the expense? The statistics themselves give one pause. Of those patients who responded, remission, as defined by a decrease in the tumor mass of approximately 50%, occurred in only 40%. The mean duration of remission was approximately 6 months.[28]

b) The second and larger question is whether or not response to chemotherapy or radiation therapy will be better if nutrition is provided to the patient to (1) stimulate his immunologic competence, (2) perhaps make the tumor grow faster so that the cells that are in the mitotic phase (traditionally the most sensitive cells of the tumor) might be more vulnerable. Clearly, this question is by far the most important and can only be addressed in a randomized, prospective double-blind study. Whether or not such studies are possible, due to the large number of variables, is moot. It is, however, a subject worthy of further investigation, and if the answer proves to be affirmative, parenteral nutrition will have a widespread usefulness in the therapy of cancer.

HEPATIC FAILURE

For the patient with hepatic insufficiency, the provision of nutrition may mean the difference between life and death. Furthermore, the patient with hepatic insufficiency poses a classic dilemma in nutrition. While adequate amounts of calories and protein are required, it is specifically the protein of which such patients are intolerant. One suspects but cannot prove that restriction to suboptimal amounts of protein, namely, 40 gm/day, may contribute to the late hepatic failure that follows portacaval shunt complicated by encephalopathy, for example.

In the urban setting of liver disease in the United States, the most common cause of which is alcoholism, we are often confronted with a patient suffering from chronic malnutrition in whom a major surgical catastrophe such as gastrointestinal bleeding has occurred. Both the disease state, e.g., variceal bleeding, and the therapy thereof, portal systemic shunt or variceal ligation, result in further aggravation of the catabolic state. Added to this is the almost inevitable hepatic deterioration that follows[93] any major stress in the patient with liver disease, and one can theoretically make a very good case for parenteral nutrition to try and break this vicious cycle. Unfortunately, these patients often do not tolerate standard forms of protein, and hepatic coma ensues.

This paradoxical situation has been one of the author's major interests, beginning in investigations in the etiology of hepatic coma. Baldessarini and Fischer, studying neurotransmitter changes in the brain, noted that there was an accumulation of serotonin, thought of as an inhibitory neurotransmitter.[10, 36] Depletion of central nervous system norepinephrine, particularly the active pool, was also noted.[24] The correlation of octopamine with the clinical state of encephalopathy has now been confirmed independently by several other laboratories.[33, 61, 69, 88] Subsequently, it became clear that the alterations in CNS neurotransmission were partially the result of alterations in plasma and thus brain-neutral amino acids, those that controlled in part the normal synthesis of adrenergic neurotransmitters. These include the aromatic amino acids phenylalanine, tyrosine and tryptophan, which compete for entry across the blood-brain barrier with the branched chain amino acids valine, leucine and isoleucine.[76] Derangements in plasma amino acid pattern in patients with hepatic decompensation are long known.[35, 53, 54, 82, 115] We were surprised to find that encephalopathy correlated, at least initially, with the ratio between the branched chain and the aromatic amino acids for competition across the blood-brain barrier.

While some patients with hepatic insufficiency will tolerate infusions of commercially available synthetic amino acid mixtures with hypertonic dextrose, patients with hepatic encephalopathy do not for the most part.[35] If, however, the deranged plasma amino acid pattern is causally related to hepatic encephalopathy, correcting this pattern might result in improvement in encephalopathy and the ability to nourish these patients properly. Toward this end, a new solution with a completely different amino acid profile — markedly reduced aromatic amino acids and increased branched chain amino acids — was proposed.[38, 39] In preliminary experiments in dogs with end-to-side portacaval shunts, whose plasma amino acid pattern is similar to that in man,[7, 38] this solution proved successful, supporting dogs indefinitely with apparent neurologic normality despite the fact that large amounts of protein were given.[38] In a recent preliminary report, patients with hepatic insufficiency associated with chronic liver disease were amply supported through the period of stress while getting large amounts of protein intravenously, coming out of coma and perhaps improving in hepatic function.[39] Subsequent investigations have confirmed initial impressions of excellent tolerance of large amounts of protein with a corrected amino acid profile. In some patients improvement in hepatic function, such as decrease in bilirubin levels, was associated with nutritional therapy only to be followed by an increase in bilirubin after cessation in therapy. This form of therapy is presently undergoing trial in a randomized prospective study. If it can be proved that patients with hepatic insufficiency demonstrate improved hepatic function and increased survival of various illnesses with nutritional supplementation, this should become a standard part of therapy of all such patients.

Patients with fulminant hepatitis differ, however, from those with chronic cirrhosis and acute decompensation by the marked elevation in plasma aromatic amino acids.[39, 87] Indeed, it has been suggested that the plasma tyrosine concentration may be prognostic. No patient with an elevation of plasma tyrosine above 600% of normal has survived.[87] It is obviously impossible to predict whether this will continue to be so, but the reasoning behind the statement is that the source of the tyrosine is the liver. Leakage of tyrosine of that magnitude indicates severe hepatic damage. In patients with fulminant hepatitis, therefore, infusional techniques are insufficient, and of late we have been combining infusional techniques with dialysis techniques to rid the patient of the tremendous loads of toxic amino acids, with promising results. Similar results have been reported by Gazzard et al.,[42] whose charcoal hemoperfusion, while originally showing promise, subsequently resulted in platelet clumping and release of large amounts of biogenic amines with hypotension and unsatisfactory results. Subsequent "laundering devices" such as hemoperfusion with a polyacrylonitrile membrane[77] may be promising. This is not a small group of patients. Cirrhosis and its complications form the 6th most common cause of death in the United States. Hepatic failure is a common mode of exitus for patients with chronic and prolonged disease and sepsis, even with previously normal hepatic function. This remains a fruitful area for investigation.

Pediatric Use of Parenteral Nutrition

The pediatric patient is often in need of nutrition during the 1st and most important developmental period, particularly if prematurity or a developmental disaster prevent adequate nutrient intake. Many problems in these patients are unique. Small size, tiny vessels, small infusion volume and immature enzyme systems lead to a degree of specialization in parenteral nutrition, especially in premature, 800-gm neonates, in whom there is minimal tolerance of error. Hyperammonemia in neonates[50] is an example of how an immature enzyme system may result in a damaging accumulation of a metabolite that is not a

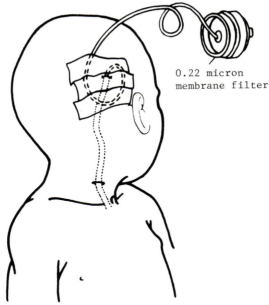

0.22 micron
membrane filter

Fig 3.—Pediatric catheter insertion. Note that in this situation the cutdown is placed in the external jugular and tunneled through the skin from the back of the neck to exit at the top of the head, where it may be kept clean. (From Heird, W. C., et al.: Pediatric Parenteral Nutrition, in Fischer, J. E., (ed.): *Total Parenteral Nutrition* [Boston: Little, Brown & Co., 1976]. Used by permission.)

problem in adults with normal hepatic function. Special insertional techniques are required. Whereas in the adult subclavian or internal jugular catheterization is performed percutaneously, an external jugular cutdown and a long subcutaneous tunnel as pictured in Figure 3 is the most efficacious way of delivering parenteral nutrition in the newborn infant. In patients aged 3 and over the subclavian approach may be attempted. Tolerance of infused volume is considerably less than in adults. Consequently, even in units where pumps are not utilized in adults, pumps are absolutely essential in the pediatric age group.

In addition, there may be an entire set of different metabolic requirements in patients who are rapidly growing.[48, 111] This will be subsequently discussed in respect to the "regrowing adult." Suffice it to say that recent evidence collected by Halliday[48] and subsequently expanded on by Winters[111] shows a remarkable similarity in the requirements of the growing infant to those of the regrowing protein-depleted adult animal. It is possible that the requirement for protein is much higher in the regrowing adult, as in the adult on maintenance alone. Thus, while the corresponding recommended requirement for optimal growth is 0.4 gm nitrogen/kg for the infant and 60 calories/kg in the growing infant, the maintenance requirement in adults is respectively approximately 0.2 – 0.24 gm nitrogen/kg and 45 calories/kg. Some have proposed pediatric solutions with a different amino acid profile.[14] More work will be necessary to verify this.

The infant also appears to differ from the more mature patient in his requirement for fat. Theoretically the requirement for phospholipid and the absolute necessity for avoiding phospholipid depletion is based on the need of the growing brain for phospholipid. Thus, while in the adult essential fatty acid deficiency may manifest itself as a skin rash and perhaps difficulties in wound healing, in the patient aged under 1 year, during which time the most rapid period of brain growth occurs, it is possible that essential fatty acid and phospholipid deficiency may result in mental retardation. Equally disturbing is the possibility that excess as well as deficiency of some critical nutrient may result in brain damage. Sufficient longitudinal follow-up simply does not exist to decide among these possibilities.

Within the surgical realm, however, clear indications for parenteral nutrition occur in these babies, especially those that are premature. Conditions causing inability to feed, as in tracheoesophageal fistula, gastroschisis, ruptured omphalocele, intractable diarrhea and developmental anomalies involving the gastrointestinal tract, all call for parenteral nutrition to tide these children over their surgical catastrophe. Whereas a detailed discussion of the nutritional requirements of children is beyond the scope of this review, the stakes in providing adequate nutrition to the pediatric patient are very gratifying. While the provision of adequate nutrition in the adult may enable a patient crippled with a chronic disease to survive a horrendous catastrophe that leaves him partially disabled, provision of adequate nutrition to a child may enable him to survive a catastrophic illness and lead a normal, productive and useful life. Rarely in the practice of medicine are the rewards as great as in pediatrics in general, and pediatric nutrition in particular.

Practical Aspects of Parenteral Nutrition

After the decision is made to start parenteral nutrition, perhaps the single most important act is catheter insertion. One purpose of a hyperalimentation team is to provide such a service. Some institutions, such as our own, do not attempt to legislate catheter insertion being carried out by members of the team. Most of the house staff and some of the visiting staff place their own catheters. We therefore attempt to protect the patient by prepackaging insertion and dressing kits and putting hyperalimentation carts at strategic intervals throughout the institution so that catheterization can be done safely, efficiently and with aseptic technique. We do not do catheterization in the operating room but carry it out in the patient's room. It is generally advantageous to have one of the hyperalimentation nurses present to make the insertion smoother and simpler and to allay the fears of patients who are understandably nervous about the procedure.

My own preference is for a subclavian catheter, despite the slightly greater incidence of technical complications. My reason for this is that dressing is made easier and the patient is generally more comfortable. Internal jugular catheters will often immobilize the neck of a patient, and some patients will complain bitterly about this. One may obviate this objection by tunneling the jugular catheter over the clavicle so that it exits in the skin in the subclavicular fossa, where secretions do not collect and dressing care is comparatively easier.

Placement of Catheters

Positioning of patients is important. The patient should be placed in the Trendelenburg position at approximately 15 degrees to aid in the filling of the subclavian veins. Arms may be positioned in relaxed fashion at the sides. Most important is the presence of a roll between the shoulder blades, throwing the clavicles back and making it easier to approach the subclavian vein. Placement of the subclavian or internal jugular catheter for hyperalimentation is never an emergency procedure; it should be carried out carefully and in the presence of adequate nursing help. In our institution 1 of the 2 nurses trained in the administration of hyperalimentation will assist in the place-

ment of the subclavian catheter. The landmark for the insertion
of the subclavian catheter is generally 1 cm inferior to the mid-
point (bend) in the clavicle. After carefully prepping the area
with acetone, iodine and alcohol, leaving the alcohol on the skin
for approximately 2 minutes, careful draping of the area should
be carried out. The inserter should be gloved, gowned and
masked. All other individuals in the room should be masked.
The skin wheal is raised with a syringe and 2% Xylocaine infiltrated in the expected path of the needle and along the periosteum of the clavicle. In general, I prefer to locate the subclavian
vein with the no. 22 needle that has been used for infiltrating
the Xylocaine. When the subclavian vein is located, a no. 14
needle used to pass the catheter may then be inserted in a similar axis, and probing with a large, potentially dangerous needle
may be avoided.

Several important technical points should be noted. First, the
subclavian vein is the most anterior structure in the thoracic
inlet (Fig 4). It runs behind the proximal third of the clavicle and
is separated from the subclavian artery by the scalenus anterior
muscle. The brachial plexus and the apex of the lung are generally posterior to the subclavian artery. Thus, if the needle is kept

Fig 4.—The subclavian vein is the most anterior structure in the thoracic inlet. If
the needle is kept anterior, it will not hit other more vulnerable structures.

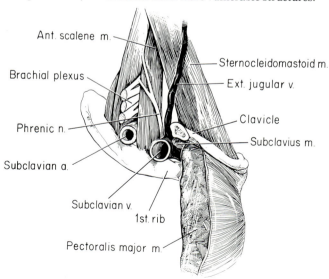

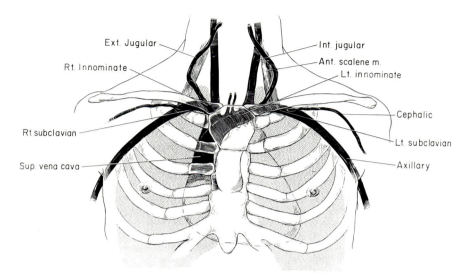

Fig 5. — The course of the subclavian and internal jugular veins in the thoracic inlet. Note that the left subclavian vein is slightly more transverse behind the medial third of the clavicle as opposed to the right subclavian. (Figs 4 and 5 from Ryan, J. A., Jr.: Complications of Parenteral Nutrition, in Fischer, J. E. (ed.): *Total Parenteral Nutrition* [Boston: Little, Brown & Co., 1976]. Used by permission.)

no more than 10 degrees to the horizontal, it is generally possible to catheterize the subclavian vein. Even if the subclavian vein is not found, potentially vulnerable structures will not be hit. Second, the direction of the subclavian on the left side is more horizontal, while on the right side it describes an arch with a shorter horizontal traverse (Fig 5). If one starts 1 cm below and 1 cm lateral to the clavicle and the point of the needle is aimed toward a spot 1 fingerbreadth above the sternal notch, one may expect to find the vein. A continuous aspirating motion on a syringe, generally a 2-ml syringe so that it may be placed horizontally without difficulty, is helpful. Usually a pop will be felt as the needle enters the subclavian vein. At this point, if aspiration is done, dark venous blood will be obtained. The patient is then asked to perform a Valsalva maneuver, the hub of the needle is tilted cephalad and the catheter inserted swiftly and smoothly. If the catheter does not thread and is not easily withdrawn, then both the needle and the catheter must be withdrawn to prevent the catheter from shearing off within the vein and perhaps migrating to the heart, in which case it must be retrieved. Blood is then aspirated with the catheter in place and an infusion of isotonic solution carried out after the dressing until the location of the tip of the catheter is confirmed on x-ray.

In placing an internal jugular catheter, a point 2 cm above the clavicle at the posterior edge of the posterior belly of the sterno-cleidomastoid is used. The internal jugular vein is lateral to the carotid artery. With the fingers on the carotid artery, displacing it medially, the internal jugular vein may be approached by aiming the needle toward the suprasternal notch with a lifting motion immediately under and in the plane of the fascia of the sternocleidomastoid. Others utilize an anterior approach in which a point 2 cm above the clavicle at the anterior edge of the anterior belly of the sternocleidomastoid is selected and inser-tion at a 30-degree angle is carried out. The internal jugular vein again may be identified with a no. 22 needle with which a skin wheal has been made and local anesthesia infiltrated, and a no. 14 needle in which the catheter may be inserted. Here again, aspiration of dark blood is followed by a Valsalva maneuver, and the catheter is inserted smoothly and swiftly. Again, no hypertonic infusion should be undertaken until the location of the tip of the catheter in the superior vena cava has been con-firmed by chest x-ray.

BEGINNING INFUSION

Infusion is generally begun at 60 ml/hour, utilizing a 23% dex-trose solution with approximately 40 gm protein/1,000 ml. This infusion in elderly patients is increased at the rate of 20 ml an hour every 36–48 hours. This is done with a careful monitoring of urinary and blood glucose because of the well-known insulin and glucose resistance during the early septic phases and early postoperative period. In younger patients the infusion may be increased more rapidly. It has been my custom to utilize insulin, 15 units/1,000 ml, in all patients over age 25. Endogenous insu-lin requirement is decreased as well as the incidence of hyper-glycemia in this group of septic patients, although hard data on this point are rare; nitrogen accumulation is also increased. In-fusion of hyperalimentation is increased until a maximum of 4,000 ml/24 hours is reached (4,500 calories), while some pa-tients, especially younger ones, may tolerate 5,000 ml/24 hours.

PROTOCOL IN THE CARE OF PATIENTS

The purpose of any protocol in the care of patients on total parenteral nutrition is the protection of these patients. The principle of such a protocol, such as the one in use at the Massachusetts General Hospital, given as an example (Table 3), is to make possible the care of such patients on a hospital-wide basis without endangering them. Since many physicians will wish to administer parenteral nutrition and may not have the expertise to be aware of some of the more complicated nuances of this form of therapy, it is appropriate that a team be established to safeguard the well-being of such patients. The main aspect of such care is the care of the catheter. The catheter must remain inviolate; it must not be used for the administration of any other materials except hyperalimentation. The dressing must be changed every 48 hours; this procedure must include an antibacterial scrub, recently shown to be of critical value,[55] and an air-occlusive dressing must be placed. Our group basically believes that catheter sepsis is the result of skin contaminants growing along the path of the catheter. To be sure, hematogenous spread must occur, but in our experience it is rare. This principle of catheter care will result in decreasing the incidence of catheter sepsis to an acceptable minimum. This has been well demonstrated in a

TABLE 3.—TOTAL PARENTERAL NUTRITION PROTOCOL

1. Infuse via new, sterile subclavian or internal jugular catheter terminating in superior vena cava, innominate or *intrathoracic* subclavian vein. X-ray confirmation mandatory (infuse D_5W at keep-open rate until x-ray confirmation).
2. Catheter should be replaced immediately in event of leak from catheter or insertion site.
3. Urinary sugar and acetone test every 6 hours.
4. Daily input and output, calorie count and A.M. weight.
5. Care of dressing (change every 48 hours) and IV tubing and filter (change every 24 hours at 6 P.M.) via nursing procedure and policy manuals.
6. *Constant* infusion rate—check every 30 minutes and *reset to rate ordered*.
7. Infuse $D_{20}W$ at the same rate if total parenteral nutrition solution unavailable (N.B.—add same amount of CZI insulin/L if patient is receiving insulin in TPN solutions).
8. Blood work: Before initiating TPN and biweekly on Monday and Thursday: HCT, WBC, differential platelets, Na, K, Cl, CO_2, TP, A-G, Ca, Mg, PO_4, osm, BUN/creatinine, glucose, Vdb, and NH_3.
9. Orders to be rewritten daily at 10 A.M. except weekends. Weekend orders to be written Friday morning.

prospective study carried out by Ryan et al. from this institution in which 355 catheters were followed in 200 consecutive patients and the catheters rated according to catheter care.[90] There was a 7-times-increased incidence of catheter sepsis in the group that received poor catheter care, i.e., in whom the catheter was violated, compared to those 275 patients in whom good catheter care was carried out, i.e., protocol was obeyed. In the latter group, a 3% incidence of sepsis is getting close to an unavoidable minimum.

We also believe that a povidone ointment is of prime importance in not selecting out fungi, as is the case with Neosporin or other antibacterial ointments.

Complications

It is probably true that any conceivable complication has occurred with parenteral nutrition, and that in due course all complications, no matter how inconceivable, will somehow occur. It is also true that complications of parenteral nutrition are almost all preventable by meticulous attention to detail. Complications can generally be discussed under 3 headings — technical, septic and metabolic. Each will be discussed in turn.

TECHNICAL COMPLICATIONS

COMPLICATIONS OF ACCESS. — These are by far the most common complications of parenteral nutrition and are generally related to the mechanical act of placing a catheter through a large-bore needle. If a subclavian approach is used, the most common complications will be (1) pneumothorax; (2) arterial laceration requiring suture (this has not to our knowledge resulted in an arteriovenous fistula, but this undoubtedly will be reported in time); (3) hemothorax, the result of leakage of blood from a subclavian vein; (4) mediastinal hematoma (this has led to the death of 1 cirrhotic patient[90]); and (5) nerve injury to the brachial plexus.

If the internal jugular approach is used, the following complications may be expected: (1) carotid artery lacerations, sometimes requiring suture; (2) phrenic nerve injury, and (3) thoracic duct injury.

As is the case with all procedures, increased experience generally leads to a decrease in the number of complications obtained, but even the most experienced placer of parenteral nutrition catheters will occasionally experience some difficulty.

RESULTS OF MALPOSITION OF CATHETER. — *1. Tip of catheter not in a large-bore vein.* — Rarely the catheter will migrate to an internal mammary vein or, when a subclavian line is placed, more commonly (a 6% incidence) the tip is diverted into the internal jugular vein. For this reason a chest x-ray must always be taken and the position of the tip of the catheter confirmed. In this way, thrombophlebitis secondary to the infusion of hypertonic solutions into a catheter tip residing in the internal jugular vein will be avoided.

2. Pleural effusions. — If the tip of the catheter lacerates the vein and terminates in the pleural space, effusions of hypertonic glucose and amino acids are generally easily recognizable. Sudden onset of chest pain, dyspnea, shock and a large pleural effusion that is positive for glucose will inform the physician that the catheter has been draining large amounts of hypertonic glucose into the pleural space. This is avoidable if, when placing the catheter, one lowers the bottle to observe reflux of blood.

There is another type of pleural effusion that is considerably less rare and may occur on the ipsilateral or contralateral side. This does not contain high amounts of glucose. In general, however, it is the result of either a mediastinal hematoma secondary to catheter placement, or thrombosis of the azygos vein or another tributary. Rarely it is unexplained. These effusions generally subside spontaneously when hyperalimentation is terminated.

LATE COMPLICATIONS

EROSION OF THE CATHETER TIP. — Erosion into the bronchus, other structures or through the tip of a venous structure has been (rarely) reported. Vigilance and the knowledge that this complication may occur is the underlying basis for expectant treatment.

THROMBOSIS. — Thrombosis of the superior vena cava or subclavian vein has been one of the least widely recognized but commonly occurring complications of parenteral nutrition. In a recent study of 34 autopsies from this institution, an incidence close to 20% was observed. Many of these patients had catheters in a short period of time, and thrombosis presumably was related to terminal low-flow states. It is clear, however, that the incidence of subclavian thrombosis, subtle as it is, is higher than we have imagined. An increase in venous tributaries along the chest wall, neck pain and slight swelling of the ipsilateral arm and the root of the neck all point to subclavian or superior vena caval thrombosis. In part this appears to be related to the material used in catheters. Polyvinyl chloride in both dogs and man is seemingly associated with a much higher incidence of subclavian thrombosis. Unfortunately, although on theoretical grounds the use of Silastic catheters would result in a lower incidence of thrombosis, satisfactory solution of engineering, fastening and other problems has not occurred. Because of this, many institutions, including our own, continue to use polyvinyl chloride catheters, which on balance appears to be safer for the patient, and less troublesome.

Septic thrombosis. — While thrombosis itself is a complication that often does not result in long-term morbidity or danger to the patient, septic thrombosis is a severe life-threatening complication. This has previously been emphasized in long lines, for example, cephalic vein septic thrombosis, especially in burn patients. Subclavian septic thrombosis, however, has not been emphasized. In the event of subclavian septic thrombosis, either as a result of staphylococcal invasion of a thrombus or, more worrisome, a yeast infection, excision, relatively easily accomplished with cephalic vein sepsis, is a technical tour de force that may jeopardize the life of an already ill patient. Under such circumstances, anticoagulation with heparin and Coumadin coupled with high-dose long-term intravenous antibiotic therapy (similar in magnitude and duration to that used in bacterial endocarditis) is indicated. A significant number of patients with septic thrombosis will die, particularly if this insult is added to the other problems of an already malnourished, debilitated patient. Prevention is much more important.

Catheter Sepsis

Sepsis is the most feared of all complications. Some confusion as to the causation of sepsis still remains, despite much evidence.[19, 27, 89, 90] While hematogenous seeding of the fibrin sleeve around catheters occurs, by far the most common cause of catheter sepsis is poor catheter technique. This has been demonstrated in a number of studies, including one from our own institution in which the incidence of sepsis was 3% when catheters received good care, despite the fact that in 84% of the patients in the study other sources of sepsis required antibiotic therapy sometime during the course of hyperalimentation.[90] Thus, while bacteremia occurs and undoubtedly on occasion seeds the fibrin sleeve around the catheter, it is uncommon. If one follows the organisms that grow from septic catheters and compares them with the organisms thought responsible for other concomitant infections, one sees that catheter sepsis is the result of contamination by skin organisms that presumably grow down the catheter entry site. These are almost always staphylococcal organisms, at least at our institution — *Staphylococcus aureus* or *epidermidis*. Unfortunately, *S. epidermidis* found on blood culture may be regarded as a skin contaminant, although once established this organism is exceedingly difficult to eradicate. It is sensitive only to vancomycin.

EPIDEMIOLOGY. — Any hyperalimentation unit dealing with sepsis control throughout an institution should focus on the epidemiology of catheter sepsis. The factors that may influence catheter sepsis include:

Patient care area. — Variables that may contribute to catheter sepsis are poor nursing technique, shortage of nursing staff and inability to do proper dressing changes, interference by physicians with the protocol and lack of adherence to protocol.

Time of year. — Although July 1975 at the Massachusetts General Hospital was not associated with an increased incidence of sepsis (Fig 6), this was the direct result of a campaign based on prior experience that the influx of new medical and nursing staff had been associated with a higher incidence of sepsis. In addition, in a non-air-conditioned institution, summer heat and contamination of the dressing by perspiration are other factors that lead to an increased incidence of sepsis during summer months.

Patients at risk. — Certain patients are more at risk for catheter sepsis, including patients on steroids,[34, 80] for some reason patients with pancreatitis during the early part of their disease,[46] and perhaps patients with inflammatory bowel disease in the absence of steroid therapy.[81, 90] Interestingly enough, debilitated patients, patients undergoing cardiac surgery[3, 110a] and

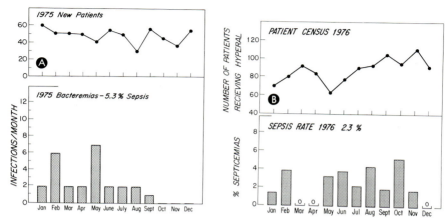

Fig 6. — **A,** the sepsis rate at the Massachusetts General Hospital in 1975. Note that there were 2 periods when sepsis seemed somewhat high. Extraordinary difficulty was experienced with filters at this point, and there was a great deal of manipulation of catheters. During the last 3 months of 1975 no bacteremias were recorded. **B,** sepsis rates during 1976 at Massachusetts General Hospital.

patients with renal failure,[1, 4, 5, 26] although theoretically at greater risk for sepsis on the basis of decreased host defenses, have not shown higher sepsis rates.

FACTORS RESPONSIBLE FOR SEPSIS. — *Duration of catheterization.* — This appears to vary from institution to institution. Whereas one of Dudrick's early publications suggested that catheters in place for greater than 30 days had an increased incidence of sepsis,[110a] this has not been borne out by our own data. Ryan's data showed a peak incidence at 2 weeks, and a decreased incidence thereafter.[90] This seeming paradox may be explained by the fact that the catheter, as a foreign body, will elicit a certain amount of tissue reaction. Once the organism "comes into symbiosis" with the foreign body and the interface becomes "locally resistant," sepsis becomes less likely and one cannot do any better by changing the catheter. This information, however, should be detailed for each institution before adopting policies for duration of catheterization.

Technique in placing catheters — Although a decreased incidence of technical complications may be expected with experi-

48   JOSEF E. FISCHER

ence in placing catheters, a relationship of technical inexperience and sepsis has not been established.

Dressing changes and catheter care.—This is probably the major determinant in catheter sepsis.[19, 28, 89, 90] Additionally, the actual skin preparation may be important. Freeman and his coworkers suggested that the mechanical scrub with iodophor was more important than the ointment utilized.[55] Our clinical impression, on the other hand, is that the incidence of fungal sepsis decreases when an iodophor ointment is used rather than Neosporin. This remains to be established.

BACTERIOLOGY.—*Contamination by skin organisms.*—This is the most common cause of sepsis. *Staphylococcus epidermidis* is most frequent. Other less frequent offenders include coliform, *Klebsiella* and other environmental organisms.

Fungal infections.—This has apparently been the scourge in several institutions.[23] Patients with fungal sepsis are sicker and die more often than patients with bacterial catheter sepsis. The reasons for the selection of fungi are many and include numerous antibiotics, steroids, poor technique in the changing of bottles and the contamination of large areas to sugar solutions which, once exposed and not refrigerated, offer excellent growth media for such organisms.

While bacterial invasion is relatively easy and straightforward, the difference between fungal colonization and actual deep-space infection, as in catheter sepsis, is sometimes a difficult judgment to make. Many patients, including those on steroids and with numerous antibiotics, will have cultures positive for fungi in sputum and urine. Indeed, the entire patient may be colonized. There is a significant difference, however, between fungal colonization and fungal invasion. Glew and co-workers suggested[45] how such a judgment may be made. While *Candida* precipitins have been advocated as a good test of fungal infection, they give false positive results at times in patients in whom invasion has not taken place. On the other hand, if *Candida* precipitins give negative results, one can be certain that actual invasion has not taken place. Crossed immunoelectrophoresis is quite accurate, however, and when positive, indicates that colonization has now progressed to invasive infection. Once the catheter is removed and the fungemia appropriately treated, this parameter will return to negative.

CLINICAL SIGNS.—There are certain clinical hints that one

may use to be suspicious of catheter sepsis. Catheter sepsis is often not sudden, but occurs gradually. The patient will often have a low-grade fever, to 100.1 or 100.2 F, for several evenings prior to development of frank catheter sepsis. Once bacteremia does occur, the fever pattern is not that of a spiking fever, but one of more constant nature as bacteria are being consistently liberated from the line and from the infected fibrin sleeve. If a patient runs a low-grade fever on several evenings and then spikes to 103 F, this is the rather classic pattern of catheter sepsis.

TREATMENT. — In many hyperalimented patients other potential sources of infection and fever are present. Thus, when a patient on parenteral nutrition spikes a sudden fever, the first step should be the removal and culture of the bottle and plastic intravenous tubing. A new bottle should be hung or, if this is unavailable, 20% dextrose and water given with a new plastic IV tubing. Blood should be drawn for culture. A thorough search should be made for obvious sources of high fever. If none is found, the line should be promptly removed and the tip promptly cultured. In individuals with high infusion rates, significant tapering can be accomplished in a very short time, i.e., 1–2 hours, so that hypoglycemia does not occur. A peripheral drip of 5% dextrose and water will help.

Use of antibiotics. — It has not been our practice to utilize antibiotics in suspected line sepsis. If the line is at fault, removal of the catheter is sufficient. If the fever does not recur and blood cultures remain negative, treatment is unnecessary. Serial blood cultures should then be drawn to rule out persistence of bacterial or fungal infections.

Restarting the line. — In suspected catheter sepsis it has been our practice to wait 24 hours before reinserting the catheter on the opposite side. In 1 patient whose line was promptly reinserted on the other side, staphylococcal infection promptly recurred. If fever persists and blood cultures remain positive, antibiotics should be utilized.

The catheter generally does not become contaminated on the opposite side once treatment has been reinstituted, but this cannot be said for patients with established fungemia. So long as hypertonic glucose solution is being infused, even if blood cultures have been negative for 4 or 5 days, cultures once again revert to positive when a high glucose infusion is restarted.

Thus, in the patient with fungemia who requires parenteral nutrition, peripheral techniques are mandatory. Treatment for fungemia involves the administration of amphotericin B or a similar agent for 6 weeks. Since this drug is toxic, the decision to treat for established fungemia should not be taken lightly, and adequate proof should be collected.

Late fungemia. — One troublesome characteristic of fungemia is its ability to lie dormant for a period of months and then appear as a fever of unknown etiology. *Candida* also has an unfortunate tendency to collect in the superior mesenteric artery, resulting in a mycotic superior mesenteric artery aneurysm with late thrombosis.

METABOLIC COMPLICATIONS

Metabolic complications may be discussed as deficiency states, a group of so-called metabolic complications due to the omission of nutrients usually present in the oral diet, and disorders of glucose metabolism.

The deficiency states include the following.
1. Hyponatremia
2. Hypokalemia
3. Hypophosphatemia
4. Hypomagnesemia
5. Zinc deficiency
6. Copper deficiency
7. Essential fatty acid deficiency
8. Chromium and other trace metal deficiencies
9. Other factors

HYPONATREMIA. — The requirement for sodium is, of course, relative. However, a certain amount of sodium is required to excrete the water load given with central TPN. With 4 L hypertonic glucose and amino acids per day, at least 100 mEq of sodium is required. This may seem somewhat paradoxical in patients with limited cardiac reserve. On the other hand, the lack of sodium administration will result in overwatering, inappropriate secretion of antidiuretic hormone (ADH) and the inability to excrete a water load, with resulting hyponatremia. Of course, certain patients will require diuretics. Certain patients, for example those with hepatic and/or renal failure, should not be given sodium at all except to replace external losses.

HYPOKALEMIA. — This generally is the result of inadequate

potassium administration, particularly during the period of rapid replenishment. Three mEq of potassium are accumulated for every gm of nitrogen retained. In addition, potassium is lost in the perspiration in rapid repletion. A limiting factor is renal function, and rapid increase in serum potassium may be one's first clue to failing renal function. Assuming normal renal function, between 100 and 160 mEq/day or greater of potassium ion are required. Failure to give adequate potassium may result in glucose intolerance.

HYPOPHOSPHATEMIA AND HYPOMAGNESEMIA. — These indicate that the requirements for phosphate and magnesium have been consistently underestimated. With the hydrolysates, a certain amount of phosphate is present in the protein that was not calculated as part of the infusion. When the synthetic amino acid solutions came into vogue, this phosphate was absent and serious hypophosphatemia was then observed. It is reasonable to assume that when serum phosphate decreases, this reflects deficiency in total body phosphorus and that partial store repletion is necessary before this is reflected in increased serum levels. Approximately 90 to 100 mEq of phosphorus are required daily.

Between 28 and 32 mEq of magnesium are required daily, particularly during anabolism. This figure may be even higher in young adults. Once the requirements for phosphate and magnesium have been met, calcium is generally not a problem and will vary with the behavior of the other 2 ions.

ZINC DEFICIENCY. — A shortage of zinc is generally associated with a deficiency in wound healing and perhaps other deleterious effects. Plasma zinc is probably not a reasonable estimate of total body zinc. As with many of the other trace metal and essential fatty acid deficiencies, zinc deficiency is not often seen in patients on short-term parenteral nutrition, i.e., patients in whom oral intake has been omitted for less than 3 or 4 weeks. It is also becoming clear that the zinc requirement is not isolated and that the zinc/copper ratio may be more important than the absolute amount of zinc itself. Zinc deficiency is associated with a characteristic rash in the perioral area and in the flexion creases as well as darkening of the skin in flexion creases.[58, 100] For reasons that are not entirely clear, zinc deficiency has been observed to a considerably greater extent in Japan.[100] This may be due to different trace metal configurations in the water or in other manufacturing processes.

COPPER DEFICIENCY. — This has recently been associated with

anemia, especially in long-term patients.[78, 103] The anemia commonly associated with parenteral nutrition is not due to copper deficiency, at least in our experience. If copper supplementation is required, 2 mg as the sulfate may be used per liter of hypertonic dextrose and amino acids without exceeding the solubility limit. For suggested trace metal intakes, see Table 2.

ESSENTIAL FATTY ACID DEFICIENCY. — As with the trace metals, essential fatty acid deficiency occurs after the patient has been on relatively long-term parenteral nutrition. Despite this, the biochemical lesion may be seen in some patients, notably depleted patients with inflammatory bowel disease, as soon as 3 days following initiation of fat-free parenteral nutrition. Essential fatty acid deficiency may be associated with phospholipid alterations in the membranes of red cells, perhaps alterations in their capacity to deliver oxygen as well as possible interference with wound healing. The characteristic biochemical lesion is the emergence of abnormal unsaturated fatty acid, eicosatrienoic acid, as well as a decrease in the normal amounts of polyunsaturated fatty acids.[72] Once linoleic acid is provided, some of the other normally occurring essential fatty acids may be synthesized. A characteristic skin rash, dry flakiness of the skin and small reddish macules are characteristic of essential fatty acid deficiency. This can be corrected by the administration of Intralipid, in which case the lesions disappear in anywhere from 3 to 7 days. The biochemical lesion takes slightly longer. Prevention of fatty acid deficiency is relatively easy by supplying as little as 4% of the total caloric source as Intralipid or by giving corn oil, safflower oil or some other polyunsaturated vegetable oil by mouth in amounts of 50 ml/24 hours. In babies some of the essential fatty acid requirement may be met by smearing the baby with the unsaturated oil but this obviously has its aesthetic shortcomings.

CHROMIUM DEFICIENCY. — Chromium deficiency has been associated with the development of a diabetic state that is corrected by the administration of chromium.[56] This again only seems to be a problem in long-term patients with no oral intake. Of course, there may be other trace metals and other factors that may be associated with deficiency states and that we are not exactly aware of. An example of this may be the peculiar skin rash that is seen in an occasional patient on synthetic amino acid infusions and disappears with the provision of the hydrolysate.[92] Whether this represents a deficiency state, some reaction to synthetic amino acids or perhaps subclinical zinc deficiency is not clear at the present time.

DISORDERS IN GLUCOSE METABOLISM. — Hyperglycemia can be very dangerous and sometimes fatal. The most common cause of hyperglycemia (Table 4) is too rapid initiation of the infusion. It is our practice to initiate the infusion at 60 ml/hour in most adults and to increase the rate of the infusion by 20 ml/hour every 24–48 hours depending on tolerance. In the young adult who is depleted it is possible to achieve a level of 4 L 23% dextrose hyperalimentation solution within 5 days after the initiation of the infusion, but this may take longer in a septuagenarian. It is not uncommon for patients to spill glucose during the first 24–48 hours because of the load delivered. Insulin by test should never be ordered unless the blood sugar is elevated as well. It has been my personal practice to include 15 units of insulin in the bottle in patients over age 30. As Wilmore has recently shown, this promotes anabolism and retention of nitrogen.[66]

Patients at risk for hyperglycemia are generally those with inadequate secretion of insulin, including patients with pancreatitis and pancreatic resection, as well as those with liver disease. Patients previously stable who suddenly develop glucose intolerance usually are septic. Hyperglycemia may antedate the development of clinical sepsis by 18–24 hours.

Diabetes, however, is not a relative contraindication to parenteral nutrition. In Ryan's recent series, a minority of patients with glucose intolerance were diabetic.[89, 90] Whether this was

TABLE 4. — COMMON CAUSES
OF HYPERGLYCEMIA

1. Rapid infusion
2. Decreased insulin output
    a) Diabetes
    b) Pancreatitis
    c) Pancreatic resection
3. "Glucose resistance"
    a) Sepsis
4. Hyperglycemic factors
    a) Steroids
    b) Liver disease (?hyperglucagonemia)
       (?decreased utilization)

due to the care in initiating parenteral nutrition in these patients or, more likely, to the release of pancreatic insulin by
amino acids is not clear. Steroids also predispose to glucose intolerance.

Hypoglycemia generally occurs when the rate of hypertonic
glucose infusion is increased and suddenly stopped. It is rare,
however, for hypoglycemia to result from abrupt termination of
the infusion, even after many weeks, when one, for example,
removes a line because of sepsis. The most common cause of
hypoglycemia is inadvertent cessation of the infusion because of
mechanical difficulties. Another less common cause is excessive
insulin administration. A very curious cause of symptomatic
hypoglycemia is the endogenous secretion of insulin that occurs
after long-term parenteral nutrition in patients getting rapid
rates of infusion. If hypoglycemia occurs in a patient with an
infusion rate of, say, 165 or 175 ml of 23% dextrose/hour, slowing
the infusion will result in disappearance of the hypoglycemia
due to endogenous insulin response.

OTHER COMPLICATIONS

Other less common complications include pancreatitis, which
we have not seen since alcohol was omitted from the infusion. In
these patients no other cause of pancreatitis was apparent; we
have not seen pancreatitis in cases in which alcohol was not utilized. Hypercalcemia is another curious complication of parenteral nutrition and may be more apparent than real, particularly in patients getting hydrolysates, when peptide-bound calcium may result in elevation of total blood calcium but the ion-
ized calcium will be normal. Other causes of hypercalcemia include vitamin D intoxication. At the present time it is our practice only to include fat-soluble vitamins on 1 day a week and to
include vitamins B and C on a daily basis. Vitamin A intoxication is similar to that described after eating polar bear liver, including jaundice, skin changes and keratitis, and has occurred
in patients on long-term parenteral nutrition who have received
excessive amounts of vitamin A.

PSYCHIATRIC COMPLICATIONS. — This area has received inadequate attention. Patients who receive parenteral nutrition are
often very ill. They undergo long periods of hospitalization and

food deprivation; severe depression is common. It is unlikely that parenteral nutrition *causes* depression, but this is being investigated. Patients hallucinate food, dream up recipes and are concerned about this preoccupation. These patients will benefit by a few kind words of reassurance.

Home or Outpatient Hyperalimentation

An increasing number of patients are candidates for outpatient parenteral nutrition. Obviously, this approach is used only as a last resort. Although it is probably not any more complicated or any more expensive than home dialysis, the resistance to the assumption of permanent home parenteral nutrition is much greater for some reason. Cost has been estimated as between $25,000 and $30,000 a year, certainly in competitive range with the cost of home dialysis programs. In addition, the patient is more often a fully rehabilitated and productive member of society than is a patient on home dialysis.[16b, 56] Thus, the reluctance of various physicians to undertake home TPN probably reflects fear of an unknown technique.

Candidates for home parenteral nutrition include patients who have undergone massive small bowel resection, some of whom may experience hypertrophy and be able to resume oral nutrition eventually,[91] and patients with inflammatory bowel disease, either secondary to repeated small bowel resections or with fistulas and nonusable bowel, among others. Other indications may involve patients with renal and hepatic failure who are incapable of taking adequate diets orally. This must be very rare in the patients with renal failure, since dialysis techniques are freely available to enable such patients to eat normal diets and be dialyzed frequently. It is possible, however, that patients with severe encephalopathy who are intolerant of gut protein may ultimately prove amenable to infusions of specific amino acid patterns recently shown to be efficacious in patients with hepatic coma.[39] An alternative use, recently suggested, is in patients with type II hypercholesterolemia who in the past have undergone end-to-side portacaval shunt after a trial of parenteral nutrition. Our own experience in patients with hypercholesterolemia suggests that parenteral nutrition is a more efficacious mechanism for lowering blood cholesterol than is the shunt. In view of the fatal nature of this illness, it is probably not unreasonable to suggest that this might be considered in patients with homozygous type II hypercholesterolemia.[96, 101]

There are 2 ways of approaching home parenteral nutrition. One technique practiced by investigators in Canada[56] and France[95] utilizes an Intralipid, 10% dextrose solution and amino acid mixture with a small halter and a cannula into a branch of the subclavian vein[95] or superior vena cava catheter. The mixture is mixed in Silastic rubber bags, which are refrigerated for 1 week and worn as a halter with a small pump. Parenteral nutrition is continuous, 24 hours a day. The American technique, pioneered by Dr. Belding Scribner among others, utilizes an amino acid-glucose infusion and overnight parenteral nutrition with a long indwelling Silastic catheter terminating in the right atrium and a long subcutaneous tunnel.[16b, 91] Such patients may be managed on an overnight basis and go about their business during the day free of encumbrances. Our own experience has been with this technique, and we find it relatively easy to carry out once the patient and his family have been trained. A 2-L pump, 2 liter bottles and specialized kits as well as instruction booklets are all available, the latter having been fabricated by Dr. Scribner in his pioneer efforts.

It is doubtful whether at the present time more than 100 patients are carried on home parenteral nutrition in this country. Nonetheless, this is a useful lifesaving technique, and probably many more patients would be candidates if acceptance were wider. In many patients this is not a permanent change but merely a technique that will serve to tide them over until the disease condition can be corrected or until bowel hypertrophy can occur and the patient once again support himself. Clearly this is a useful adjunct whose full potential has not yet been exploited.

Ancillary Techniques in Parenteral Nutrition

ADMINISTRATION OF PERIPHERAL AMINO ACIDS: "PROTEIN SPARING," ETC.

It is of interest that attempts at parenteral nutrition began with this therapeutic mode, casein hydrolysates with hypocaloric or inadequate amounts of dextrose. Dudrick in his classic experiments began using casein hydrolysates and 5% glucose in an attempt to support his experimental animals and found that he could not. Thus, the administration of peripheral protein was largely abandoned until reemphasized through the efforts of Blackburn, Flatt and their collaborators.[12, 13] Briefly, Blackburn, Flatt et al. suggested that the use of peripheral amino acids, namely 3% Freamine in water, could result in the retention of lean body mass ("protein sparing") as opposed to the traditional technique of 5% dextrose in water. There are several aspects of the "Blackburn-Flatt hypothesis":

1. Administration of 90 gm crystalline amino acids in water/24 hours.

2. That under these circumstances, the administration of 90 gm of 3% amino acids and water would result in nitrogen equilibrium and in some cases positive nitrogen balance.[13]

3. The mechanism of this therapeutic mode was the adaptation to the "starved state" in which the body utilized its own fat stores for energy, and utilized less endogenous protein for gluconeogenesis.

4. Since the promotion of lipolysis was desirable and insulin inhibited lipolysis, carbohydrates should be strictly avoided as they tended to increase insulin and inhibit lipolysis.[12, 13]

5. That under such circumstances visceral protein synthesis would be promoted at the expense of lean body mass protein synthesis (which is the principal fate of amino acids given with hypertonic dextrose).

Since the initial publication of this hypothesis, a number of studies have attempted to confirm or deny it. The emphasis on the importance of protein as the central building block and the essential portion of the body composition that must be retained is most welcome. However, granted nitrogen losses are halved, the efficacy of giving amino acids as opposed to 5% dextrose in water remains theoretical. As with much of parenteral nutrition, it has not yet been demonstrated that a superior outcome follows this therapeutic mode as routine postoperative therapy in most patients. In an era of increased cost consciousness, it goes without saying that the adoption of a form of therapy 3 times as expensive as the routine form of therapy (on which most patients without complications do perfectly well) will require the demonstration of efficacy. Let us now review the evidence that exists for each of the points as previously stated.

1. It has clearly been demonstrated that there is decreased net nitrogen loss in the routine postoperative patient treated with 3% amino acids and water as opposed to 5% dextrose and water and electrolytes. This amounts to approximately 5 or 6 gm nitrogen/24 hours. It is important to point out that while nitrogen excretion in the patients receiving 3% amino acids in water is higher than that in patients treated with dextrose and water, the administration of amino acids in excess results in nitrogen retention. This cumulative nitrogen retention is what is referred to as "protein sparing."[13, 40, 47, 52, 113]

2. It has not been confirmed that nitrogen equilibrium results. Subsequent papers from a variety of laboratories have demonstrated that the mean nitrogen excretion in postoperative patients treated with 3% Freamine and water is a net 3–4 gm negative/24 hours.[40, 47, 52, 113]

3. While ketosis suggests an adaptation to the starved state and occurs in patients receiving 3% Freamine and water, this does not appear to be the mechanism of such nitrogen sparing. As originally pointed out, the adaptation to starvation takes between 10 and 14 days and it is unlikely to be the mechanism by which nitrogen sparing occurs.[17, 32] Secondly, it has recently been demonstrated that giving hypocaloric amounts of fat or glucose with amino acids or amino acids alone results in no significant difference in nitrogen excretion in the 3 groups of patients, all of whom retain more nitrogen than do patients receiving 5% dextrose alone.[47] The hormonal set, namely insulin and glucagon, appears to be determined by the caloric source, insulin being high when glucose is furnished, low when fat is furnished.[47] On the other hand, insulin levels do not seem to affect nitrogen balance. Subsequent investigations have suggested that the addition of 150 gm of glucose, i.e., 600 calories/24 hours, results in greater nitrogen retention than amino acids alone[113] in normal volunteers.

4. The argument that visceral protein is retained at the expense of the synthesis of peripheral lean body mass has little data to support it. On the other hand, Shizgal and his co-workers have reported that, using total potassium space as a measurement, lean body mass is protected by the administration of amino acids as opposed to the administration of glucose alone.[92b] The same techniques have not been applied to the administra-

tion of hypocaloric glucose and amino acids as opposed to amino acids and water.

The status of this important theoretical consideration remains moot at the present time. It is appropriate to consider this form of therapy as an intermediate step in the preservation of some lean body mass for short-term situations where oral intake is doubtful for several days. It is not, however, a substitute for the repletion of patients using hypertonic dextrose and amino acids by the central technique. Its exact place in the armamentarium remains to be defined.

ADMINISTRATION OF ALPHA-KETO ACIDS

The use of alpha-keto analogues in nutritional support reflects a quantum jump in our understanding of intermediary catabolism. Previously various investigators have been concerned with the provision of amino acids as the essential building blocks. In a series of investigations dating back to 1950, Walser and his co-workers realized that it is the carbon skeleton of the essential amino acids that the body cannot synthesize and that this is primarily responsible for the division of amino acids into essential and nonessential categories. Ample stores of available nitrogen exist in many disease states, including uremia and hepatic failure, either in the form of urea, free ammonia, the ammonia ion or bound to an ammonia acceptor such as glutamate in glutamine. Reasoning that if the body could not synthesize the carbon skeleton, it should be possible to promote utilization of endogenous waste nitrogen by giving the carbon skeleton in the form of the alpha-keto analogue of the essential amino acids, Walser and his co-workers have published a series of cases of uremia[106, 108] and of patients with chronic hepatic insufficiency in whom such nutritional support seems appropriate.[68] The mechanism in the 2 groups seems to differ slightly, however.

In uremia, urea is theoretically an end product. It is, however, excreted into the gut and split by gut bacteria to ammonia, which is then reabsorbed and transaminated. While this has been the underlying theoretical framework of the Giordano-Giovanetti diet, Walser and his co-workers estimate that nitrogen reutilization or urea reutilization plays only a small role in the alpha-keto efficacy in uremia.[107, 108] Rather, they focus on the protein-sparing effect of the alpha-keto acids, which may be more potent than the amino acids themselves, for reasons poorly understood. Thus, the administration of alpha-keto acids in patients with chronic uremia appears to decrease the frequency of dialysis and maintains nutritional support.[107, 108] Unfortunately, in these studies caloric intake was not well controlled.

With respect to liver disease, in a small series a few patients, but not all, with encephalopathy appear to have been improved.[68] Glutamine and not ammonia is the principal nitrogen donor. Glutamine is increased in cerebrospinal fluid in patients in hepatic coma, and it is possible that this is a beneficial effect. Other possible beneficial effects are the alterations in plasma amino acid pattern, including tyrosine and glycine, amino acids that had not been given. This suggests that a principal effect of the alpha-keto acids is decreased muscle catabolism, recently proposed as being extremely important in the therapy of hepatic coma.[87] Here again, caloric intake was not controlled,[68] and it is possible that variations in efficacy may be due to variations in caloric intake, suboptimal caloric intake being associated with failure of therapy.

Several problems prevent the widespread usage of alpha-keto acids in patients with hepatic and/or renal insufficiency. This is unfortunate, as the author believes that for the patient with hepatorenal syndrome, for example, alpha-keto acids are theoretically the best form in which amino acids can be given. While expense is widely thought of as being a hindrance to the widespread use of alpha-keto acids, it appears only a matter of time before a reasonable manufacturing process becomes generally available and the substances become less expensive. A greater problem is the requirement for large quantities of sodium and calcium for administration of the acids in the salt form. There does not appear to be an easy solution to this problem, and much work will be necessary before these acids are available for general usage.

The Use of the Gastrointestinal Tract

A long dissertation on the use of the gastrointestinal tract is beyond the scope of this review. Nonetheless, it should be noted that where the gastrointestinal tract is available and can accept

2,000–3,000 calories/24 hours, it is the preferable route of nutritional support. This, of course, will depend on the individual physician's preference. It should be pointed out, however, that recent studies[16c] have suggested greater efficacy when the gut is used than when the same number of calories are given intravenously. Another argument for the use of parenteral nutrition is that the solutions are specialized, but this becomes less important as similar synthetic amino acid formulations become available for enteral use, as in renal or hepatic failure.

To a certain extent less has been done in enteral nutrition than in parenteral nutrition to date. For example, what is the most efficacious form of peptide absorption, dipeptides or synthetic amino acids, and how does this relate to clinical usage? The absorption of fat as opposed to carbohydrate and the fate of such nutrients has not been fully investigated. Suffice it to say that if one wishes to use the enteral route in a very depleted patient, even most enthusiasts for this route will start with a parenteral supplement, since it does take a matter of days before a significant caloric intake is achieved. Too rapid initiation of enteral nutrition with hyperosmolar solutions will result in diarrhea, electrolyte wasting, fluid loss and hyperosmolar coma. Thus, in any institution in which a nutrition unit exists, there should be the capacity to go in either direction, either enterally or parenterally, or a combination of both, to provide the best choice as far as any given patient is concerned.

There is little question that the use of enteral nutrition in the form of elemental diets is efficacious in patients with inflammatory bowel disease, for example, as a midway step between parenteral nutrition and a normal diet. In addition, several institutions have reported large series of patients with fistulas in whom respectable rates of closure have been achieved with an enteral diet.[83, 105] Bowel rest achieved with an enteral diet, however, is less complete than with intravenous parenteral nutrition, as one would expect.[112]

The Future

In view of all the accomplishments of parenteral nutrition, it is difficult to recall that the field is less than a decade old in the United States and slightly older in western Europe. Much remains to be done. We are just beginning to understand the different nutritional requirements for different disease states. With regard to caloric source, we still have no idea as to whether fat, carbohydrate or both may be more appropriate for certain situations. Preliminary data seem to indicate that fat will not be utilized under certain high-stress or traumatic situations, but this is by no means proved, and many persist in using fat in seemingly ill-advised fashion under these circumstances. The amino acid requirements remain to be elucidated. While it is clear that diseases with abnormalities in nitrogen metabolism require different amino acid formulations, subsequent data, notably those of Halliday,[48] recently emphasized by Winters,[111a] and some of our own preliminary data suggest that protein-depleted patients have different amino acid requirements from those patients one is merely trying to maintain. Indeed, the entire aspect of amino acids and their measurements have been thrown into confusion by the recent important work of Vinnars, Kinney and their co-workers, who suggest that plasma amino acid levels, although easily accessible, may not accurately reflect the muscle free amino acid pool (that available for protein synthesis), which, after all, is what one is attempting to promote.[104]

The field of parenteral nutrition has attracted many investigators whose specialized training and biochemical knowledge have invited widespread collaboration with different areas of scientific investigation and endeavor. Knowledgeable individuals are returning to the bedside and engaging in meaningful clinical research. Clearly, the next decade will be an exciting one in this area.

REFERENCES

1. Abbott, W. M., Abel, R. M., and Fischer, J. E.: Treatment of acute renal insufficiency after aortoiliac surgery, Arch. Surg. 103:590, 1971.
2. Abbott, W. M.: Indications for Parenteral Nutrition, in Fischer, J. E. (ed.): *Total Parenteral Nutrition* (Boston: Little, Brown & Co., 1976).
3. Abel, R., Fischer, J. E., Buckley, M. J., Barnett, G. O., and Austen, W. G.: Effects of prophylactic total parenteral nutrition in the early postoperative period following cardiac surgery, Arch. Surg. In press.
4. Abel, R. M., Abbott, W. M., and Fischer, J. E.: Intravenous essential L-amino acids and hypertonic dextrose in patients with acute renal failure: Effects on serum potassium phosphate and magnesium, Am. J. Surg. 123:632, 1972.
5. Abel, R. M., Beck, C. H., Jr., Abbott, W. M., Ryan, J. A., Barnett, G. O.,

and Fischer, J. E.: Improved survival from acute renal failure following treatment with intravenous essential L-amino acids and glucose, N. Engl. J. Med. 288:695, 1973.

6. Abel, R. M., Shih, V. E., Abbott, W. M., Beck, C. H., and Fischer, J. E.: Amino acid metabolism in acute renal failure: Influence of intravenous essential L-amino acids on hyperalimentation therapy, Ann. Surg. 180: 350, 1974.

7. Aguirre, A., Yoshimura, N., Westman, T., and Fischer, J. E.: Plasma amino acids in dogs with two experimental forms of liver damage, J. Surg. Res. 16:339, 1974.

8. Aguirre, A., Fischer, J. E., and Welch, C. E.: The role of surgery and hyperalimentation in therapy of gastrointestinal-cutaneous fistulae, Ann. Surg. 180:393, 1974.

9. Anderson, G. H., Patel, D. G., and Jeejeebhoy, K. N.: Design and evaluation by nitrogen balance and blood aminograms of an amino acid mixture for total parenteral nutrition of adults with gastrointestinal disease, J. Clin. Invest. 53:904, 1974.

10. Baldessarini, R. J., and Fischer, J. E.: Serotonin metabolism in rat brain after surgical diversion of the portal venous circulation, Nature, New Biology 254:25, 1973.

11. Bergstrom, J., Bucht, H., Furst, P., Hultman, E., Josephson, B., Noree, L. O., and Vinnars, E.: Intravenous nutrition with amino acid solutions in patients with chronic uraemia, Acta Med. Scand. 191:359, 1972.

12. Blackburn, G. L., Flatt, J. P., Clowes, G. H. A., and O'Donnell, T. E.: Peripheral intravenous feeding with isotonic amino acid solutions, Am. J. Surg. 125:447, 1973.

13. Blackburn, G. L., Flatt, J. P., Clowes, G. H. A., O'Donnell, T. E., and Hensle, T. E.: Protein-sparing therapy during periods of starvation with sepsis or trauma, Ann. Surg. 177:588, 1973.

14. Borreson, H. Ch.: Clinical Applications in Pediatric Surgery and Pediatrics, in Lee, H. (ed.): *Parenteral Nutrition in Acute Metabolic Illness* (New York: Academic Press, Inc., 1974).

15. Brennan, M. F., Aoki, T. T., Muller, W. A., et al.: The role of glucagon as a catabolic hormone, Surg. Forum 25:74, 1974.

16. Brennan, M. F., Fitzpatrick, G. F., Cohen, K. H., et al.: Glycerol: Major contributor to the short term protein sparing effect of fat emulsions in normal man, Ann. Surg. 182:386, 1975.

16a. Brennan, M. F.: Personal communication.

16b. Broviac, J. W., and Scribner, B. H.: Prolonged parenteral nutrition in the home, Surg. Gynecol. Obstet. 139:24, 1974.

16c. Bury, K. D., Grayston, M., and Kanarens, J.: Comparative weight gain in animals receiving total nutrition by either the intravenous or intragastric routes, J. Surg. Res. In press.

17. Cahill, G. F., Herrera, M. G., Morgan, A. P., et al: Hormone fuel interrelationships during fasting, J. Clin. Invest. 45:1751, 1966.

18. Chalmers, T. C.: Randomized Controlled Trials in Disease of the Liver, in Popper, H., and Schaffner, F. (eds): *Progress in Liver Disease* (New York: Grune & Stratton, Inc., 1976), Vol. V.

19. Copeland, E. M., MacFadyen, B. V. J., McGown, C., et al: The use of hy-

peralimentation in patients with potential sepsis, Surg. Gynecol. Obstet. 138:377, 1974.

20. Copeland, E. M., MacFadyen, B. V. J., and Dudrick, S. J.: Effect of intravenous hyperalimentation on established delayed hypersensitivity in the cancer patient, Ann. Surg. 184:60, 1976.

21. Culebras, J. M., Brennan, M. F., Fitzpatrick, G. F., et al: Nitrogen sparing in normal man. Effect of glycerol and amino acids given peripherally, Surg. Forum 27:37, 1976.

22. Curreri, P. W., Wilmore, D. W., Mason, A. D., Jr., Newsome, T. W., Asch, M. J., and Pruitt, B. A., Jr.: Intracellular cation alterations following major trauma: Effect of supranormal caloric intake, J. Trauma 11:390, 1971.

23. Curry, C. R., and Quie, P. G.: Fungal septicemia in patients receiving parenteral hyperalimentation, N. Engl. J. Med. 285:1221, 1971.

24. Dodsworth, J. M., Cummings, M. G., James, J. H., and Fischer, J. E.: Depletion of brain norepinephrine in acute hepatic coma, Surgery 75: 811, 1974.

25. Dudrick, S. J., Wilmore, D. W., Vars, H. M., and Rhoads, J. E.: Can intravenous feeding as a sole means of nutrition support growth in the child and restore weight loss in an adult? An affirmative answer, Ann. Surg. 169:974, 1969.

26. Dudrick, S. J., Steiger, E., and Long, J. M.: Renal failure in surgical patients: Treatment with intravenous essential amino acids and hypertonic dextrose, Surgery 68:180, 1970.

27. Dudrick, S. J., MacFadyen, B. V., Van Buren, C. T., Ruberg, R. L., and Maynard, A. T.: Parenteral hyperalimentation, metabolic problems and solutions, Ann. Surg. 176:259, 1972.

28. Dudrick, S. J.: Hyperalimentation in the cancer patient. Presented at Symposium on Parenteral Nutrition, Maastricht, Holland, Sept. 1976. In press.

29. Edmunds, L. H., Jr., Williams, G. M., and Welch, C. E.: External gastrointestinal fistulas arising from the gastrointestinal tract, Ann. Surg. 152:445, 1960.

30. Elman, R.: *Parenteral Alimentation in Surgery* (New York: Paul B. Hoeber, Inc., 1948).

31. Escourrou, J., James, J. H., Hodgman, J. M., et al.: Effect of branched chain amino acids on plasma and brain amino acids and brain neurotransmitters, Gastroenterology 71:(a-11) 904, 1976.

32. Felig, P.: Intravenous nutrition: Fact and fancy, N. Engl. J. Med. 294: 1455, 1976.

33. Fischer, J. E., and Baldessarini, R. J.: False neurotransmitters and hepatic failure, Lancet 2:75, 1971.

34. Fischer, J. E., Foster, G. S., Abel, R. M., Abbott, W. M., and Ryan, J. A.: Hyperalimentation as primary therapy for inflammatory bowel disease, Am. J. Surg. 125:165, 1973.

35. Fischer, J. E., Yoshimura, N., James, J. H., Cummings, M. G., Abel, R. M., and Deindoerfer, F.: Plasma amino acids in patients with hepatic encephalopathy: Effects of amino acid infusions, Am. J. Surg. 127:40, 1974.

36. Fischer, J. E.: False Neurotransmitters and Hepatic Coma, in *Brain Dysfunction in Metabolic Disorders,* ARNMD Series 53:53 (New York: Raven Press, 1974).

37. Fischer, J. E.: The Management of High-Output Intestinal Fistulas, in Longmire, W. P., Jr. (ed.): *Advances in Surgery* (Chicago: Year Book Medical Publishers, Inc., 1975), Vol. 9.

38. Fischer, J. E., Funovics, J. M., Aguirre, A., James, J. H., Keane, J. M., Wesdorp, R. I. C., Yoshimura, N., and Westman, T.: The role of plasma amino acids in hepatic encephalopathy, Surgery 78:276, 1975.

39. Fischer, J. E., Rosen, H. M., Ebeid, A. M., James, J. H., Keane, J. M., and Soeters, P. B.: The effect of normalization of plasma amino acids on hepatic encephalopathy in man, Surgery 80:77, 1976.

40. Freeman, J. B., Steginck, L. D., Irg, L. K., Sherman, B. M., and Den-Besten, L.: Evaluation of amino acid infusions as protein sparing agents in normal adult subjects, Am. J. Clin. Nutr. 28:477, 1975.

40a. Freund, H., Yoshimura, N. and Fischer, J. E.: Role of the branched chain amino acid in protein sparing. Submitted for publication.

41. Gamble, J. L.: Physiological information gained from studies on the life raft ration, Harvey Lect. 42:247, 1946.

42. Gazzard, B., Weston, M. S., Murray-Lyon, I. M., et al.: Charcoal hemoperfusion in the treatment of fulminant hepatic failure, Lancet 1:1301, 1974.

42a. Gibbons, G. W., Blackburn, G. L., Harken, D., Valdes, P., and Moorehead, D.: Hyperalimentation in the treatment of cardiac cachexia, J. Surg. Res. 20:439, 1976.

43. Giordano, C.: Use of exogenous and endogenous urea for protein synthesis in normal and uremic subjects, J. Lab. Clin. Med. 62:231, 1963.

44. Giovannetti, S., and Maggiore, Q.: A low-nitrogen diet with protein of high biological value for severe chronic uraemia, Lancet 1:1000, 1964.

45. Glew, R. H., Buckley, H. R., Rosen, H. M., Moellering, R. C., and Fischer, J. E.: Value of prospective candida precipitins in fungemia in patients with hyperalimentation, Surg. Forum 26:113, 1975.

46. Goodgame, T. J., and Fischer, J. E.: Parenteral nutrition in the treatment of acute pancreatitis: Effect on complications and mortality, Ann. Surg. In press.

47. Greenberger, G. R., Marliss, E. B., Anderson, G. H., et al.: Protein sparing therapy in postoperative patients, N. Engl. J. Med. 294:1411, 1976.

48. Halliday, M.: Personal communication.

49. Halmagyi, M. P. B.: Parenteral nutrition in trauma. Presented at Symposium for Nutritional Care of the Critically Ill, Maastricht, Holland, Sept. 1976. In press.

50. Heird, W. C., Nicholson, J. F., Driscoll, J. M., Jr., Schullinger, J. N., and Winters, R. W.: Hyperammonemia resulting from intravenous alimentation using a mixture of synthetic L-amino acids: A preliminary report, J. Pediatr. 81:162, 1972.

51. Holter, A. R., and Fischer, J. E.: The effects of perioperative hyperalimentation on complications in patients with carcinoma and weight loss, J. Surg. Res. In press.

52. Hoover, H. C., Jr., Grant, J. P., Gorschboth, C., et al.: Nitrogen-sparing

intravenous fluids in postoperative fluids, N. Engl. J. Med. 293:172, 1975.

53. Iber, F. L., Rosen, H., Levenson, S. M., and Chalmers, T. C.: The plasma amino acids in patients with liver failure, J. Clin. Lab. Med. 50:417, 1957.

54. Iob, V., Coon, W. W., and Sloan, M.: Altered clearance of free amino acids from plasma of patients with cirrhosis of the liver, J. Surg. Res. 6: 233, 1966.

55. Jarrard, M., and Freeman, J. B.: The effects of antiseptics and ointments on the skin flora beneath subclavian catheter dressings during total parenteral nutrition, J. Surg. Res. In press.

56. Jeejeebhoy, K. N., Langer, B., Tsallas, G., et al.: Total parenteral nutrition at home: Studies in patients surviving 4 months to 5 years, Gastroenterology 71:943, 1976.

57. Jeejeebhoy, K. N., and Phillips, R. J.: Isolated mammalian hepatocytes in culture, Gastroenterology 71:1086, 1976.

57a. Jeejeebhoy, K. N.: Relationship of energy input to nitrogen retention and substrate hormone profile. Presented at Symposium on Parenteral Nutrition, Maastricht, Holland, Sept. 1976. In press.

58. Kay, R. G., Tasman-Jones, C., Pybus, J., et al.: A syndrome of acute zinc deficiency during total parenteral alimentation in man, Ann. Surg. 183: 331, 1976.

59. Kinney, J. M., Long, C. L., and Duke, J. H., Jr.: Carbohydrate Metabolism after Injury, in R. Porter and J. Knight (eds.): *Energy Metabolism in Trauma* (London: J. & A. Churchill, Ltd., 1970). Presented at CIBA Conference, London, Feb. 1970.

60. Kinney, J. M.: Energy Requirements for Parenteral Nutrition, in Fischer, J. E. (ed.): *Total Parenteral Nutrition* (Boston: Little, Brown & Co., 1976).

61. Lam, K. C., Tall, A. R., Goldstein, G. B., et al.: Role of a false neurotransmitter, octopamine, in the pathogenesis of hepatic and renal encephalopathy, Scand. J. Gastroenterol. 8:465, 1973.

62. Landau, R. L., and Lugibihl, H.: Effect of glucagon on concentrations of several free amino acids in plasma, Diabetes 20:834, 1971.

63. Lee, H. A., Sharpstone, P., and Ames, A.: Parenteral nutrition in renal failure, Postgrad. Med. J. 43:18, 1967.

64. Lee, H.: Parenteral nutrition in renal failure. Presented at Symposium on Parenteral Nutrition, Maastricht, Holland, Sept. 1976. In press.

65. Long, J. M., Wilmore, D., Mason, A. D., et al.: Fat-carbohydrate interactions: Effect on nitrogen sparing in total intravenous feedings, Surg. Forum 25:61, 1974.

66. Long, J. M., III, Wilmore, D. W., Mason, A. D., et al.: Comparison of carbohydrate and fat as caloric sources, Surg. Forum 26:108, 1975.

67. MacFadyen, B. V., Jr., and Dudrick, S. J.: Management of gastrointestinal fistulae with parenteral hyperalimentation, Surgery 74:100, 1973.

68. Maddrey, W. C., Weber, F. L., Coulter, A. W., et al.: Effects of keto-analogues of essential amino acids in portal systemic encephalopathy, Gastroenterology 71:190, 1976.

69. Manghani, K. K., Lunzer, M. R., Billings, B. H., et al.: Urinary and se-

rum octopamine in patients with portal systemic encephalopathy, Lancet 2:943, 1975.
70. Mattson, W. J., Jr., Iob, V., Sloan, M., Coon, W. W., Turcotte, J. G., and Child, C. G., III: Alterations of individual free amino acids in brain during acute hepatic coma, Surg. Gynecol. Obstet. 130:263, 1970.
71. McEnany, R. J., Vang, J. H., and Drapanas, T.: Amino acids and α-keto acid concentrations in the plasma and blood of the liverless dog, Am. J. Physiol. 209:1046, 1965.
72. Meng, H. C.: Fat Emulsions in Parenteral Nutrition, in Fischer, J. E. (ed.): *Total Parenteral Nutrition* (Boston: Little, Brown & Co., 1976).
73. Moore, F. D.: *The Metabolic Care of the Surgical Patient* (Philadelphia: W. B. Saunders Company, 1959).
74. Munro, H. N.: A General Survey of Pathological Changes, in Munro, H. N., and Allison, J. B. (eds.): *Protein Metabolism* (New York: Academic Press, Inc., 1970).
75. Oddessey, R., and Goldberg, A. L.: Oxidation of leucine by rat skeletal muscle, Am. J. Physiol. 223:1376, 1972.
76. Oldendorf, W. H.: Brain uptake of radiolabelled amino acids, amines and hexoses after arterial injection, Am. J. Physiol. 221:1629, 1971.
77. Opolon, P., Rapin, J. R., Huguet, C., et al.: Hepatic failure coma (HFC) treated by polyacrylonitrile membrane (PAN) hemodialysis (HD), Trans. Am. Soc. Artif. Intern. Organs 22:701, 1976.
78. Palmisano, D. J.: Nutrient deficiencies after intensive parenteral alimentation, N. Engl. J. Med. 291:799, 1974.
79. Parkes, J. D., Sharpstone, P., and Williams, R.: Levo-dopa in hepatic coma, Lancet 2:1341, 1970.
80. Reilly, J., Ryan, J. A., Strole, W., and Fischer, J. E.: Hyperalimentation in inflammatory bowel disease, Am. J. Surg. 131:192, 1976.
81. Reilly, J.: Inflammatory Bowel Disease, in Fischer, J. E. (ed.): *Total Parenteral Nutrition* (Boston: Little, Brown & Co., 1976).
82. Richmond, J., and Girwood, R. H.: Observations on amino acid absorption, Clin. Sci. 22:301, 1962.
83. Rocchio, M. A., Cha, C. M., Haas, K. F., and Randall, H. T.: Use of chemically defined diets in the management of patients with high output gastrointestinal fistulas, Am. J. Surg. 127:148, 1974.
84. Rocha, D. M., Faloona, G. R., and Unger, R. H.: Glucagon stimulating activity of 20 amino acids in dogs, J. Clin. Invest. 51:2346, 1972.
85. Rose, W. C., Coon, M. J., and Lambert, G. F.: The amino acid requirements of man: The role of the caloric intake, J. Biol. Chem. 210:331, 1954.
86. Rose, W. C., and Wixom, R. L.: The amino acid requirements of man. XVI. The role of the nitrogen intake, J. Biol. Chem. 217:997, 1955.
87. Rosen, H. M., Yoshimura, N., Hodgman, J. M., and Fischer, J. E.: Plasma amino acids in hepatic encephalopathy of differing etiology, Gastroenterology 72:483, 1977.
88. Rossi-Fanelli, F., Cangiano, C., Attik, A., et al.: Octopamine plasma levels and hepatic encephalopathy: A reappraisal of the problem, Clin. Chim. Acta 67:255, 1976.
89. Ryan, J. A., Jr.: Complications of Total Parenteral Nutrition, in Fischer,

J. E. (ed.): *Total Parenteral Nutrition* (Boston: Little, Brown & Co., 1976).

90. Ryan, J. A., Jr., Abel, R. M., Abbott, W. M., Hopkins, C. C., Chesney, T. McC., Colley, R., Phillips, K., and Fischer, J. E.: Catheter complications in total parenteral nutrition: A prospective study of 200 consecutive patients, N. Engl. J. Med. 290:757, 1974.

91. Scheflan, M., Galli, S. J., Perrotto, J., et al.: Intestinal adaptation after extensive resection of the small intestine and prolonged administration of parenteral nutrition, Surg. Gynecol. Obstet. 143:757, 1976.

92. Schlappner, O. L. A., Shelley, W. B., Ruberg, R. L., et al.: Acute papulo-pustular acne, J.A.M.A. 219:877, 1972.

92a. Sheldon, G. F., Gardiner, B. N., Way, L. W., et al.: Management of gastrointestinal fistulas, Surg. Gynecol. Obstet. 113:490, 1971.

92b. Shizgal, H. M., Spanier, A. H., and Kurtz, R. S.: Effect of parenteral nutrition on body composition in the critically ill patient, Am. J. Surg. 131:156, 1976.

93. Soeters, P. B., and Fischer, J. E.: Insulin, glucagon, amino acid imbalance, and hepatic failure, Lancet 2:880, 1976.

93a. Soeters, P. B., and Fischer, J. E.: In preparation.

94. Soeters, P. B., Weir, G., Ebeid, A. M., et al.: Changes in insulin and glucagon with onset of hepatic encephalopathy, J. Surg. Res. In press.

95. Solassol, C., and Joyeux, H.: Ambulatory Parenteral Nutrition, in Fischer, J. E. (ed.): *Total Parenteral Nutrition* (Boston: Little, Brown & Co., 1976).

96. Starzl, T. E., Putnam, C. E., Chase, H. P., et al.: Portacaval shunt in hyperlipoproteinemia, Lancet 2:940, 1973.

97. Starzl, T. E., Francavilla, A., Halgrimson, C. G., Francavilla, F. R., et al.: Origin, hormonal nature and action of hepatotrophic substances in portal venous blood, Surg. Gynecol. Obstet. 137:179, 1973.

98. Steffe, C. H.: Studies in amino acid utilization determination of minimal daily essential amino acid requirements in protein depleted adult male albino rats, J. Nutr. 40:483, 1950.

99. Steiger, E., Oram-Smith, J., Miller, E., Kuo, E., and Vars, H. M.: Effects of nutrition on tumor growth and tolerance of chemotherapy, J. Surg. Res. 18:455, 1975.

100. Takagi, Y., Itakura, T., Okada, A., et al.: A clinical analysis of zinc deficiency during hyperalimentation, Jap. J. Surg. 33:427, 1975.

101. Torsvik, H., Fischer, J. E., Feldman, H. A., and Lees, R. S.: Effects of intravenous hyperalimentation on plasma-lipoproteins in severe familial hypercholesterolaemia, Lancet 1:601, 1975.

102. Unger, R. H.: Glucagon and the insulin/glucagon ratio in diabetes and other catabolic illnesses, Diabetes 20:834, 1971.

103. Vilter, R. W., Bozian, R. C., Hess, E. V., et al.: Manifestations of copper deficiency in a patient with systemic sclerosis or intravenous hyperalimentation, N. Engl. J. Med. 291:188, 1974.

104. Vinnars, E., Bergstrom, J., and Furst, P.: Influence of the postoperative state on the intracellular free amino acids in human muscle tissue, Ann. Surg. 182:665, 1975.

105. Voitk, A. J., Echave, V., Brown, R. A., McArdle, A. H., and Gurd, F. N.:

Elemental diet in the treatment of fistulas of the alimentary tract, Surg. Gynecol. Obstet. 137:68, 1973.

106. Walser, M., Sapir, D. G., and Maddrey, W. C.: The Use of Alpha-Keto Analogues of Essential Amino Acids, in Fischer, J. E. (ed.): *Total Parenteral Nutrition* (Boston: Little, Brown & Co., 1976).

107. Walser, M., and Bodenlos, L. J.: Urea metabolism in man, J. Clin. Invest. 38:1617, 1959.

108. Walser, M., Dighe, S., Coulter, A. W., and Crantz, F. R.: The effect of keto-analogues of essential amino acids in severe chronic uremia, J. Clin. Invest. 52:678, 1973.

109. Wilmore, D. W., Lindsey, C. A., Moylan, J. A., Jr., Faloona, G. R., Pruitt, B. A., Jr., and Unger, R. H.: Hyperglucagonemia in burns, Lancet 1:73, 1974.

110. Wilmore, D. W., and Pruitt, B. A., Jr.: Parenteral Nutrition in Burn Patients, in Fischer, J. E. (ed.): *Total Parenteral Nutrition* (Boston: Little, Brown & Co., 1976).

110a. Wilmore, D. W., and Dudrick, S. J.: Safe long-term venous catheterization, Arch. Surg. 98:256, 1969.

111. Winters, R. W., and Hasselmeyer, E. G. (eds.): *Intravenous Nutrition in the High Risk Infant* (New York: John Wiley & Sons, Inc., 1975).

111a. Winters, R. W.: Lessons learned from the pediatric patient, Arch. Surg. In press.

112. Wolfe, B. M., Keltner, R. M., and Willman, V. L.: Intestinal fistula output in regular elemental and intravenous nutrition, Am. J. Surg. 124: 803, 1972.

113. Wolfe, B. M., Culebras, J. M., Fitzpatrick, G. F., et al.: Nitrogen sparing in man: The effect of carbohydrate calories added to intravenous amino acid infusions. Presented at Tripartite meeting, Philadelphia, Sept. 27, 1976.

114. Wretlind, A.: Complete intravenous nutrition: Theoretical and experimental background, Nutr. Metab. [Suppl.] 14:1, 1972.

115. Wu, C. J., Bollman, J. R., and Butt, H. R.: Changes in free amino acids in the plasma during hepatic coma, J. Clin. Invest. 37:845, 1955.

Surgical Aspects of Ulcerative Colitis and Crohn's Disease of the Large Bowel

J. C. GOLIGHER

University Department of Surgery, the General Infirmary at Leeds, England

In this account of ulcerative colitis and Crohn's disease of the large bowel as they concern the surgeon, it seemed appropriate to consider ulcerative colitis first of all and then to examine in what ways the presentation and surgical management of Crohn's colitis differ from those of ordinary colitis.

Ulcerative Colitis

Though the surgical treatment of ulcerative colitis is now to a large extent stereotyped, there are still a few outstanding issues, and in the description that follows particular note will be taken of these controversial points.

THE FORM THAT SURGICAL TREATMENT TAKES

Colectomy and Ileorectal Anastomosis

I should like to start with a question that always provokes a great deal of discussion, at any rate in Britain, and that is the role of colectomy and ileorectal anastomosis. This procedure

71

involves keeping virtually the whole of the rectum and carrying out an end-to-end or side-to-end anastomosis between the terminal ileum and the top of the rectal stump. It has the great attraction that it spares the patient a permanent ileostomy. Unfortunately, in ulcerative colitis the rectum is almost invariably affected by the disease, so this operation means keeping and using a diseased distal segment of large bowel, which would seem to be flying in the face of reason. However, sometimes after an ileorectal anastomosis the inflammation in the retained rectal stump resolves or, even if it does not, the patient may manage to obtain a very good functional result. In other cases the severe recurrent proctitis plagues the patient with intractable diarrhea and passage of blood and mucus, or complications arise, such as the development of an abscess or fistula, a stricture or even a carcinoma. There is a considerable difference of opinion as to how frequently unsatisfactory results of this kind occur and how often it is necessary for the patient subsequently to undergo rectal excision and conversion to an ileostomy. Aylett[5-7], Turnbull[63] and Watts and Hughes[67] paint a very rosy picture of the results of colectomy and ileorectal anastomosis for ulcerative colitis. The experiences of many other surgeons have been a good deal less impressive.[1, 2, 4, 8, 18, 26] Certainly, until recently the average surgical opinion in Britain and America has been distinctly unfavorable to this operation, but in the past 2 or 3 years a few British surgeons have been giving it a cautious trial again.[27, 54]

Unfortunately, surveys of patients treated by colectomy and ileorectal anastomosis have not revealed any clear guidelines as to which patients may be anticipated to do well with this operation and which badly.[8] Perhaps it is good policy to reserve the operation for patients with relatively mild changes in the rectum. It would also seem to be a wise precaution to follow Aylett's[7] advice and routinely establish a temporary defunctioning loop ileostomy immediately proximal to the ileorectal anastomosis to lessen the morbidity resulting from anastomotic dehiscence, which in his experience has not been uncommon. The ileostomy is maintained till the anastomosis is soundly healed and the patient has made a good recovery from the initial operation.

Ileostomy and Complete Proctocolectomy (or Subtotal Colectomy)

The operation most surgeons prefer for patients ill enough to require surgical treatment is ileostomy and proctocolectomy. A 1-stage ileostomy and complete proctocolectomy is ideal insofar as it eliminates in 1 step all the diseased tissue, and, if the surgeon is accustomed to using the synchronous combined approach to rectal excision,[22, 31, 41] the whole operation can be performed very easily and expeditiously. If the surgeon is not familiar with the synchronous combined technique for removing the rectum or has relatively little experience of colitis surgery, or if the patient is undergoing an urgent or emergency operation during a severe exacerbation of the disease, it may be wiser to do an ileostomy and subtotal colectomy in the 1st instance. In this operation the rectum and distal end of sigmoid colon are retained and the end of the sigmoidorectal stump is brought up to the anterior abdominal wall in the suprapubic or left iliac region as a mucous fistula (or, rarely, closed by suture if the tissues of the colon wall are strong enough to permit secure stitching). Ileostomy and subtotal colectomy has the additional advantage that it keeps open the possibility of a secondary ileorectal anastomosis if the inflammation in the rectum should subside sufficiently in the next 6–12 months or later. More usually, however, though the patient achieves a good recovery of general health, such changes in the rectum persist that a subsequent anastomosis is unwise. Indeed, continued troublesome discharge of blood and pus from the rectal remnant may necessitate its removal within a few months. In any event, if the rectum is not used for ileorectal anastomosis, it should eventually be excised because of the risk of malignant change (or kept under close supervision with rectal biopsies every 6–12 months to detect signs of so-called precancer).

The feature about a proctocolectomy that proves so daunting to the patient is of course the ileostomy. When first contemplated by the average lay person, particularly a young woman or teenager, an ileostomy seems a revoltingly unnatural arrangement, calculated to put an end to all romantic aspirations or even to imperil the integrity of a well-established marriage. Unquestionably the best way to overcome the patient's initial revulsion is to arrange for her or him to have a heart-to-heart talk with an ileostomy patient of the same sex, age and social background. It is no exaggeration also to say that the success of the operation is largely dependent on the surgeon's ability to provide the patient with a good ileostomy and the patient's capacity to learn to manage it in a trouble-free manner.

ILEOSTOMY TECHNIQUE. — In the construction of the ileostomy the first consideration — and a vitally important one — is the siting of the stoma, bearing in mind that the patient is going to wear an adherent bag on the skin immediately surrounding the stoma. To make sure of having a smooth, flat skin surface to which to affix the appliance, it is best to make the ileostomy at a separate circular or "trephine" wound, away from the main incision and not too close to the umbilicus, the anterior superior iliac spine or the groin — in fact, in the sort of locations shown in Figure 1, probably best at the lower site (B). The higher site (A) lies at the waistline and, though that helps in holding the appliance securely with a belt, it is inconvenient in other ways. It is ruinous to a woman's figure if she is wearing a tightly fitting dress, and it is a nuisance to a man if, as is increasingly popular, he uses a belt instead of suspenders to support his trousers. A very good plan is to choose tentatively the place for the ileostomy the day before the operation and to make the patient wear

Fig 1. — Diagram showing sites for separate trephine wounds for an ileostomy.

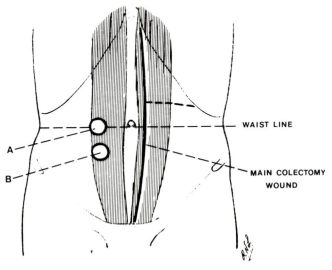

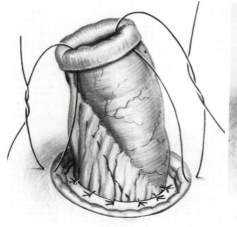
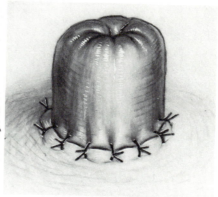

Fig 2 (left). – Technique of ileostomy. The ileal stump has been fixed by a circumferential row of 3–0 silk sutures between the anterior rectus sheath and the ileal wall and mesentery, leaving 5–7 cm of ileum projecting beyond the skin. The cut end of the bowel is then sutured to the edge of the skin wound by further fine silk or catgut stitches to produce eversion and mucocutaneous apposition.

Fig 3 (above). – Completed ileostomy. (Figs 2 and 3 from Goligher, J. C.[19]).

an adherent bag at that site for 24 hours or so while fully ambulant, if possible, to demonstrate any disadvantages of the position. This site is then marked for the guidance of the surgeon at the operation.

The actual operative technique for making an ileostomy now used by virtually all surgeons is immediate eversion and primary mucocutaneous suture, as described by Brooke.[10] This obviates the staggeringly high incidence (almost 50%) of ileostomy dysfunction that occurred when the ileostomy was made by simply leaving the terminal ileum projecting beyond the abdominal skin with the serosa exposed.[15, 64] The exact way in which I practice the eversion technique is portrayed in Figures 2 and 3. It should be stressed that the silk sutures fixing the inner tube of bowel pass between the anterior rectus sheath and the ileal wall itself, not just the leaf of the mesentery as advised by Brooke[10] and many others. However, the bite of the stitch in the bowel wall is relatively superficial, just through the serosa and muscularis, so that if necrosis occurs it will not lead to the development of an intestinal fistula. I have used this method of fixation without untoward results in several hundred patients. The bowel is then everted by suture of its cut end to the skin, producing a projecting stoma. It is probably wise to aim to have the completed ileostomy project 2.5–3.5 cm beyond the skin, which means that before the ileal stump is everted, it should extend at least 5–7 cm beyond the skin level.

STOMAL CARE. — In regard to stomal care, the great innovation was the introduction of the adherent bag by Koenig and Rutzen.[61] This was a rubber bag stuck to the skin by a cement or a double-sided adhesive plaster. Quite a number of my patients who have had ileostomies for several years still use this type of bag and are very satisfied with it. But, as with so many other things in life at present, the trend is toward the use of disposable plastic substitutes, and the fashionable ileostomy appliances

Fig 4.—A, Hollister plastic disposable ileostomy bag, back view. **B,** frilly, colored cloth bag to cover the Hollister appliance.

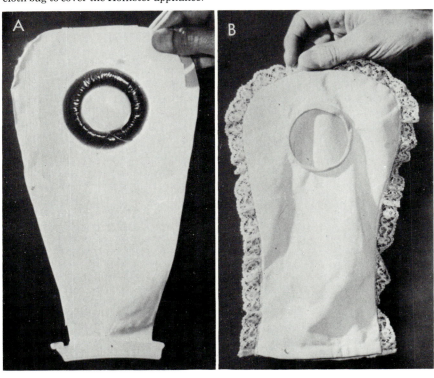

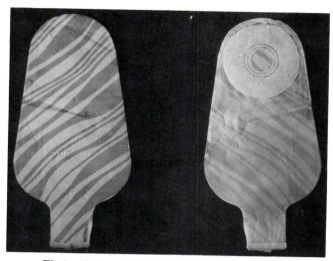

Fig 5. — Patterned Coloplast plastic disposable bag.

nowadays are plastic. A popular bag at the moment is the Hollister appliance (Fig 4,A). One criticism often leveled at it is that the feces are visible through the translucent plastic material, which embarrasses some patients. But it does not require too much ingenuity or expertise to make an attractive frilly covering of cloth to overcome this objection (Fig 4,B). Alternatively, a patterned type of plastic bag may be preferred (Fig 5).

The other great advance in stomal care has been the evolution of the so-called enterostomal therapist. We owe this largely to the vision and drive of Rupert Turnbull of Cleveland, Ohio, and the superb example of his colleague, Norma Gill, who has now trained several hundred enterostomal therapists. Though a surgeon can look after all details of stomal management himself, as used to be done, it is a great convenience on a busy surgical service to have available an experienced enterostomal therapist familiar with the various types of appliances on the market for ileostomies, colostomies and urinary stomas and knowledgeable about all the problems that may arise in connection with their use.

COMPLICATIONS. — Of the various complications that can occur with an ileostomy, unquestionably the commonest is soreness of the peristomal skin, for which there may be several causes.

Rarely it is due to a sensitivity to the material of the appliance or the adhesive. More usually it is caused by leakage of ileal contents between the appliance and the skin, with resultant cutaneous digestion. Such leakage may be caused by inadequate attention on the part of the patient to the details of application of the bag, by very liquid feces (as after resection of some of the terminal ileum along with the large bowel) or by structural imperfections of the stoma itself.

However the skin soreness originates, once it is present it makes it difficult to secure firm fixation of the appliance to the abdominal wall. Leakage is thus liable to occur, with further excoriation of the skin. A vicious circle is established, which used to present a very difficult problem in management. But now we have 2 agents that are invaluable aids in dealing with this situation – karaya gum, either as a powder or a washer, and Stomahesive squares (E. R. Squibb). With these preparations one can stick the appliance to a raw, oozing skin surface; the agents also exercise a soothing and healing effect on the inflamed skin. Some patients continue to use karaya or Stomahesive indefinitely; others are able to return to their ordinary routine of management after a few weeks, but with greater attention to detail.

If the feces are very loose or liquid, it is helpful as a rule to prescribe codeine phosphate (60–120 mg 4 times daily) or Lomotil (2 tablets 4 times daily). Some patients find it useful to persist indefinitely with such medication, possibly at reduced dosage.

If the stoma itself shows major structural imperfections – fixed inadequate protrusion, sliding recession, prolapse, fistulation of the ileal spout, peristomal herniation – or is badly sited, it may be necessary to consider refashioning or resiting it. The fact that the stoma is not perfectly made or sited or shows one or more of these complications does not automatically mean that a further operation is required. On the contrary, if the patient is able to compensate for structural inadequacy by particular attention to ileostomy care, probably employing the special measures listed earlier, there is no need to reoperate. But if these measures fail, a reconstruction of the stoma at the same or another site can be a gratifying maneuver.[19, 22] In some patients a badly functioning or complicated ileostomy has been converted to a reservoir ileostomy, often with very satisfactory results.

RESERVOIR ILEOSTOMY. — N. G. Kock of Gothenburg, Sweden, has described several ingenious techniques[32-35] for preparing a so-called reservoir ileostomy, in which the 45 or 50 cm of ileum immediately proximal to the stoma is folded on itself, opened and anastomosed to form a pouch or sump in which the feces can accumulate until evacuated by the passage of a tube through the stoma into the reservoir. In this way the patients are spared the necessity of wearing an external appliance, which makes this an attractive idea to them. Originally it was hoped that the method of constructing the reservoir would result in an aperistaltic intestinal sac that would exhibit no proclivity to expel feces between intubations. Unfortunately, further experience showed that for complete continence it was necessary to intussuscept the base of the exit conduit of bowel into the reservoir to produce a nipple valve, thus mimicking the effect of an unspillable inkwell. Furthermore, it was soon discovered that there is a great tendency for the nipple valve to be extruded from the reservoir in time, with resultant loss of continence and difficulty in passing the tube.[23, 34, 35] The main problem with the reservoir ileostomy is, indeed, how to construct the valve in such a way that it will remain in position.

Formerly[33] Kock made the nipple valve in the way depicted in Figure 6. As a preliminary, the serosal surface of the 8–10-cm segment of ileal exit conduit that was to be used for constructing the valve was diathermized. Then this diathermized piece of bowel was drawn into the reservoir as a 4–5-cm intussusception, while the walls of the entering and leaving segments of the valve were sutured together by 2 or 3 rows of through-and-through stitches of fine silk. Though this technique secured good apposition of the 2 bowel walls over most of their circumference, inevitably at the sector corresponding to the entering and leaving mesentery no sutures could be inserted, leaving a gap in this location. Kock[34, 35] believes that it is through this gap that most valve extrusions take place (Fig 7).

Recently[34, 35] Kock has adopted a new technique for construction of the valve. The mesentery of the piece of ileum to be used for the intussusception valve is split into 2 halves corresponding to the future entering and leaving segments of bowel (Fig 8,A). Next, 1 or 2 Lembert sutures of fine silk are inserted on 1 side of the piece of ileum that will be the entering layer in the completed valve, and are passed through the mesenteric split, to be

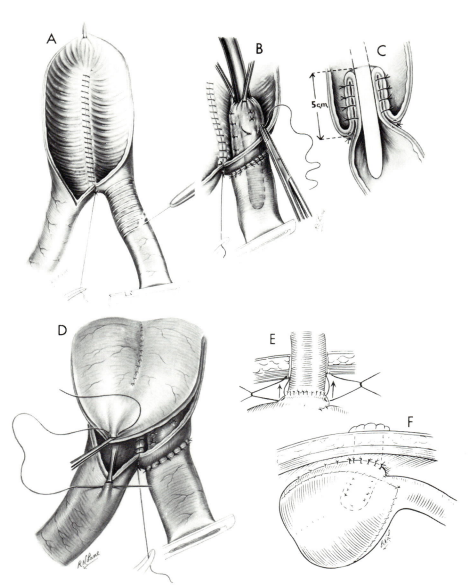

Fig 6. – Construction of reservoir ileostomy. **A,** loop of ileum has been joined by suture and opened up to form an oval plate. On the terminal unopened part that will form the exit conduit connecting the reservoir to the surface, the serosal surface of the proximal 8 – 10 cm is being scored with diathermy preparatory to making the nipple valve. **B,** part of the exit conduit has been drawn into the uncompleted reservoir to form the nipple valve and is being sutured in position by 2 or 3 rows of through-and-through silk stitches (**C**). **D,** opened bowel is folded over and sutured to close the reservoir. **E,** exit conduit is brought out through the abdominal wall and sutured to the skin while the reservoir around the base of the conduit is firmly secured by sutures to the anterior parietal peritoneum (**F**). (From Goligher, J. C., and Lintott, D.[23])

80

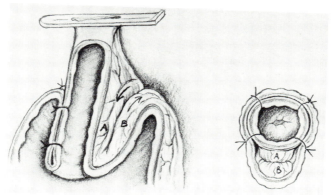

Fig 7. — Diagram to show the wide mesenteric gap left by the technique described in Figure 6, through which valve extrusion probably takes place.

inserted on the opposite side of the future leaving layer. As the intussusception is drawn into the lumen of the reservoir, tying these sutures has the effect of rotating the bowel, so that the 2 parts of the mesentery in the finished valve do not coincide but lie at different points on the bowel circumference (Fig 8,B). Fur-

Fig 8. — Technique of constructing nipple valve with partial rotation of ileum as it is intussuscepted to separate the mesentery of the ingoing from that of the outgoing bowel. **A,** mesentery is split at a point corresponding to the apex of the future nipple valve, and silk Lembert sutures are passed from one side of the bowel to the other through the mesenteric split. **B,** when the bowel is intussuscepted, tying of these and similarly placed sutures secures a rotation and separation of the 2 halves of the mesentery, the result being 2 small mesenteric gaps instead of 1 large one (**C**). (Figs 7 and 8 after Kock.[34])

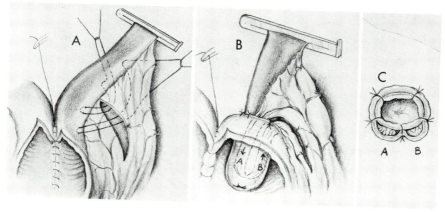

ther silk Lembert sutures can then be placed around the base of the valve, with such a distribution as to leave 2 small mesenteric gaps rather than a single large one (Fig 8,C). In this technique the preliminary application of diathermy to the serosa of the bowel is carried out as in the previous method, and the peritoneal leaves and some of the fat of the portion of mesentery corresponding to the diathermized piece of ileum are dissected away. The numerous deep silk sutures through both layers of bowel in the valve are avoided, because in some patients Kock[34, 35] has found that they lead to the development of fistulas through the valve, with resulting loss of continence.

The precise value of this new method of preparing the nipple valve remains to be established by further experience, but the results to date are encouraging, according to Kock,[35] with few subsequent extrusions. This compares favorably with the frequent valve extrusions that occurred after the previous method and which, together with other complications such as abscess formation and fistulation, necessitated 2d and even 3d or 4th operations in no less than 30–40% of patients.[9, 23, 34, 35]

As for the place of the reservoir ileostomy in the overall pattern of contemporary surgery for ulcerative colitis, caution must be exercised in making pronouncements at present. Obviously this type of operation carries intrinsic risks of leakage and infection that scarcely apply at all to a conventional ileostomy. As such hazards are likely to be increased during acute phases of the disease, consideration of this procedure should be reserved exclusively for patients whose colitis is in complete remission and who are in reasonably good general condition. Even these patients should be left in no doubt that the choice of a reservoir ileostomy increases somewhat the hazards of operation. It has also been necessary, until recently at least, to stress that it is difficult to guarantee that complete continence will be obtained without a possible further intervention. Unquestionably the most satisfactory type of patient to be considered for a reservoir ileostomy is the patient who has already had a proctocolectomy and conventional ileostomy and because of persistent problems in relation to the ileostomy is anxious to try a reservoir type of operation. Finally, it should be emphasized that unless a surgeon is doing a lot of ileostomies, it is unlikely that he will be finding enough indications for reservoir ileostomy to enable him to become really competent at the technically quite challenging task of constructing a continent reservoir. Until the difficulties and uncertainties of the operation are clearly seen to be in large measure resolved, reservoir ileostomy will be better avoided by the occasional ileostomy surgeon.

INDICATIONS FOR SURGERY

Elective Operation

CHRONIC INVALIDISM AND FAILURE OF MEDICAL TREATMENT. — This is probably the commonest reason for elective surgical treatment. Sometimes the indication is only too evident, as in the patient with a history of severe colitis for several years who presents in a state of extreme emaciation with gross extensive changes in the large bowel on sigmoidoscopic and radiologic examination, and often with local or systemic complications as well.

In other patients with less severe symptoms and disability the decision for or against surgery may be extremely difficult. To a large extent it depends on the patient's own assessment of the relative handicap imposed by the continued colitis against the risks, discomfort and subsequent inconvenience of an operation involving a permanent ileostomy. Clearly it is of paramount importance that he or she be given the opportunity to talk to other patients who have had an ileostomy to form a clear impression of how compatible ileostomy under modern management is with a really full and active life. From the surgeon's point of view an important consideration will be the radiologic extent of the disease, for there is no doubt that total or subtotal colitis is much more serious than is a more limited colitis as regards the possible occurrence of additional severe attacks of the disease, the development of malignant change or other complications.

RISKS OR ACTUAL DEVELOPMENT OF MALIGNANT CHANGE. — That long-standing extensive colitis carries a risk of cancerous change is now well established, and avoidance of this serious complication is important in the management of patients with total or subtotal colitis.[22] At one time it was my practice to urge prophylactic proctocolectomy on such patients who had had colitis for 10 or more years. Now Morson and Pang[48] have claimed to be able to select the colitis patients particularly prone to carci-

noma by the finding of epithelial dysplasia on rectal biopsy.
There is at present in Britain a trend, in which we have partici-
pated, to use this screening device in the conservative management of patients with extensive colitis to indicate which ones
should be urged to undergo proctocolectomy. It remains to be
seen how reliable this method of selection is, particularly if extended to include colonoscopic biopsies.[39]

Unfortunately, one still sees a certain number of colitis patients who have harbored the disease for 14–20 years without
too much inconvenience and then present with an evident carcinoma of the colon or rectum. This provides a clear indication for
operation, unless, as is frequently the case, the growth is already obviously inoperable.

POSSIBLE RETARDATION OF GROWTH AND DEVELOPMENT. — In
children or adolescents the possibility of physical retardation
due to continued colitis must also be seriously considered and
may be an additional reason for advising radical operation. It has
to be remembered, too, that the risk of malignant change applies
particularly to patients whose colitis commenced in childhood,
so that operation in these young patients may have a double
prophylactic objective. Misgivings have often been expressed
about the infliction of an ileostomy on children. My experience is
that they tolerate this operation well and with good management quickly adapt to the stoma.

LOCAL ANORECTAL COMPLICATIONS. — Though anorectal abscesses and fistulas in connection with colitis may need some
local surgical treatment, this should be as conservative as possible, for there is a great tendency for these complications to improve as the underlying bowel condition undergoes remission. It
is only rarely that such complications contribute to the overall
indication for radical bowel surgery.

SYSTEMIC COMPLICATIONS. — Though systemic complications,
such as arthritis, skin lesions and iritis, may subside largely or
completely as the bowel condition improves, they may persist
till radical surgical treatment is undertaken. They are thus occasionally a factor in the indications for surgery.

Urgent or Emergency Operation

During a severe attack of ulcerative colitis, when medical
treatment fails or major complications occur, the surgeon may

TABLE 1.—OPERATIVE MORTALITY IN
ULCERATIVE COLITIS ACCORDING TO
URGENCY OF SURGICAL INTERVENTION

	PATIENTS TREATED	MORTALITY (%)
Elective operation	420	3
Urgent and emergency operations	135	16
All operations	555	6

be asked by the internist to undertake a lifesaving operation. Unfortunately, surgical interventions of this kind have not infrequently failed to save life, because they tend to carry a much higher mortality than elective operations (Table 1). In this connection it is convenient to distinguish between urgent and emergency operations.

URGENT OPERATION. — In treating a severe attack of ulcerative colitis with intensive steroid therapy and other supportive measures, it is the expectation of the internist that spontaneous remission will occur. The question is how long conservative measures should be continued in this hope. Opinions differ, but many experienced clinicians would accept that, if clear signs of commencing remission are not evident within 7 days, it is unlikely to occur, and continued conservative treatment beyond that point may simply expose the patient to an increased risk of toxic megacolon and colonic perforation. Certainly our experience (see Table 2) would suggest that a lower mortality may be

TABLE 2.—OUTCOME OF SEVERE ATTACKS OF COLITIS
ACCORDING TO DURATION OF MEDICAL TREATMENT
BEFORE RESORT TO SURGERY*

OUTCOME	MEAN PERIOD OF MEDICAL TREATMENT	
	14 DAYS (% OF 124 ATTACKS, 1955–63)	7 DAYS (% OF 134 ATTACKS, 1964–69)
Remission	52.4	46.3
Resort to surgery	32.3	53.0
Deaths		
Under medical treatment	4.8	0.7
Operative	20.0	7.0
Total	11.3	4.5

*From Goligher et al.[20]

obtained if a maximum period of medical treatment of 7 days is accepted instead of 14 days. But it is wise for the internist to have some set period in mind and, if remission fails to commence in that time, to resort fairly rapidly to what might be termed an urgent operation.

EMERGENCY OPERATION. — A patient who is undergoing intensive medical treatment of a severe attack needs to be watched with particular vigilance for the occurrence of any development that might indicate the necessity for an immediate or emergency operation. One such development would be suspected perforation of the colon. This could reveal itself by the occurrence of classic abdominal and constitutional signs of bowel perforation; but if the patient is under heavy steroid medication, which tends to mask signs, these abdominal manifestations may be less definite or entirely absent. In the latter event the diagnosis and decision to intervene have to depend on a sudden deterioration in the general condition.

Another complication demanding emergency intervention is toxic megacolon, which can quickly lead to perforation. To detect the development of this preperforation state at the earliest possible moment, it is a good plan to insist on a plain radiograph of the abdomen every day while the patient is undergoing medical treatment for a severe attack of colitis. Extremely rarely, profuse continued bleeding from the large bowel may be the indication for an emergency operation.

TYPE OF OPERATION TO BE PERFORMED IN URGENT OR EMERGENCY INTERVENTIONS. — Until recently most surgeons have favored an ileostomy and subtotal colectomy (or proctocolectomy) as the operation to be performed during severe attacks of colitis. But if, as happens in only a proportion of these patients, toxic megacolon has developed, this operation may be technically quite difficult. In 1970 Turnbull et al.[62] suggested as an alternative in patients with megacolon the performance of a simple loop ileostomy with a decompressing transverse (and/or sigmoid) colostomy. Results with this method were certainly impressive, with only 1 death in 26 patients so treated, an experience that has since been considerably extended with an almost equally favorable outcome.[64] Patients for whom this method would seem to be especially indicated are those with a toxic megacolon and a colonic perforation that has sealed itself off by adherence of the affected part of the colon, say the sigmoid, to the abdominal wall, for if a formal colectomy is carried out in these patients, the perforation is reopened with resultant contamination of the general peritoneal cavity. These, in fact, are the only patients in whom I personally have used the Turnbull technique. For patients with toxic megacolon without perforation or with an open perforation that has already drained freely into the abdominal cavity, and for patients with severe attacks of colitis without megacolon, I have performed subtotal colectomy (or proctocolectomy) and ileostomy. Even in patients with a sealed perforation, it is often possible with brisk use of a sucker or possibly the excision of a disk of anterior parietal peritoneum along with the adherent colon to avoid major peritoneal contamination.

Crohn's Disease of the Large Intestine

Crohn's disease (regional enteritis or granulomatous disease) may present in many ways and may occur anywhere from the mouth to the anus, or even very rarely may manifest itself entirely outside the alimentary tract.[22, 49] But from the practical point of view it is convenient to recognise 2 main forms of the condition:

1. Terminal ileitis (less commonly jejunitis or jejunoileitis), which not infrequently spreads distally into the cecum or ascending colon. This is of course the classic presentation, as described by Crohn et al.[16] If it comes to surgical treatment, this lesion has usually been dealt with by terminal ileectomy (often with less or more right hemicolectomy). Over the past 45 years most general surgeons have become thoroughly familiar with the entity and its treatment and know only too well that on prolonged follow-up after operation recurrence unfortunately takes place in at least 60–80% of the patients.[22] It is not proposed to consider further classic Crohn's disease in this article.

2. Crohn's disease mainly or entirely of the large bowel. We owe the recognition and clear description of this form of the disease to Pugh,[56] Wells,[68] Brooke,[11] Marshak et al.,[46] Cornes and Stecher,[14] Lindner et al.,[40] and above all to Lockhart-Mummery and Morson.[42, 43] As these writers have shown, Crohn's disease can occur in the colon and rectum exclusively or with less or more involvement of the small intestine. During the past 17 years this form of the disease has been increasingly frequently encountered, and at the present time in areas where colitis is

common, when a patient is referred to hospital with this diagnosis, there is at least an even chance that the condition will turn out to be Crohn's colitis rather than ordinary ulcerative colitis. Crohn's disease of the large bowel has thus become a major interest of gastroenterologically minded internists and surgeons.

Clinical Features and Diagnosis of Crohn's Disease Mainly or Entirely in the Colon and Rectum

At first sight Crohn's colitis and ordinary ulcerative colitis resemble each other quite closely, but there are a number of dissimilarities that enable the 2 conditions to be distinguished clinically, radiologically and pathologically in at least 90% of cases. Because of differences in the prognosis and possibly in the indications for and type of surgical treatment required, it is desirable if possible to make a differential diagnosis before embarking on definitive therapy. The pathologic and clinical differentiation between the 2 diseases is well discussed by Lockhart-Mummery and Morson.[42, 43] Some of the more significant features on which a clinical differentiation is based are listed in Table 3. It will be appreciated that a few of these points, such as the highly characteristic appearance of Crohn's proctitis or the absence of rectal involvement in Crohn's colitis, provide an absolute distinction, as does a positive rectal or anal biopsy for this condition or a barium enema examination showing "skip lesions" in the colon or extensive ileal disease together with con-

TABLE 3.–POINTS IN FAVOR OF A CROHN'S COLITIS
RATHER THAN ORDINARY ULCERATIVE COLITIS

1. Diarrhea less severe, often only diurnal rather than diurnal and nocturnal as in ulcerative colitis
2. Bleeding less common
3. On sigmoidoscopy, rectum appears normal or shows a patchy proctitis
4. Biopsy of any rectal lesion may show typical histologic appearances of Crohn's disease – but biopsy is only as good as the pathologist!
5. Anal fissure, abscess or fistula more common in Crohn's colitis but not infrequent in ulcerative colitis; biopsy may help
6. Perianal edema, discoloration and ulceration highly characteristic of Crohn's disease[44]; biopsy may confirm
7. Barium enema examination may suggest Crohn's colitis from distribution of disease – "skipping," sparing of rectum, extensive implication of terminal ileum – or from nature of radiologic appearances – spiculation, asymmetry, stricture
8. Small-bowel meal examination shows considerable involvement of ileum or jejunum

siderable involvement of the large bowel. Other points, such as the severity of the alteration of bowel habits or the presence or absence of overt rectal bleeding, merely add collectively to the likelihood of one or the other diagnosis.

SURGICAL TREATMENT

It should be emphasized that Crohn's disease of the large bowel often responds well, at any rate for a time, to conservative treatment with steroids, salicylazosulfapyridine (Salazopyrin) and other supportive measures, as used in ordinary ulcerative colitis, and certainly seems to be more amenable to such management than is Crohn's disease of the small intestine. I have had many patients with extensive Crohn's colitis who have been maintained in reasonable or very good health on an expectant regime of this kind for several years or indefinitely. During this period they have usually had several recurrent attacks, which have been dealt with by further courses of intensive steroid therapy and often a period of hospitalization.

In the long run, however, patients with Crohn's colitis often come to radical surgical treatment for the same sort of reasons that lead to surgery for ulcerative colitis. Most prominent among the indications is continued invalidism and intractability alone or combined with systemic or local complications, gross perianal sepsis or ulceration being a fairly frequent accompaniment. Though there is some evidence to suggest that long-standing Crohn's disease (more particularly of the small bowel) predisposes to malignant change,[17, 22, 29, 55, 58, 71] opinion on the subject is divided, and so far the possibility of a complicating carcinoma has not been seriously taken into account in deciding on the need for surgical treatment. However, retardation of physical development is a well-recognized effect of severe extensive Crohn's disease in children, which does need to be borne in mind in considering a resort to surgery in these young patients. Lastly, it cannot be stressed too strongly that some patients with Crohn's disease of the large bowel have a dramatically acute form, exactly like severe attacks of ulcerative colitis, and may exhibit toxic dilatation or perforation of the colon.[22] Sometimes in these patients with severe exacerbation of the disease there are clinical indications (as, for example, the presence of perianal disease with an uninvolved rectum) that the condition is Crohn's colitis; at other times the clinical features are indistinguishable from those of an acute episode of ordinary colitis, and it is only on pathologic examination of the operative specimen after urgent ileostomy and colectomy that the true nature of the complaint is revealed.

CHOICE OF OPERATION. — Rarely, localized lesions of Crohn's disease of the large intestine can be treated by limited resection with anastomosis or, if the condition is restricted to the rectum, by abdominoperineal excision with permanent iliac colostomy. Much more often the disease in the large bowel is extensive and calls for one of the standard procedures of colitis surgery — an ileostomy with proctocolectomy (or subtotal colectomy) or a colectomy and ileorectal or ileosigmoid anastomosis. Frequently these operations have to be combined with a variable amount of terminal ileal resection if there is associated involvement of the ileum. Oberhelman et al.'s suggestion[52] that Crohn's colitis could often be made to resolve by temporary ileostomy, which might eventually be dispensed with, has not been confirmed by other observers[12] or indeed by Oberhelman's own subsequent experience,[53] and this procedure has not enjoyed any substantial support.

Outcome of Surgery

OPERATIVE MORTALITY. — The hospital mortality of operations for Crohn's disease mainly of the large bowel is very similar to that of operations for ulcerative colitis. Thus, in a series of 197 patients with this form of Crohn's disease treated surgically, the immediate mortality of nonurgent operations was 3.5% and that of urgent or emergency procedures 31%,[24] which is very similar to the respective mortalities for elective and urgent operations for ulcerative colitis (Table 2). Similar mortality figures have been recorded by Williams[69] and Krause et al.[37]

SUBSEQUENT RECURRENCE. — Soon after Crohn's disease of the large bowel was recognised as a definite entity, the idea rapidly gained wide credence that the incidence of recurrence after surgical treatment, and particularly after ileostomy and proctocolectomy, was probably going to be much less than after surgical resection of classic ileal or ileocolic Crohn's disease.[14, 30] During the years that have elapsed, surgeons and physicians heavily involved in the management of this disease have been very in-

TABLE 4. – RECURRENCE OF CROHN'S DISEASE
AFTER LARGE BOWEL EXCISION AND ILEOSTOMY
OR COLOSTOMY

AUTHOR	PATIENTS FOLLOWED	INCIDENCE OF RECURRENCE (%)
Nugent et al.[51] Boston, Mass.	28	3.6
Ritchie and Lockhart-Mummery[57] London	80	6.2
Steinberg et al.[60] Birmingham, England	70	33.0
Korelitz et al.[36] New York	67	46.0
Goligher[24] Leeds, England	167	10.2

terested to see whether this initial impression has been borne out or not. Several careful studies of the medium- and long-term results of surgery, especially of ileostomy and complete proctoco-lectomy (with or without terminal ileectomy), for Crohn's disease have now been published with widely divergent findings as regards the frequency of recurrence (Table 4).

It is certainly difficult to explain these differences in results,

Fig 9. – Cumulative risk of recurrence after ileostomy and proctocolectomy (or sub-total colectomy) for Crohn's disease. (From Goligher, J. C.[24])

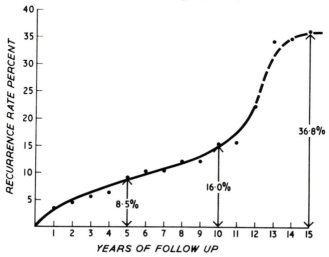

for one of the longest-followed series was that of Nugent et al.,[51] who had the lowest incidence of recurrent disease. In my series[24] the overall incidence of recurrence was also reasonably low, but when the cumulative frequency of recurrence was determined at various periods after operation, as shown in Figure 9, it is seen that there was a steady increase in the number of recurrences with continued follow-up, the incidence being 8.5% at 5 years, 16% at 10 years and 36.8% at 15 years. The resulting curve of incidence, if prolonged beyond that point, would seem to indicate a progressive increase in recurrence, perhaps reaching 100% in 25 or 30 years, but there is such a falling off in the numbers of our patients available for study after 12 years that it is difficult to feel confident of the reliability of the graph beyond that point.

Recurrence was almost as common in patients whose original disease had been confined to the large bowel as in those who had extension into the small bowel. By far the commonest site for

Fig 10. — X-ray plate after barium progress meal, showing narrowing of ileum just proximal to ileostomy due to recurrent Crohn's disease. (From Goligher, J. C.[21])

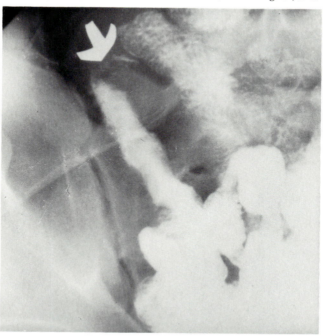

recurrence was immediately above the ileostomy (Fig 10), comparable to usual recurrence just proximal to the anastomosis after an anastomotic type of operation. What is encouraging is that re-resection of a recurrence together with the ileostomy and establishment of a new ileostomy at the same or another site was often followed by a good symptomatic result for a further period of some years.[25]

Recurrence after colectomy and ileorectal or ileosigmoid anastomosis. — In perhaps 30% or more of the patients suffering from Crohn's disease confined mainly or entirely to the large bowel, the rectum or rectum and distal sigmoid are uninvolved. In such cases, if surgical treatment becomes necessary, there is a strong incentive to the surgeon to perform a colectomy with ileorectal or ileosigmoid anastomosis, and the immediate results of this operation can be quite good.[38] Unfortunately, recurrence is much more frequent after this operation than after ileostomy and proctocolectomy, the usual site of the recurrent disease being in the ileum just proximal to the anastomosis.[1, 25, 57, 60, 69]

PROFUSELY ACTING ILEOSTOMY. — Because often a certain amount of terminal ileum is resected along with the colon in ileostomy and proctocolectomy or subtotal colectomy for Crohn's disease, a profusely acting ileostomy may result, possibly generating special problems in stomal management from leakage and soreness of the peristomal skin. Of a group of 132 recently surveyed patients who had had ileostomy for Crohn's disease, 25% were found to be taking codeine phosphate or Lomotil regularly to control the looseness of their feces, and 11% had occasional trouble with skin soreness requiring special attention.[25] But it should be added that only 3% of the patients found that the soreness was of such severity or persistence as to constitute a major inconvenience.

PREDISPOSITION TO CHOLELITHIASIS. — The ileum normally plays an important role in the reabsorption of bile acids from the intestinal tract. If this segment of the intestine is diseased or subjected to partial resection, the loss of these acids from the body may lower their concentration in the bile, with a resulting tendency for cholesterol to come out of solution and form nonopaque gallstones.[28] Incidentally, another effect of ileal resection if the continuity of the small intestine with the large bowel is restored by anastomosis, as after right hemicolectomy or ileosigmoid or ileorectal anastomosis, is that the unabsorbed bile acids pass into the colon and by their irritation may provoke considerable diarrhea. This may be a factor in producing the frequent bowel actions often experienced after these operations. The administration of cholestyramine, which prevents this irritating effect, is sometimes helpful in mitigating the diarrhea.

DELAYED HEALING OF THE PERINEAL WOUND AND FORMATION OF SINUSES. — The healing of the perineal wound after rectal excision or proctocolectomy for ulcerative colitis and even more so for Crohn's disease is notoriously liable to be prolonged and to result in the development of a persistent perineal sinus. In 82 consecutive patients of mine submitted to proctocolectomy for Crohn's disease, the perineal wound healed *per primam* in 20%, in less than 3 months in 22%, in more than 3 and less than 6 months in 27% and in more than 6 months in 21%. It remained permanently unhealed in 10%. No less than 20% of these patients were subjected to reoperations to lay open and curette the granulating areas.

These experiences immediately beg the question as to the best way to manage the perineal wound in connection with rectal excision for inflammatory bowel disease. In the patients just referred to the perineal dissection was performed in roughly the same way as for carcinoma, but no special effort was made to keep wide of the bowel. If at the conclusion hemostasis was good and there had been no gross fecal or purulent contamination during the operation, the perineal wound was closed completely by suture of the skin and fat and the pelvic cavity was drained by 2 closed suction drains of Redivac type inserted extraperitoneally from the suprapubic region. If, on the other hand, there had been much soiling of the perineal wound as a result of perforation or tearing of the rectum or if satisfactory hemostasis had not been obtained, the middle third of the perineal wound was left open and a rubber drain was inserted through it, or if necessary the wound was packed with dry gauze to control oozing.

Other surgeons adopt different tactics. Some prefer to use the sort of dissection just described but leave the perineal wound partly open as a routine. Others, like Lyttle and Parks,[45] keep the perineal excision small and dissect up in the plane between the internal and external sphincters. Turnbull[63] also makes a small circumcision around the anus and keeps very close to the anal canal in his dissection, but removes the sphincters. It is fair to say that the precise value of these alternative techniques remains to be established.

As for the management of established perineal sinuses, more elaborate maneuvers than the laying open and curetting described have been favored by some surgeons. Thus, Silen and Glotzer[59] have employed a method that involves excision of the coccyx and possibly the terminal 2 pieces of the sacrum and turning in a flap of skin to provide a partial lining for part of the saucerized wound. They claim very good results in hitherto intractable cases. Anderson and Turnbull[3] advocate the application of split-skin grafts 2 or 3 days after the sinus has been saucerized, the patient being maintained on ACTH at a dose of 40 units/day throughout the period in the hospital. They report some encouraging experiences with this method.

DISTURBANCES OF SEXUAL FUNCTION. — Young people with inflammatory bowel disease requiring ileostomy and proctocolectomy are naturally concerned about the possible effects of this operation on their sexual function. Most women and many men fear that the ileostomy may make them less desirable to the opposite sex, and in a recent postal survey of married ileostomists by Burnham et al.,[13] some degree of marital tension as a result of the stoma was mentioned by 10% and actual breakdown of the marriage in 2%. On the other hand, in interviews with a group of my female ileostomists, the majority claimed enhanced sexual relations since the operation due to the great improvement in their general health,[65] and I know that many of my unmarried female patients who come to ileostomy seem to experience little difficulty in acquiring boyfriends, getting married and having children.

In women removal of the rectum for inflammatory bowel disease leads to some degree of dyspareunia in a proportion of cases — 8%[65] to 30%[13] — due to perineal sinuses or to vaginal stenosis or tenderness. In men the consequences of rectal excision for this condition are more serious. Thus 11 of 41 male patients interrogated by Watts et al.[66] had some impairment of sexual function (failure of ejaculation in 2; temporary impotence in 2 and permanent impotence in 7). However, as found also in the surveys of May[47] and Burnham et al.,[13] the major disorders of sexual function were largely confined to older men.

COMMENT. — No surgeon can feel anything like satisfied with the progressive tendency to recurrence after operation for Crohn's disease, even of the large bowel alone, and with the lack of an obvious solution to this disappointing state of affairs. But the picture is not one of unrelieved gloom, for many patients derive substantial, sometimes dramatic, temporary benefit from surgical intervention, often for many years. In fact, the main objective of the surgeon should be not cure of the disease, which is to be regarded as an occasional bonus, but relief of symptoms by means of operation and reoperation as required. Viewed in this light, surgery has quite a lot to offer until more effective medical treatment has been evolved.

REFERENCES

1. Adson, M. A., Cooperman, H. M., and Farrow, G. M.: Ileorectostomy for ulcerative disease of the colon, Arch. Surg. 104:424, 1972.
2. Anderson, A. F.: Colectomy and ileorectal anastomosis in surgical treatment of ulcerative colitis, Aust. NZ J. Surg. 30:107, 1960.
3. Anderson, R., and Turnbull, R. B., Jr.: Grafting the unhealed perineal wound after coloproctectomy for Crohn's disease, Arch. Surg. 111:335, 1976.
4. Ault, G. W.: Selective surgery for ulcerative colitis, Proc. R. Soc. Med. 52:11, 1960.
5. Aylett, S. O.: Diffuse ulcerative colitis and its treatment by ileorectal anastomosis, Ann. R. Coll. Surg. Engl. 27:260, 1960.
6. Aylett, S. O.: Three hundred cases of diffuse ulcerative colitis treated by total colectomy and ileorectal anastomosis, Br. Med. J. 1:1001, 1966.
7. Aylett, S. O.: Delayed ileorectal anastomosis in the surgery of ulcerative colitis, Br. J. Surg. 57:812, 1970.
8. Baker, W. N. W.: The results of ileorectal anastomosis at St. Mark's Hospital from 1953 to 1968, Gut 11:235, 1970.
9. Beahrs, O. H.: Personal communication, 1976.
10. Brooke, B. N.: The management of ileostomy, Lancet 2:102, 1952.
11. Brooke, B. N.: Granulomatous disease of the intestine, Lancet 2:745, 1959.
12. Burman, J. H., Williams, J. A., Thompson, H., and Cooke, W. T.: The effect of diversion of intestinal contents on the progress of Crohn's disease of the large bowel, Gut 12:11, 1971.
13. Burnham, W. R., Lennard-Jones, J. E., and Brooke, B. N.: The incidence and nature of sexual problems among married ileostomists, Gut. In press.
14. Cornes, J. S., and Stecher, M.: Primary Crohn's disease of colon and rectum, Gut 2:189, 1961.
15. Counsell, P. B., and Goligher, J. C.: The surgical treatment of ulcerative colitis, Lancet 2:1045, 1952.
16. Crohn, B. B., Ginzburg, L., and Oppenheimer, G. D.: Regional ileitis: A pathologic and clinical entity, J.A.M.A. 99:1323, 1932.

17. Darke, S. G., Parks, A. G., Grogono, J. L., and Pollocks, D. J.: Adenocarcinoma and Crohn's disease, Br. J. Surg. 60:169, 1973.
18. Goligher, J. C.: Surgical treatment of ulcerative colitis, Br. Med. J. 1:
151, 1961.
19. Goligher, J. C.: Ileostomy reconstruction, Br. J. Surg. 50:259, 1963.
20. Goligher, J. C., Hoffman, D. C., and de Dombal, F. T.: Surgical treatment
of severe attacks of ulcerative colitis, with special reference to the advantage of early operation, Br. Med. J. 4:703, 1970.
21. Goligher, J. C.: Ileal recurrence after ileostomy and excision of the large
bowel for Crohn's disease, Br. J. Surg. 59:253, 1972.
22. Goligher, J. C.: Surgery of the Anus, Rectum and Colon (3d ed.; London:
Baillière, Tindall, & Cox, 1975).
23. Goligher, J. C., and Lintott, D.: Experience with 26 reservoir ileostomies,
Br. J. Surg. 62:893, 1975.
24. Goligher, J. C.: The results of excision of the large bowel with ileostomy (or
colostomy) for Crohn's disease, with particular reference to the incidence
of recurrence, Dis. Colon Rectum 19:584, 1976.
25. Goligher, J. C.: Unpublished data, 1976.
26. Griffen, W. O., Lillehei, R. C., and Wangensteen, O. H.: Ileoproctostomy in
ulcerative colitis: Long-term follow-up extending in early cases to more
than 20 years, Surgery 53:75, 1963.
27. Hawley, P. R.: Personal communication, 1975.
28. Hill, G. L., Mair, W. S. J., and Goligher, J. C.: Gallstones after ileostomy
and ileal resection, Gut 16:932, 1975.
29. Jones, J. H.: Colonic cancer and Crohn's disease, Gut 10:651, 1969.
30. Jones, J. H., Lennard-Jones, J. E., and Lockhart-Mummery, H. E.: Experience in the treatment of Crohn's disease of the large intestine, Gut 7:448,
1966.
31. Kirschner, M.: Das synchrone kombinierte Verfahren bei der Radikalbe-
handlung des Mastdarmkrebses, Arch. Klin. Chir. 180:296, 1934.
32. Kock, N. G.: Intra-abdominal reservoir in patients with permanent ileostomy, Arch. Surg. 99:223, 1969.
33. Kock, N. G.: Continent ileostomy in progress, Surgery 12:180, 1973.
34. Kock, N. G.: The present status of the continent ileostomy: Surgical revision of the malfunctioning ileostomy, Dis. Colon Rectum 19:200, 1976.
35. Kock, N. G.: Personal communication, 1976.
36. Korelitz, B. I., Present, D. H., Alpert, L. I., Marshall, R. H., and Janowitz,
H. D.: Recurrent regional ileitis after ileostomy and colectomy for granulomatous colitis, N. Engl. J. Med. 287:110, 1972.
37. Krause, U., Bergman, L., and Norlen, B. J.: Crohn's disease: A clinical
study on 186 patients, Scand. J. Gastroenterol. 6:97, 1971.
38. Lefton, H. B., Farmer, R. G., and Fazio, V.: Ileorectal anastomosis for
Crohn's disease of the colon, Gastroenterology 69:612, 1975.
39. Lennard-Jones, J. E., Parrish, J. A., Ritchie, Jean, Swarbrick, E. T., and
Williams, C. B.: Prospective study of outpatients with extensive colitis,
Lancet 1:1065, 1974.
40. Lindner, A. E., Marshak, R. H., Wolf, B. S., and Janowitz, H. D.: Granulomatous colitis: A clinical study, N. Engl. J. Med. 269:379, 1963.

41. Lloyd-Davies, O. V.: Lithotomy-Trendelenburg position for resection of rectum and lower pelvic colon, Lancet 2:74, 1939.
42. Lockhart-Mummery, H. E., and Morson, B. C.: Crohn's disease of the intestine and its distinction from ulcerative colitis, Gut 1:87, 1960.
43. Lockhart-Mummery, H. E., and Morson, B. C.: Crohn's disease of the large intestine, Gut 5:493, 1964.
44. Lockhart-Mummery, H. E.: Anal lesions of Crohn's disease, Clinics in Gastroenterology 1:377, 1972.
45. Lyttle, J. A., and Parks, A. G.: Intersphincteric excision of the rectum in benign inflammatory conditions, Gut. In press.
46. Marshak, R. H., Wolf, B. S., and Eleasoph, J.: Segmental colitis, Radiology 73:767, 1959.
47. May, R. E.: Sexual function following rectal excision for ulcerative colitis, Br. J. Surg. 53:29, 1966.
48. Morson, B. C., and Pang, L. S. C.: Rectal biopsy as an aid to cancer control in ulcerative colitis, Gut 8:423, 1967.
49. Mountain, J. C.: Cutaneous ulceration in Crohn's disease, Gut 11:18, 1970.
50. Muir, E. G.: The results of ileo-rectal anastomosis: Anglo-American Conference on Proctology, Proc. R. Soc. Med. (Suppl.) 25, 1959.
51. Nugent, F. W., Veidenheimer, M. C., Meissner, W. A., and Haggitt, R. C.: Prognosis after colonic resection for Crohn's disease of the colon, Gastroenterology, 65:298, 1973.
52. Oberhelman, H. A., Jr., Taylor, K. B., and Kivil, R. M.: Diverting ileostomy in the surgical management of Crohn's disease of the colon, Am. J. Surg. 115:231, 1968.
53. Oberhelman, H. A., Jr., and Kohatsu, S.: Diversion by Ileostomy for Crohn's Disease of the Colon, in *Skandia Symposium on Regional Enteritis (Crohn's Disease)* (Stockholm: Nordiska Bokhandels Forlag, 1971).
54. Parks, A. G.: Personal communication, 1975.
55. Perrett, A. D., and Truelove, S. C.: Crohn's disease and carcinoma of the colon, Brit. Med. J. 2:468, 1968.
56. Pugh, H. L.: Regional enteritis, Ann. Surg. 132:845, 1945.
57. Ritchie, J. K., and Lockhart-Mummery, H. E.: Gut 14:263, 1973.
58. Shiel, F. O'M., Clarke, C. G., and Goligher, J. C.: Adenocarcinoma associated with Crohn's disease, Brit. J. Surg. 55:53, 1968.
59. Silen, W., and Glotzer, D.: The prevention and treatment of the perineal sinus, Surgery 75:535, 1974.
60. Steinberg, D. M., Allan, R. N., Thompson, H., Brooke, B. N., Alexander-Williams, J., and Cooke, W. T.: Excisional surgery with ileostomy for Crohn's colitis with particular reference to factors affecting recurrence, Gut 15:845, 1974.
61. Strauss, A. A., and Strauss, S. F.: Surgical treatment of ulcerative colitis, Surg. Clin. North Am. 24:211, 1944.
62. Turnbull, R. B., Jr., Weakley, F. L., Hawk, W. A., and Schofield, P.: Choice of operation for the toxic megacolon phase of non-specific ulcerative colitis, Surg. Clin. North Am. 50:1151, 1970.
63. Turnbull, R. B., Jr.: Discussion of paper by Anderson and Turnbull, 1976.[3]
64. Turnbull, R. B., Jr., Weakley, F. L., and Hawk, W. A.: Choice of Operation

for the Tonic Megacolon Phase of Nonspecific Ulcerative Colitis, in Kremer, K., and Kivelitz, H. (eds.): *Colitis Ulcerosa* (Stuttgart: Georg Thieme, 1977).

65. Warren, R., and McKittrick, L. S.: Ileostomy for ulcerative colitis: Technique complications and management, Surg. Gynecol. Obstet. 93:55, 1951.
66. Watts, J. McK., de Dombal, F. T., and Goligher, J. C.: Long-term complications and prognosis following major surgery for ulcerative colitis, Br. J. Surg. 53:1014, 1966.
67. Watts, J. McK., and Hughes, E. S. R.: Ulcerative colitis and Crohn's disease: Result after colectomy and I.R.A., Br. J. Surg. 64:77, 1976.
68. Wells, C. A.: Ulcerative colitis and Crohn's disease, Ann. R. Coll. Surg. Engl. 11:105, 1952.
69. Westerman, I. R., and Pena, A. S.: The long-term prognosis of ileorectal anastomosis and proctocolectomy in Crohn's disease, Scand. J. Gastroenterol. 11:185, 1976.
70. Williams, J. A.: The place of surgery in Crohn's disease, Gut 12:739, 1971.
71. Wyatt, A. P.: Regional enteritis leading to carcinoma of the small bowel, Gut 10:924, 1969.

Monitoring the Critically Ill Surgical Patient

C. JAMES CARRICO

*Department of Surgery, University of Washington School of Medicine,
Seattle, Washington*

AND

JOEL H. HOROVITZ

*Department of Surgery, Cornell University Medical College,
New York, New York*

The goals of supportive management to ensure survival of the severely ill patient are (1) to preserve the function of vital organs and (2) to prevent further organ injury due to the patient's disease or secondary to our treatment. To achieve these goals, it is necessary to have some measure of the functioning of vital organs and of the effects of various treatments. Although these concepts are hardly new, they are becoming more formalized as increased use of technology yields progressively more precise measurements of physiologic functions. The sometimes formidable title of "monitoring" has been applied to observations directed toward these goals. In its strictest sense, "to monitor" means "to observe" and implies minimal disturbance of the system under observation.

Principles of Patient Monitoring

To accomplish these goals, 2 types of measurements are required. Measurements of organ function, which assure maintenance of adequate perfusion, oxygenation and nutrition, serve as the *baseline* of adequate treatment. A second group of measurements are needed to provide an *upper limit*. These indicate lack of response to or potential deleterious effects of a particular manipulation. The physician treating the patient attempts to stay in the "safe zone" between these 2 limits. For some physiologic systems 1 parameter may serve as both an upper and lower limit (e.g., the arterial Pco_2 as a measure of ventilation). For the cardiovascular system, for example, the distinctions are sharp (e.g., evidence of adequate perfusion being the lower limit and filling pressures being the upper limit). Emphasis is placed on monitoring the most "vital" physiologic systems, including hemodynamic (cardiovascular), pulmonary and renal, as well as the central nervous system.

Monitoring techniques applied on the basis of these principles can produce significant benefits. However, complications can occur and generally fall into 3 categories: (1) separation of the patient from personnel responsible for his care; (2) errors in data collection and misinterpretation of data, and (3) direct complications of the techniques themselves.

Maloney[53] has emphasized the potential dangers of interposition of electronic devices between the patient and those responsible for his care. The techniques described in this chapter are intended to augment, not to replace, bedside observation of critically ill patients by skilled physicians, nurses and therapists.

In each section, potential sources of error are described. Errors are suspected when 1 piece of data does not seem compatible with the clinical situation or the remainder of the monitoring data. Misinterpretation or misapplication of data can occur when confusion exists between upper and lower limits, for example, when a patient is transfused "until his CVP is 10 cm H_2O" despite the presence of clinical evidence of adequate perfusion.

Some technical complications can be avoided, while others can be limited by patient selection. Ideally, the instrumentation used for monitoring should be noninvasive and unobtrusive. Unfortunately, the present state of the art does not allow reliable and accurate measurement of many bodily functions without access to the system under consideration. Any invasive technique has the potential for introducing complications of its own. Therefore, the risk-to-benefit ratio must be evaluated by the physician prior to insertion of intravascular catheters, sensors, and so on. If the patient's condition warrants the risk of possible complications from instrumentation, the benefits to be derived must outweigh the risks.

PATIENT SELECTION. — As we can see from this discussion, every patient requires monitoring. The data required and the techniques used depend on the clinical situation and may vary from routine vital signs to the use of extensive invasive measurements. There is a group of patients who are at high risk for complications and can be considered for extensive monitoring. This group includes patients with:

1. Significant sepsis
2. Prolonged hypotension
3. Significant preexisting cardiovascular, pulmonary or renal disease
4. Severe multisystem injury
5. Multiple transfusions of stored blood
6. Strong possibility of pulmonary or cardiac injuries

Monitoring Hemodynamic Function

It is customary after all operative procedures to assess hemodynamic stability. This is traditionally done by the frequent recording of the heart rate, systemic blood pressure, ECG and urine output. These basic measurements are very valuable but have limitations. Their chief advantage is that they can be obtained without invasion of the vascular system. However, these parameters may be inadequate when needed most, for example, in a patient with a complicated shock or fluid problem. Under these circumstances, more sophisticated monitoring devices are required. These are listed in Table 1.

TABLE 1. — HEMODYNAMIC MONITORING

1. Arterial catheter
2. Central venous pressure catheter
3. Pulmonary artery catheter
4. Cardiac output
5. Blood volume

ARTERIAL CATHETERS

Arterial cannulation has become a relatively commonplace technique in the modern intensive care unit. It is useful for obtaining continuous blood pressure readings as well as arterial blood for blood gas determination and the measurement of cardiac output. Rarely is the insertion of an arterial line justified on the basis of arterial pressure study alone. However, it may be very useful in the unstable patient because it is frequently impossible to obtain accurate arterial pressure measurements or reliable arterial blood in the patient who may suddenly become hypotensive. Frequent arterial punctures may cause greater patient discomfort than arterial cannulation. An arterial cannula allows repeated arterial sampling without disturbing the steady state, and so avoids the acute changes in blood gas tensions that may confuse the interpretation of results obtained by intermittent puncture. The importance of obtaining pure arterial blood has been demonstrated by Doty and Mosely.[20] Due to the shape of the oxyhemoglobin dissociation curve, admixture of a small volume of venous with arterial blood may produce a disproportionately large drop in the partial pressure of oxygen (Pa_{O_2}). For example, 0.5 ml venous blood with a Pa_{O_2} of 31 mm Hg, mixed with 4.5 ml arterial blood with a Pa_{O_2} of 86 mm Hg, will result in a final mixture with a Pa_{O_2} of 56 mm Hg.

The sites of cannulation and the methods of insertion of the catheter vary. Commonly used arteries for long-term cannulation include the radial, brachial and femoral vessels. It is the opinion of the authors that the radial artery is the vessel of choice for continuous arterial cannulation. The risk of accidental obstruction of the blood supply to the hand is minimal if certain simple precautions are taken. Fixation of the catheter is secure, and it is easy to apply effective pressure to the puncture site to minimize hematoma formation. Table 2 details the most common complications associated with the use of a radial artery catheter. Major complications occur infrequently, with an overall incidence of less than 1%.[23, 40] Mortensen[60] reported no major complications in 500 patients. Minor complications, predominantly hematoma formation and a decrease in peripheral pulsation, occur quite commonly.[8, 9, 90] Atherosclerosis, hypertension, the use of anticoagulants and failure to adhere to simple guidelines predispose to both major and minor complications.[59]

TABLE 2.—COMPLICATIONS OF RADIAL
ARTERY CATHETERIZATION

MAJOR	MINOR
Local obstruction with distal ischemia	Pain
External hemorrhage	Ecchymosis (common)
False aneurysm	Temporary loss of pulse
Massive ecchymosis	Arteriospasm
Dissection	Infection (rare)

The material of choice for the arterial catheter at present is Teflon.[7] Bedford has recently published a study comparing polypropylene and Teflon catheters. He found that only 10% of Teflon catheters compared to 70% of polypropylene catheters resulted in prolonged arterial occlusion over the same time period.[4] Chemically, Teflon is more inert and less likely to cause tissue reaction.[34, 44]

An Allen test should be performed to assess the ulnar palmar circulation.[32] The test is performed by compressing the radial artery at the wrist while the patient forcibly opens and closes the hand a few times. Normally, a slight transitory ischemia will be seen, which disappears quickly when the hand is kept still and compression maintained. When the ulnar artery does not adequately support the palmar circulation, persistent signs of ischemia will be seen. During the final part of the examination, the fingers should not be hyperextended, since this may result in a false positive reaction.[18, 65] If Doppler instruments are available, they may be used to test completeness of the palmar circulation.[58]

Whether percutaneous or cutdown techniques are used for insertion of the catheter, aseptic technique is mandatory. If the palmar arch is intact, the diameter of the catheter is probably not critical. However, a smaller catheter size relative to the artery is probably associated with a lower risk of thrombus formation.[29] Intermittent high-volume irrigation of radial artery catheters may result in distal and proximal (even cerebral) embolization and should be avoided. With continuous low-flow irrigation, distal embolization to the terminal digital vessels is less likely[22] and proximal embolization to the central circulation is not possible.[48, 56] Removal of the cannula should be followed by compression of the puncture site for 5–10 minutes.[16, 52] During unexplained septic periods, the cannula should be removed and the tip cultured. With meticulous care, the arterial catheter may be safely kept in for 48–72 hours. Since thrombotic complications increase with time after 30 hours, the catheter should be removed as soon as it is no longer necessary.

CENTRAL VENOUS CATHETERS

Central venous pressure (CVP) monitoring is now a widely accepted guide for the regulation of fluid and blood replacement in the seriously ill patient. It is a valuable method if measuring errors or misinterpretation are avoided. Table 3 lists normal values for pressure measurements on both sides of the circulation. A properly positioned CVP catheter should be within the superior vena cava (SVC). The catheter may be inserted either through an antecubital fossa vein or into the subclavian or internal jugular veins and advanced to the SVC. Proper placement should be verified by x-ray studies. It is important to establish a zero reference level (midaxillary line = right atrium) and to use this level for all subsequent measurements.

The CVP measurement is a reflection of right ventricular end-diastolic pressure and is related to the efficacy of the right ventricle in handling the venous return. Since the CVP is a measure of the dynamic interrelationship among cardiac action, vascular tone and blood volume, it is obvious that one cannot determine volume status from a single CVP reading. In the case of nondisparate ventricular function, serial CVP values are valuable in assessing the patient's response to a fluid challenge. Table 4 outlines several common causes of incorrect CVP val-

TABLE 3.–NORMAL SYSTEMIC AND
PULMONARY PRESSURES

	SYSTOLIC	END-DIASTOLIC	MEAN
Right atrium	–	–	4
Right ventricle	25	0–4	15
Pulmonary artery	25	8–10	15
Pulmonary artery (wedge)	–	–	8
Left atrium	–	–	8
Left ventricle	90–140	0–5	–
Aorta	90–140	60–90	–

TABLE 4.—CAUSES OF INACCURATE CVP READINGS

1. Incorrect zero reference
2. Change in position of patient
3. Coughing or straining during a reading
4. Positive-pressure ventilation
5. Incorrect placement of catheter

ues. Attention to detail will obviate all of these. For example, all measurements of filling pressure are obtained with the patient off a ventilator if his condition permits. Table 5 outlines several guidelines to the safe use of the CVP catheter.

PULMONARY ARTERY CATHETERS

Swan and his associates introduced a method for measuring the pulmonary artery (PA) pressure and pulmonary capillary wedge pressure (PCWP) for monitoring purposes. [85, 86] The pulmonary artery catheter used is shown schematically in Figure 1. Insertion is accomplished by inflating a soft balloon at the catheter tip, which allows the flow of blood to carry it into the PA (for normal pressures, see Table 3). The catheter can be easily positioned with the aid of a pressure monitor, oscilloscope and ECG. With the balloon inflated and the catheter advanced to a "wedge" position, a static column of blood is created, which al-

TABLE 5.—GUIDELINES TO THE SAFE USE OF THE CVP CATHETER

1. Carry out surgical skin preparation for all cannulations.
2. Assure proper adapter-catheter fit prior to insertion.
3. Place the patient's head down when inserting subclavian or jugular catheters to avoid air embolism.
4. When subclavian puncture is unsuccessful, obtain x-ray of chest before attempting puncture on the contralateral side.
5. Use only radiopaque catheters. Do not bevel catheter tips. Remeasure after removal.
6. Whenever the catheter does not advance through the needle with ease, remove needle and catheter together. Never attempt to withdraw the catheter through the needle.
7. Obtain chest x-ray routinely after catheter insertion to assure location of catheter tip and the absence of a pneumothorax.
8. Remove catheter for unexplained fever, local inflammation or at the earliest date that catheter does not contribute to patient's care.
9. Submit the distal catheter tip for culture.
10. Expend every effort to locate and retrieve lost catheters.

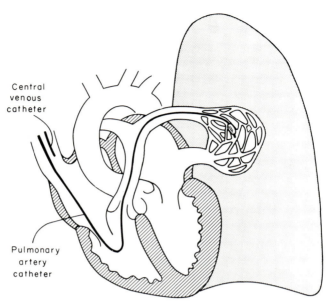

Fig 1.—Pathway of pulmonary artery catheter used to measure pulmonary artery and pulmonary capillary wedge pressures.

lows estimation of the pressure level and pressure changes in the left atrium. In the absence of valvular heart disease the PCWP will be a good estimate of left ventricular end-diastolic filling pressure.[19, 25, 26, 30]

In diseases characterized by differences in the function of the 2 ventricles, disparities between CVP and PCWP should be anticipated. Forrester and co-workers[27] studied patients after myocardial infarction and found that the CVP did not correlate well with left ventricular filling pressure, PCWP or x-ray evidence of congestive heart failure. Rapaport and Scheinman[71] found CVP values less than 10 cm H_2O in 30% of postinfarction patients with acute left ventricular failure and pulmonary edema. Referring to Figure 2, it may also be seen that if pulmonary vascular resistance is abnormally elevated, PCWP has the advantage of measuring left atrial pressure more accurately than the CVP. In patients with normal cardiac reserve and normal pulmonary vascular resistance, however, the CVP will reflect the ability of the myocardium to pump the volume presented to it. Properly applied, the CVP remains a useful clinical tool.

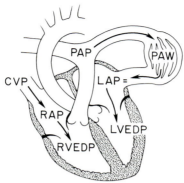

Fig 2. — Cardiovascular pressures measured in hemodynamic monitoring. CVP, central venous pressure; RAP, right atrial pressure; RVEDP, right ventricular end-diastolic pressure; PAP, pulmonary artery pressure; PAW, pulmonary artery (wedge); LAP, left atrial pressure; LVEDP, left ventricular end-diastolic pressure.

The advantages of using a pulmonary artery catheter must be weighed against the added risk to the patient. Table 6 lists those patients in whom the authors feel the risk-to-benefit ratio justifies its use. Other uses of the Swan-Ganz catheter are listed in Table 7. Alone, these rarely serve as adequate indication for catheter insertion. The importance of obtaining true mixed venous blood for the assessment of the shunt fraction has been demonstrated.[36] If central venous blood is used in critically ill patients, it will lead to an overestimation of the shunt fraction.

Table 8 lists the complications associated with central venous and pulmonary artery catheters. The guidelines of safety used for CVP catheters are also applicable for the PA catheter. In addition, during and after insertion, repeated evaluation of the

TABLE 6.—INDICATIONS FOR USING PULMONARY
ARTERY CATHETERS

1. Increased pulmonary resistance (chronic obstructive lung disease)
2. Coronary artery disease requiring complicated intravenous fluid regimen
3. Cardiac surgery and trauma
4. Decreased left ventricular function secondary to anoxia, acidosis or electrolyte imbalance
5. Decompensated cirrhosis, severe pancreatitis, generalized peritonitis and severe multisystem trauma
6. Massive transfusions
7. High CVP in the presence of underperfusion of peripheral tissues
8. Suspected disparate ventricular function

TABLE 7. – ADDITIONAL USES OF
PULMONARY ARTERY CATHETERS

1. Bedside pulmonary angiogram in cases of pulmonary emboli
2. Mixed venous blood sampling
3. Injection of indicators for cardiac output study and determination of pulmonary venous resistance
4. Administration of medication

character of the pressure tracing is important. Loss of the characteristic pulse may indicate unintentional catheter wedging,[14, 75] with the possibility of pulmonary infarction.[13] Frequent chest x-rays should be obtained in the first 24 hours to detect tightening of the catheter loop, which indicates peripheral movement.[24] In the original description of the flow-directed balloon-tipped catheter, Swan and co-workers suggested advancing the catheter 1 – 3 cm further after the initial wedge position had been obtained.[86] It is now felt that this may lead to rupture of a pulmonary vessel in some patients.[31, 43] If, on repeated balloon inflations, a wedge pressure is obtained with less than the recommended volumes (0.8 ml with a no. 7 French catheter), it is probable that the catheter has advanced too far and should be partially withdrawn.[24] Before wedge determinations, withdrawal of the catheter a short distance and inflation of the balloon in small increments will minimize the chances of perforation of the PA. If the pulmonary artery end-diastolic pressure is less than 20 mm Hg and pulmonary edema is not present, a wedge pressure is not necessary, since mean left atrial pressure is almost certain to be lower than pulmonary artery end-diastolic pressure.[76] Intracardiac knotting of the catheter can be prevented by allowing the catheter to advance itself while the tip remains in the right atrium or ventricle.[14] Continuous dilute heparin infusions should be used to maintain paten-

TABLE 8. – COMPLICATIONS OF CV
AND PA CATHETERS

BOTH	PA ONLY
Infection	PA perforation
Loss of catheter	Ischemic lung lesion
Thromboembolism	Catheter kinking
Perforation of right ventricle	Heart murmurs

cy in all intravenous monitoring cannulas. By adhering to these guidelines, the incidence of complications can be minimized.

CARDIAC OUTPUT

The determination of cardiac output (CO)(flow) is valuable but not essential in the postoperative management of the injured patient. Methodology is more cumbersome and expensive than that of the previously outlined hemodynamic tests. The dye dilution technique is still the most common method for measuring CO, although more recent techniques are gaining in popularity. Indocyanine green dye estimations are subject to at least a 10-15% error under most conditions, this being increased by extremely low or high CO.[10, 64] Ganz et al.[28] have simplified the thermal dilution method of CO detection by incorporating thermistors in a pulmonary artery catheter. This allows measurement of a change in temperature of a bolus of cold saline injected into the SVC and sampled in the PA. The CO is then inversely proportional to the fall in temperature. The advantages of this method are: (1) a "physiologic" indicator is used; (2) blood withdrawal is not required, and (3) no recirculation of the indicator occurs (a pure right heart CO is obtained). Extensive use of this method in man has recently been reported,[93] and it is becoming the most frequently used clinical method in many centers.

Another modification of the Swan-Ganz catheter has allowed a virtually continuous estimate of CO without the use of an indicator or sampling. A small fiberoptic oximeter attached to the tip of a PA catheter is able to measure oxygen saturation in the mixed venous blood. Mixed venous oxygen saturation is directly proportional to the CO if oxygen consumption is unchanged and the position of the hemoglobin-oxygen dissociation curve is constant. This method is still experimental, but does have a great deal of appeal because of its simplicity. The range of error in work done to date in man is about the same as that for the dye-dilution method.[39]

BLOOD VOLUME

A direct measure of the circulating blood volume may be very helpful in the management of fluid balance problems. To date, these measurements have remained almost exclusively a research tool. The indicator dilution principle is utilized, the marker most commonly used being a radioactive-tagged element of the blood. Swan and Nelson[87] have written an excellent review of the theory and practice of blood volume determinations. By means of chromium-tagged erythrocytes, the red cell mass can be measured. Total blood volume can be determined either by adding the estimated plasma volume[35] or by using the corrected hematocrit. The red cell volume is the most accurate because the label resides exclusively in the intravascular fluid space.

A commercially available device (Volemetron) is available for clinical measurement of blood volume. Its major disadvantages are that its error increases during acute changes in volume status and that "normal" values are subject to wide individual variation.

The use of CO and blood volume estimates depends upon the financial and technical resources of the hospital. Effective hemodynamic monitoring can be done without measuring these parameters in most patients. Cardiotonic and vasoactive drugs are administered only after an accurate hemodynamic assessment has been made. This approach helps avoid the administration of drugs deleterious to a particular patient's circulation and organ perfusion in the treatment of complicated circulatory problems.

Monitoring Renal Function

Damage to the kidney may result from ischemia, the extent of damage varying with the severity and duration of the insult.[44] The incidence of primary acute oliguric renal failure has decreased due to improved fluid resuscitation and immediate corrective surgery.[5, 6] Less severe forms of renal failure, with normal or increased urine output, are now being recognized more frequently. Table 9 lists the time-honored classification of renal impairment. Adequate monitoring must supply information as to the effective plasma volume perfusing the kidneys. Similarly, any suggestion of postrenal obstruction must be investigated by means of retrograde pyelography.

A useful bedside test for the quick differentiation of prerenal and renal failure is the measurement of urine electrolyte con-

TABLE 9.—CAUSES OF
RENAL FAILURE

1. Prerenal: decreased effective plasma volume
2. Renal: intrinsic disease or ischemia
3. Postrenal: obstruction

centration and specific gravity. In the former, the sodium concentration is usually greater than 20 mEq/L, and the specific gravity is less than 1.018 and fixed.[45] These readily obtained test results may be extremely useful in the rapid differentiation of prerenal from renal dysfunction when more elaborate tests are unavailable.

The blood urea nitrogen (BUN) and serum creatinine are considered the preferred screening methods for assessing glomerular function.[41] Tissue trauma and multiple transfusions do not lead to azotemia or hypercreatinemia in patients with normal renal function. Persistent minimal elevations of BUN or serum creatinine are uniformly associated with a significant loss of renal function (at least 70%).[82] Normal tubular function alters the amount of water and the concentration of dissolved materials in the urine, making it different from plasma. Urine-to-plasma ratios approaching unity, therefore, are diagnostic of tubular damage.

Table 10 lists those tests that have been proposed as good determinants of renal damage. Careful interpretation is indicated in injured patients, who may have twofold and threefold increases of endogenous creatinine clearances (C_{cr}).[42] Changes in muscle metabolism following severe trauma cause increased loads of creatinine to be presented to the kidney. Apparently normal values of C_{cr} may lead to a false sense of security, when, in fact, the glomerular filtration rate may be reduced by a factor of 2–3. Free water clearance, calculated as the difference between urine output and osmolar clearance, has been proposed as a use-

TABLE 10.—TESTS OF RENAL FUNCTION

1. Urine sodium concentration
2. Urine specific gravity
3. C_{cr} (clearance of creatinine)
4. C_{urea} (clearance of urea)
5. C_{osm} (osmolar clearance)
6. Urine-to-plasma (U/P) urea ratio
7. U/P creatinine
8. U/P osmolality
9. Free water clearance

ful test of early renal impairment.[2] Complete loss of concentrating ability of the kidney is characterized by free water clearance values near zero. The return of free water clearance toward normal marks the functional recovery of the tubular cells. However, in a recent study, patients with the most severely damaged kidneys demonstrated positive free water clearances, as did patients with septic infection.[78] Therefore, care must be taken in interpreting the results of positive free water clearance in the acutely ill patient.

Simultaneous measurement of urine and plasma concentration of solutes is important. Clearance studies in the unstable patient tend to be difficult because of the need for prolonged urine collections.[41] Because of the variability of individual dissolved materials, the most useful measurement appears to be the urine-to-plasma osmolar ratio.[78] This method indicates the ratio of the concentrations of all dissolved materials in the urine. If an osmometer is not readily available, the urine-to-plasma urea ratio may be determined. The finding of identical concentrations of dissolved material in both plasma and urine is proof of a loss of the concentrating ability of the kidney and substantiates the diagnosis of acute renal failure in the oliguric patient.

Oliguric renal failure is a well-recognized complication. It is less well recognized that renal failure may occur without an observed period of oliguria.[78] Renal insufficiency without oliguria is important from the standpoint of recognition. Table 11 lists the main features of the 2 syndromes. The chief danger in the nonoliguric type of renal failure lies in lack of recognition.

TABLE 11.—TYPES OF RENAL FAILURE

OLIGURIC	NONOLIGURIC
1. Persistent oliguria after circulatory stabilization	1. Normal or increased urine output
2. Chemical evidence of uremia	2. Chemical evidence of uremia
3. Progressive rise in urine volume after several days to several weeks	
Gradual restoration of excretory plus concentrating functions of the kidney	

TABLE 12.— TESTS FOR MONITORING RENAL FUNCTION

GENERAL	SPECIFIC RENAL FUNCTION
1. Arterial pressure	1. Urinalysis
2. Central venous pressure	2. Specific gravity
3. ECG	3. Urine electrolytes
4. Strict intake and output	4. Urine/plasma osmolar ratio
5. Serum electrolytes	5. Serum BUN and creatinine

This may allow the rapid progression of hyperkalemia from the administration of potassium salts with the threat of cardiac arrest. In addition, mild azotemia may be converted to severe renal failure by the inadvertent administration of nephrotoxic drugs. Similarly, drugs that normally do not demonstrate toxicity may do so in the face of reduced renal function.

In summary, the monitoring of renal function requires an assessment of the adequacy of plasma volume, specific renal function tests and the exclusion of obstruction. Table 12 lists the parameters that should be routinely monitored in the severely ill patient to assure adequate renal function and to alert the physician to the fact that alterations in therapy may be required.

Monitoring Pulmonary Function

ASSESSMENT OF PULMONARY FUNCTION

Assessment of the adequacy of pulmonary function begins immediately after operation in those patients at risk for adult respiratory distress syndrome (ARDS). Endotracheal tubes inserted for airway control during surgery are usually left in place for 4–5 hours postoperatively in high-risk patients. This additional 4–6 hours of intubation will usually be sufficient to allow the physician to determine that ARDS is not a threat. If any suspicion of defective pulmonary function is present after this interval, extubation is delayed until adequate lung function has been demonstrated.

If several days of intubation are contemplated, a nasotracheal tube may be substituted for the endotracheal tube in the operating room. This will allow for greater patient comfort and acceptance.

A prerequisite for optimal lung function is normal cardiovascular status. Hemodynamic monitoring, therefore, should be instituted routinely. This usually includes recording of heart rate, arterial pressure, ECG and CVP. PAP measurement is included in patients with indications listed in Table 6. Serial body weight, intake and output balance, bacteriologic studies, coagulation profile and chest x-ray are other important data to be obtained.

Monitoring of pulmonary function can be conveniently divided into three general areas: evaluation of oxygenation, ventilation and lung-thorax mechanics. Table 13 details the most easily obtained tests, with normal values included. As a general principle, isolated determinations are not as valuable as serial measurements obtained at regular intervals. Hypoxemia is often detected in apparently normal patients who appear to be doing well clinically.

The partial pressure of oxygen in the arterial blood (Pa_{O_2}) is the hallmark of determining the adequacy of oxygenation. This must be considered in the light of the inspired oxygen concentration (FI_{O_2}). A simple means of establishing a measurable relationship between Pa_{O_2} and FI_{O_2} is their ratio. Ratios between 350 and 500 are considered adequate, while a value of less than 250 is definitely abnormal. This ratio provides the clinician with a gross estimation of the efficacy of oxygenation at the bedside

TABLE 13.— ASSESSMENT OF PULMONARY FUNCTION

	ACCEPTABLE	INSTITUTE THERAPY
Oxygenation		
1. Partial pressure O_2 arterial blood	$Pa_{O_2} > 90$ mm Hg on 40% FI_{O_2}	< 90 mm Hg on 40% FI_{O_2} or decreasing
2. Ratio of partial pressure O_2 arterial blood to fraction inspired O_2	$Pa_{O_2}/FI_{O_2} > 350$	< 300
3. Alveolar-arterial O_2 gradient (breathing 100% O_2 for 10–15 min)	50–200 mm Hg	> 200 mm Hg or increasing
Ventilation		
1. Partial pressure CO_2 arterial blood	35–40 mm Hg	30 or decreasing
2. Minute volume	< 12 L/min	increasing
Mechanics		
1. Rate	12–25/min	25 or increasing
2. Effective compliance	50 ml/cm H_2O	50 or decreasing

during rapid changes in therapy. It appears to be most reliable when the FI_{O_2} is between 0.2 and 0.5.[37]

The alveolar-arterial oxygen difference $(A-aD_{O_2})$, with the patient breathing pure oxygen for 10–15 minutes, may allow rapid differentiation of the cause of hypoxemia. Of the 4 causes of hypoxemia (hypoventilation, diffusion defects, ventilation-perfusion abnormalities and pulmonary shunt) only the pulmonary shunt is theoretically refractory to oxygen administration. In general this relationship holds true. However, the $A-aD_{O_2}$ is affected by cardiac output, oxygen consumption, the position of the hemoglobin-oxygen dissociation curve and the magnitude of the pulmonary shunt. If the 3 other variables are constant, then the $A-aD_{O_2}$ is a good reflection of the amount of pulmonary shunting. Despite its theoretical advantages, measurement of $A-aD_{O_2}$ using pure oxygen is usually not recommended for clinical monitoring, since it adds little to simple determinations and the use of high concentrations of oxygen, even for short periods of time, may be deleterious.[21, 73, 84]

The adequacy of ventilation is determined by the arterial partial pressure of carbon dioxide (Pa_{CO_2}). By definition, hypoventilation is present when the Pa_{CO_2} is elevated; ARDS is usually associated with hypocarbia (hyperventilation). Therefore, the patient with both a decreased Pa_{CO_2} and Pa_{O_2} probably has ARDS. Tidal volume (V_T) (the amount of air breathed during 1 respiratory cycle) is another indication of the adequacy of ventilation. This is readily measured with a modestly priced respirometer. Tidal volume multiplied by the respiratory rate is called the minute ventilation. This value is easily derived, but by itself is only a rough guide to adequate ventilation. In many postinjury patients high minute ventilations are recorded. It is not established whether this is a compensatory response or a result of pathologic changes.

The effective compliance (C_{eff}) may be quite valuable as an assessment of the ease of distensibility of lung and thoracic cage. This derived value is obtained by dividing the V_T by the peak airway pressure. Effective compliance indicates the "stiffness" of the lungs, i.e., how difficult they are to ventilate (low C_{eff} means increased stiffness). A decreased C_{eff} may indicate increased extravascular lung water, airway constriction or increased chest wall resistance (impaired bellows activity). Low values are usually found in patients with ARDS.

An adequate assessment of pulmonary function can be achieved by serial measurement of arterial blood gases, V_T, minute ventilation and C_{eff}. Several other monitoring devices have been advocated. The work of breathing is almost always increased in ARDS; this value is a measure of the mechanical cost of achieving adequate ventilation. Peters et al. have reported on the efficacy of the work of breathing measurement in predicting the need for ventilatory support.[66] The major disadvantage of this test is that it requires an intraesophageal balloon to measure transthoracic pressure and the availability of an analogue computer for usable results.[62] Although highly desirable, the work of breathing is difficult to obtain in the critically ill patient.

Although sophisticated and expensive equipment is available to monitor arterial and venous blood gases and other pulmonary function tests continuously, these have not been shown to improve patient survival significantly.[17, 67, 88]

ASSESSMENT OF ADEQUACY OF VENTILATORY TREATMENT

There are no universal guidelines for the institution of ventilatory support. The indications outlined in Table 13 have been found to be reliable in treating a large number of patients. The most common indication for beginning ventilatory therapy is hypoxemia. If the Pa_{O_2} is less than 65 mm Hg, initial management includes increasing the FI_{O_2} both as a diagnostic test and as a temporary relief of hypoxemia. For effective therapy, control of the airway must be achieved. The most rapid and reliable way to do this is the insertion of an endotracheal or nasotracheal tube. Mechanical ventilation may then be applied. Since a defect in the matching of ventilation to perfusion is present, therapy is directed at trying to maintain ventilation to marginally ventilated alveoli and the recruitment of collapsed or partially occluded alveoli. This is assessed by observation of the arterial P_{O_2}, as described later.

The choice of the type of respiratory support will be dictated by the patient's respiratory function and the physician's preference.[69, 74, 77] The volume ventilator is the device most often chosen in the treatment of ARDS and will be used for illustrative purposes. The initial tidal volume setting may be 10–15 ml/kg body weight at a rate of 12–14 breaths/minute with an inspiration:expiration ratio of 1:2.[68] An F_{IO_2} of 0.4 is applied initially and blood gas determinations will indicate the efficacy of this treatment. Blood gases are checked within 10–20 minutes of beginning respiratory treatment to determine the patient's response. If hypoxemia persists on 40% oxygen, a trial of increasing the V_T still further may be warranted in an effort to increase the functional residual capacity (FRC). The effect of this maneuver is best assessed by following serial compliance changes. If the C_{eff} is improving, then benefit from increased V_T may be expected. If C_{eff} decreases with an increase in V_T, then too much volume is being given to the patient. Lower tidal volume ventilation will then be required to minimize the risk of complications of ventilatory therapy. The compliance curve is shaped somewhat like the Starling curve of cardiac function, i.e., a plateau is reached, after which any increase in volume is achieved only at the expense of a marked increase in airway pressure.

Maintenance of Oxygenation – Use of Upper and Lower Limits

Acceptable levels of Pa_{O_2} are between 65 and 80 mm Hg. If this cannot be achieved with the treatment outlined, there are 2 alternatives.

MANIPULATION OF F_{IO_2}. – The F_{IO_2} may be increased to higher levels. This is unlikely to be of significant benefit and, in fact, may be detrimental to the patient. Pulmonary shunting is caused by continued perfusion of nonventilated alveoli. As Powers[70a] has stated, "It is not important what gas is not ventilating parts of the lung." In addition, washout of nitrogen from poorly ventilated alveoli will make them more susceptible to collapse, thus converting low gas volume/blood volume (V/Q) areas to areas of shunt resulting in more atelectasis. McAslan et al. have reported on the deleterious effect of pure oxygen on the shunt fraction in trauma patients.[49] Although there is still controversy over the role of oxygen toxicity in the genesis of ARDS, the literature clearly indicates that prolonged use of high oxygen concentrations can produce a clinical picture similar to ARDS.[77] More than 50% oxygen is required to produce deleterious effects in patients with normal lungs, depending upon the amount of time that alveolar hyperoxia is maintained. The higher the oxygen concentration, the less time is required to produce damage. Therefore, every effort should be made to limit the FI_{O_2}.

POSITIVE END-EXPIRATORY PRESSURE. — The 2d alternative is to recruit collapsed or partially collapsed alveoli with some modification of ventilatory therapy. This can be done by applying continuous positive end-expiratory pressure (PEEP) to the airway. Although the technique was first published in 1938, by Barach,[3] the use of PEEP in treating ARDS was emphasized by Ashbaugh in 1967.[1] Since that time a large number of articles have appeared concerning the uses and abuses of PEEP.[69, 70, 77]

Positive end-expiratory pressure may be achieved by either inserting an airflow resistance during expiration or using a ventilator with an end-expiratory plateau of positive pressure. Providing positive pressure throughout the respiratory cycle prevents alveolar and small airway collapse and may recruit lung units that were previously collapsed. The commonly used volume ventilators have the capability of instituting PEEP without modifying the equipment. Although there is some controversy about the absolute level required, incremental increases in pressure are advocated. The usual beginning level is 5 cm H_2O of PEEP. Cardiorespiratory monitoring is done after 10–15 minutes to assess the effects. If no beneficial effect is noted, further increases in PEEP follow in increments of 3–5 cm H_2O pressure. There may be a variable response to PEEP.[38] While some patients respond with an immediate increase in Pa_{O_2}, others may not show improvement for 30–60 minutes or longer. Therefore, absence of immediate response should not be interpreted as an absolute failure of PEEP.

A relatively new concept is that of "best PEEP." Suter et al. have defined "best PEEP" as that pressure giving the maximal oxygen transport (cardiac output multiplied by oxygen content of arterial blood.).[84] Each patient may have a different but demonstrable optimal PEEP level that correlates well with the highest compliance. Thus, a practical bedside monitor of the effectiveness of PEEP may be the C_{eff}. In patients with more complicated disease and those requiring more than 10 cm H_2O, PEEP monitoring of cardiac output (using thermodilution) after each increase in end-expiratory pressure is desirable.

Gastrointestinal Monitoring (Prevention of Stress Ulcer)

Stress ulceration with upper gastrointestinal hemorrhage is being encountered with increasing frequency. About 50% of all stress ulcer patients who bleed will require surgery, and the overall surgical mortality remains between 35 and 40%.[60] Table 14 lists the factors that predispose to stress bleeding.[12] In general, the more severe the illness, the greater the risk of stress ulceration.[83] The most frequently associated factor is the presence of sepsis. It has been estimated that at least 70% of patients with stress ulceration have some form of significant infection.[15] The etiology and pathogenesis of the syndrome remain unclear. Factors that have been implicated include hypersecretion of acid and pepsin,[47, 61] breakdown of the gastric mucosal barrier with back diffusion of acid,[58, 78, 81] reflux of bile and enzymes, alteration in quality and quantity of mucus production[72] and development of disseminated intravascular coagulopathy.[54, 57]

In the management of the severely ill patient, emphasis is placed on prevention of this serious complication. Table 15 outlines a general plan of management. Most patients at risk will have a nasogastric tube inserted for both decompression of the stomach and instillation of antacids. Although the value of antacids has not been proved conclusively in clinical trials, animal experiments strongly support their use.[80] The general feeling is that whatever the pathogenesis of stress ulceration, the presence of acid in the stomach contributes to ulcer formation and, therefore, neutralization should be of benefit.[46, 55, 89] In postoperative cardiac and thoracic surgery patients, a significant reduction in stress ulcer occurrence has been shown with the administration of antacids. There is little documentation in the literature as to the type or dose of antacids to be used. Anti-

TABLE 14.—CONDITIONS WITH
GREATEST RISK OF STRESS BLEEDING

1. Severe multisystem trauma
2. Major surgery
3. Major intracranial injury or surgery
4. Shock
5. Burns
6. Infection
7. Renal insufficiency
8. Respiratory insufficiency

TABLE 15.—MEANS OF PREVENTING STRESS
ULCERATION IN POSTINJURY PATIENTS

1. Nasogastric tube
2. Antacids
3. Anticholinergics
4. Coagulation studies
5. Careful monitoring for precipitating causes
   Infection
   Renal or respiratory insufficiency
6. Support for healing or protective processes
   Hyperalimentation
   Vitamin A

cholinergics may be beneficial to patients suffering severe intra-cranial injury or having major neurosurgical procedures.[63, 91, 92]

Careful monitoring of the coagulation status and an aware-ness of precipitating causes that may develop postoperatively are important. It appears that maintaining good nutritional sta-tus with hyperalimentation[33] and the administration of vitamin A may aid in preventing stress ulceration. Vitamin A adminis-tered parenterally in doses of 100,000 units twice daily in adults and 50,000 units twice daily in children increases the regenera-tion of gastric mucus cells and the production of gastric mucus.[11]

With careful monitoring of precipitating factors, the adminis-tration of antacids (and anticholinergics when indicated), the maintenance of good nutrition and supplemental vitamin A administration, the incidence of stress ulceration has been sig-nificantly reduced. The development of pH-sensitive monitoring devices that can be inserted as part of or along with a nasogas-tric tube may greatly facilitate the monitoring and management of these patients.

Summary

This review has focused on several aspects of monitoring the critically ill patient. A few of the more commonly used monitor-ing devices have been discussed to emphasize that their use car-ries some risk. Because of this, proper indications, based on the benefits to be achieved, must be available before they are used. Guidelines for the safe use of these devices have been outlined. We have dealt with hemodynamic assessment, renal insufficien-cy, pulmonary monitoring and stress ulceration. Guidelines and specific examples have been presented to illustrate the prevention, early diagnosis and management of problems.

REFERENCES

1. Ashbaugh, D. G., et al.: Continuous positive-pressure breathing (CPPB) in adult respiratory distress syndrome, J. Thorac. Cardiovasc. Surg. 57:31, 1969.
2. Baek, S. M., Brown, R. S., and Shoemaker, W. C.: Early prediction of acute renal failure and recovery, Ann. Surg. 177:253, 1973.
3. Barach, A. L., et al.: Positive pressure respiration and its application to the treatment of acute pulmonary edema, Arch. Int. Med. 12:754, 1938.
4. Barr, P. O.: Percutaneous puncture of the radial artery with a multipurpose Teflon catheter for indwelling use, Acta Physiol. Scand. 51:343, 1973.
5. Baxter, C. R., and Maynard, D. R.: Prevention and recognition of surgical renal complications, Clin. Anesthesiol. 3:322, 1968.
6. Baxter, C. R., Zedletz, W. H., and Shires, G. T.: High output acute renal failure complicating traumatic injury, J. Trauma 4:567, 1964.
7. Bedford, R. E.: Percutaneous radial-artery cannulation: Increased safety using Teflon catheters, Anesthesiology 42:220, 1975.
8. Berneus, B., Carlsten, A., Holmgren, A., et al.: Percutaneous catheterization of peripheral arteries as a method for blood sampling, Scand. J. Clin. Lab. Invest. 6:217, 1954.
9. Brown, A. E., Sweeney, D. B., and Lumley, J.: Percutaneous radial artery cannulation, Anesthesia 24:532, 1969.
10. Carey, J. S., et al.: Accuracy of cardiac output computers, Ann. Surg. 174:762, 1971.
11. Chernov, C. S., Cook, F. B., Wood, M., et al.: Stress ulcer: A preventable disease, J. Trauma 12:831, 1972.
12. Chernov, C. S., Hale, H. W., and Wood, M.: Prevention of stress ulcers, Am. J. Surg. 122:674, 1971.
13. Chun, G. M. H., and Ellestad, M. H.: Perforation of the pulmonary artery by a Swan-Ganz catheter, N. Engl. J. Med. 284:1041, 1971.
14. Civetta, J. M., and Gabel, J. C.: Flow-directed pulmonary artery catheterization in surgical patients, Ann. Surg. 176:753, 1972.
15. Colman, R. W., Robboy, S. J., and Minna, J. D.: Disseminated intravascular coagulation, Am. J. Med. 52:679, 1972.
16. Control of infections from intravenous infusions, Med. Lett. Drugs Ther. 15:105, 1973.
17. Dardik, H., et al.: On-line in vivo measurements of partial pressures of oxygen and carbon dioxide of blood, tissue and respired air by mass spectrometry, Surg. Gynecol. Obstet. 131:1157, 1970.
18. De Gowin, E., and De Gowin, R.: Bedside Diagnostic Examination (2d ed.; New York: Macmillan Company, 1969).
19. DeLaurentis, D. A., Hayes, M., Matsumoto, T., et al.: Does central venous pressure accurately reflect hemodynamic and fluid volume patterns in critical surgical patients? Am. J. Surg. 126:415, 1973.
20. Doty, D. B., and Mosely, R. V.: Reliable sampling of arterial blood, Surg. Gynecol. Obstet. 219:701, 1970.

64. Oriol, A., et al.: Limitations of indicator-dilution methods in experimental shock, J. Appl. Physiol. 23(4):605, 1976.
65. Paaby, H., and Stadil, F.: Thrombosis of the ulnar artery, Acta Orthop. Scand. 39:336, 1968.
66. Peters, R. M., et al.: Objective indications for respiratory therapy in post-trauma and postoperative patients, Am. J. Surg. 124:262, 1972.
67. Peters, R. M., and Stacy, R. W.: Automatized clinical measurement of respiratory parameters, Surgery 56:44, 1964.
68. Petty, T. L.: Intensive and Rehabilitative Respiratory Care (2d ed.; Philadelphia: Lea & Febiger, 1974).
69. Pontoppidan, H., et al.: Acute respiratory failure in adults, N. Engl. J. Med. 287:690, 1972.
70. Pontoppidan, H., Laver, M. B., and Geffin, B.: Acute Respiratory Failure in the Surgical Patient, in Advances in Surgery (Chicago: Year Book Medical Publishers, Inc., 1970), Vol. 4.
70a. Powers, S. R., Jr.: Pulmonary Complications of Fluid and Electrolyte Imbalance. Paper presented at American College of Surgeons Fourth Annual Spring Meeting, April 29, 1976, Boston, Mass.
71. Rapaport, E., and Scheinman, M.: Rationale and limitations of hemodynamic measurements in patients with acute myocardial infarction, Mod. Concepts Cardiovasc. Dis. 38:55, 1969.
72. Robbins, R., Idjahi, F., Stahl, W. M., et al.: Studies of gastric secretions in stressed patients, Ann. Surg. 175:555, 1972.
73. Sachner, M. A., et al.: Pulmonary effects of oxygen breathing, Ann. Intern. Med. 82:40, 1975.
74. Schmidt, G. B., O'Neill, W. W., Kotto, K., Hioang, K. K., Bennett, E. J., and Bomback, C. T.: Continuous positive airway pressure in the prophylaxis of the adult respiratory distress syndrome, Surg. Gynecol. Obstet. 143:613, 1976.
75. Scott, M. L., Weber, D. R., Arers, J. F., et al.: Clinical applications of a flow-directed balloon-tipped cardiac catheter, Am. Surg. 38:690, 1972.
76. Sharefkin, J. B., and MacArthur, J. D.: Pulmonary artery pressure as a guide to the hemodynamic status of surgical patients, Arch. Surg. 105:699, 1972.
77. Shires, G. T., Carrico, C. J., and Canizaro, P. C.: Shock: Major Problems in Clinical Surgery (Philadelphia: W. B. Saunders Company, 1973), Vol. XIII, chap. IV.
78. Shires, G. T., Carrico, C. J., and Canizaro, P. C.: Shock: Major Problems in Clinical Surgery (Philadelphia: W. B. Saunders Company, 1973), Vol. XIII, chap. III.
79. Skillman, J. J.: Acute gastroduodenal stress ulceration: Barrier to disruption of varied pathogenesis, Rev. Surg. 59:478, 1970.
80. Skillman, J. J., Gould, S. A., Chung, R. J. K., et al.: The gastric mucosal barrier: Clinical and experimental studies in critically ill and normal man and in the rabbit, Ann. Surg. 172:564, 1970.
81. Smith, B. M., Skillman, J. J., Edwards, B. G., et al.: Permeability of the human gastric mucosa: Alteration by acetylsalicylic acid and ethanol, N. Engl. J. Med. 285:716, 1971.
82. Stahl, W. M., and Stone, A. M.: Prophylactic diuresis with ethacrynic

acid for prevention of postoperative renal failure, Ann. Surg. 172:361, 1970.

83. Stremple, J. F., Mori, H., Lev, R., et al.: The Stress Ulcer Syndrome, *Current Problems in Surgery* (Chicago: Year Book Medical Publishers, Inc.), April, 1973.

84. Suter, P. M., Fairley, H. B., and Schlobohm, R. M.: Shunt lung volume and perfusion during shunt periods of ventilation with oxygen, Anesthesiology 43:617, 1975.

85. Swan, H. J. C., Ganz, W., Forrester, J., et al.: Catheterization of the heart in man with the use of a flow-directed balloon tipped catheter, N. Engl. J. Med. 283:447, 1970.

86. Forrester, J. S., Diamond, G., Chatterjee, K., and Swan, H. J. C.: Medical therapy of acute myocardial infarction by application of hemodynamic subsets, N. Engl. J. Med. 295:1356, 1976.

87. Swan, H., and Nelson, S. W.: Blood volume, Ann. Surg. 173:481, 1971.

88. Turney, S. Z., et al.: Respiratory monitoring; recent developments in automatic monitoring of gas concentration, flow, pressure and temperature, Ann. Thor. Surg. 16:184, 1973.

89. Wangensteen, S. L., and Golden, G. T.: Acute stress ulcers of the stomach: A review, Am. Surg. 1973.

90. Ward, R. J., and Green, H. D.: Arterial puncture as a safe diagnostic aid, Surgery 57:672, 1965.

91. Watts, C. C., and Clark, K.: Effects of an anticholinergic drug on gastric acid secretion in the comatose patient, Surg. Gynecol. Obstet. 130:61, 1970.

92. Watts, C. C., and Clark, K.: Gastric acidity in the comatose patient, J. Neurosurg. 30:107, 1969.

93. Weisel, R. D., et al.: Measurements of cardiac output by thermodilution, N. Engl. J. Med. 292:682, 1975.

Problems with Postoperative Drug Therapy*

FRANK J. COLGAN

Departments of Anesthesiology and Medicine, University of Rochester Medical Center, Rochester, New York

Many problems associated with the surgical experience complicate postoperative drug therapy. The purpose of this report is to review some of these problems and their management in relation to current concepts of drug dosage, monitoring and metabolism.

Drug History of the "New" Surgical Patient

Patients requiring surgery often present themselves as virtual unknowns, having been referred by another physician or hospital emergency room or frequently without referral. Knowledge of current drug intake and past drug experience is an important aspect of proper patient evaluation and management, since the effects of some drugs may be prolonged for days. The patient is the best and frequently the only source of information on drug intake. A careful history may reveal specific drug names, and many patients will have brought medications with them. Identification may be aided by referral to full-color reproductions of most currently available drugs.[1] Labels of prescription drugs include the generic name of the drug, if requested by the prescribing physician. This practice should be encouraged

*Supported in part by USPHS Grant HL-09609.

for all prescription drugs, particularly with drugs like tricyclic antidepressants, known to induce drug interaction, or antibiotics, which induce allergic reactions. Recall of specific illnesses evoked by careful history taking should prompt inquiry into responses to drugs frequently used in treatment or diagnosis: iodides associated with contrast studies, sulfa-containing drugs with genitourinary infections, analgesics with operative procedures and tranquilizers or antidepressants in patients with emotional problems.

The referring physicians' records from previous hospital admissions and information from the patient's family provide ancillary sources of drug intake information. Patients frequently stop taking prescribed drugs, however, alter dosage up or down depending on desirable or undesirable sequelae or may even substitute proprietary drugs of their own choosing, all without their families' or referring physicians' knowledge. A proper understanding of each patient's current and historical experiences with drugs is thus the first step toward reducing problems in drug therapy.

Effects of Environmental Changes

The surgical patient rarely finds the hospital routine similar to that at home. The diabetic admitted for elective surgery and well stabilized on insulin may find that changes in physical activity, the hospital timing of meals and changes in sleep patterns may seriously alter insulin requirements, in spite of conscientious mimicking of the home diet.

Anxiety, a frequent problem with the hospitalized patient facing surgery, may prompt the physician to prescribe sedatives or other mood ameliorators for the first time. These drugs are frequently responsible for in-hospital problems. Delirium due to drug ingestion can be caused by many commonly used drugs, such as diazepam, chlordiazepoxide, atropine, antacids, trihexyphenidyl (Artane) and the tricyclic antidepressants.[2, 3]

Elderly patients are particularly vulnerable to environmental changes. Some are not capable of coping with the loss of daily routines and the familiar social pleasantries that were suddenly removed by sickness and hospitalization. Windowless rooms or stalls, which prevent measuring time by light, significantly add to the likelihood of mental problems in hospitalized patients.[4, 5]

Any agitation and confusion is more likely to increase at night when loss of orientation is greatest. This exhausting behavioral pattern may complicate the postoperative course. Differentiation from toxic delirium due to anticholinergic intoxication may be safely made using intravenous physostigmine.[6] Similar symptoms due to alcoholic withdrawal often appear in the early postoperative period in patients who have had an unchallenged source of alcohol suddenly cut off by their hospital experience.[7] Many toxicology laboratories now perform blood levels of diazepam, which has a half-life of up to several days. Blood levels may be of considerable help in the differential diagnosis of delirium. Thus, while hospitalization allows for greater control of drug therapy, the change in environment and its new restrictions may produce many new drug problems not encountered by the ambulatory patient residing at home.

Effects of Surgery and Anesthesia on Drug Therapy

Frequently patients receive such drugs as oxygen, antibiotics, narcotics or diuretics for the first time in the immediate postoperative period. Recognition of any untoward reaction to these drugs induced by disease, genetic factors or drug interaction may easily be overlooked during a rapidly changing postoperative course. Other drugs that the patient may have taken by oral ingestion preoperatively may be temporarily discontinued or given parenterally by one of several routes, resulting in altered serum levels.

Gut function is routinely suppressed following abdominal surgery. Loss or suppression of gastric motility and mixing will induce variable rates of absorption of drugs commonly taken by mouth. Fasting or reduced diets following surgery may increase absorption of some drugs that tend to form nonabsorbable complexes when taken with foods, while other drugs may be rendered relatively inactive by excess gastric acids. The bioavailability of a drug taken orally can also be altered by means of fortuitous inactivation by other substances taken orally. For example, absorption of lincomycin was found to be effectively blocked by concomitant use of a cyclamate-containing diet drink.[8] Absorption of drugs like digoxin may also be affected more by a change in oral form (liquid or tablet) than by dose. Changes in blood pH induced by gastric suction can affect not only the proof the abdominal aorta, in whom prolonged renal hypoxia is a common factor, may experience acute oliguric renal failure.[16] Therapeutic control of such drugs as lidocaine, procainamide, digoxin, nitroprusside and diuretics when given intravenously becomes difficult. Serum radioimmunoassay and more recently, enzyme-multiplied immunoassay* of drugs such as digitalis and antiepileptics in patients with fluctuating renal function have proved useful in avoiding toxic drug concentrations.[17]

Transient or permanent renal damage may follow the prolonged inhalation of methoxyflurane. Renal damage is characterized by high-output renal failure and dehydration. Induced renal damage in the immediate postoperative period may be overlooked because of polyuria. Those drugs dependent on renal function for excretion that are themselves nephrotoxic, such as gentamicin and polymyxin, may cause additional problems in the postoperative period.

Both methoxyflurane and enflurane, a more recently introduced halogenated anesthetic, are metabolized to inorganic fluoride, the former, however, to a much greater extent.[18] The extent of early renal damage is related to the level of inorganic fluoride in the blood, while the intratubular deposition of oxalate crystals, should it occur, may account for permanent renal damage. Patients who have received other drugs known to cause enzyme induction in the liver may experience rapid biotransformation of these inhalation agents with resulting renal damage, even though inspired concentrations have been kept low.[19]

Quite apart from these renal toxic effects of anesthetics on renal function, most commonly used inhalation anesthetics, including nitrous oxide with pentothal, directly induce some renal vasoconstriction and antidiuresis. Renal function, upon which most drug therapy is dependent, should be carefully watched in high-risk patients undergoing anesthesia. These include those with already impaired renal function, elderly patients with obstructive jaundice and those who have undergone prolonged cardiopulmonary bypass and aortic resective surgery. Hemorrhage and hypotension, often prolonged, may be experienced in patients having these operations.

Anesthesia, paradoxically, will induce renal vasodilatation in

*Syva Corporation, Palo Alto, CA

the presence of significant hemorrhage and hypotension in contrast to the intense renal ischemia that occurs in conscious man.[20] While this protective aspect of anesthesia should be considered in evaluating the etiology of postoperative renal failure, significance should also be given to the return of the patient to consciousness and the further increase in renal vasoconstriction that may occur in the presence of a relative hypovolemia.

Postoperative renal insufficiency usually impairs drug excretion because of a reduction in the glomerular filtration rate. Elimination of drugs given before or during anesthesia may be significantly prolonged, resulting in an extended recovery period. Prolonged postoperative muscle paralysis, for example, may occur in patients who have received gallamine triethiodide, a muscle relaxant that is totally dependent on the kidney for excretion.[21] d-Tubocurarine is also excreted by the kidney. In the presence of impaired renal function, elevated plasma levels will persist until the biliary route of excretion, which normally accounts for 15% of excretion, can reduce plasma levels and any persistent muscle paresis. The elimination of pancuronium bromide, a widely used relaxant during anesthesia and in intensive care areas, is markedly diminished in patients with poor renal function. The problem of postoperative recurarization is likely to occur in these patients, particularly if acid-base abnormalities and dehydration develop or if large doses of narcotic analgesics have been used.[22]

Morphine and meperidine, frequently given intravenously during and following anesthesia, may themselves cause a reduction in glomerular filtration rate. In the presence of underlying renal disease, cardiovascular and respiratory depression may persist for more than 6 days following administration.[23] Successful reversal with naloxone is possible but is dependent on an awareness of the importance of impaired renal function in elimination of narcotics. The use of large doses of narcotics for certain types of cardiac surgery has led to postoperative respiratory problems, even in the presence of normal renal function. Patients having mitral valve replacement who receive 0.5 mg/kg morphine sulfate and nitrous oxide anesthesia require significantly longer periods of mechanical ventilation than patients who receive halothane and nitrous oxide anesthesia. The dead space/tidal volume ratio may also be elevated for 2–3 days

EFFECT OF HEPATIC DISEASE ON POSTOPERATIVE DRUG METABOLISM

There is little evidence that one or another inhalation anesthetic is better tolerated than others in patients with liver disease. Nitrous oxide and cyclopropane have minimal effect in the liver and do not appear to undergo biotransformation. Halogenated anesthetics undergo various degrees of biotransformation in the liver, and some are enzyme inducers, yet no direct evidence exists that these agents per se will cause further hepatic damage and interfere with postoperative drug metabolism.

Narcotics, however, are probably contraindicated both during and following surgery in patients with significant disease. Glucuronic acid synthesis is depressed even in mild liver disease and, as a consequence, conjugation with morphine is retarded. Because meperidine (Demerol) undergoes hydrolysis and demethylation in the liver, its use is also discouraged. In patients with underlying liver disease, either drug may precipitate a postoperative hepatic encephalopathy heralded by progressive confusion, headache, lassitude and asterixis.[37, 38]

The liver, healthy or diseased, is more vulnerable than the kidney to transient episodes of hypoxia, hemorrhage and hypotension. The low-pressure portal circulation, its principal blood supply, normally carries blood that is only 60–75% saturated. Marked intraoperative hemorrhage or hypoxia can be expected to induce vasoconstriction in the splanchnic vascular bed, causing not only local ischemic changes but also markedly curtailing blood flow to the liver, resulting in organ damage. In addition, hypercapnia, ganglionic blockade and excessive use of antihypertensive agents can affect liver blood flow and precipitate hepatic failure, influencing drug metabolism.

Known hepatotoxic drugs given in the presence of compromised liver function can also lead to liver failure. Thus the postoperative patient with previous liver disease who may have experienced intraoperative hypotension or hypoxia or received hepatotoxic drugs either before or during surgery should be carefully watched for signs of liver failure. Frequently the kidney experiences damage from the same insults and the clinical picture, the so-called hepatorenal syndrome, presents as persistent oliguria possibly progressing to complete anuria. While the kidneys of patients dying from the hepatorenal syndrome frequently are grossly and histologically normal and have been used successfully as donor kidneys, even temporary renal shutdown complicates drug excretion in the patient with liver damage.[39] Progressive malaise, anorexia, fever, delirium, hypoalbuminemia and jaundice characterize hepatic involvement.

Many drugs, including narcotics, enjoy 2 routes of excretion: detoxification within the liver and direct excretion via the kidneys. When both routes of elimination have been blocked, narcotic antagonists may be used to reduce the likelihood of further hepatic injury from circulating narcotic.

Treatment of hepatic failure includes withdrawal or substitution of all drugs known to be hepatotoxic. In spite of a probable hypoalbuminemia, complete protein restriction is initially necessary to reduce ammonia production in the gut and kidney. Intravenous hyperalimentation, however, may be helpful in supplying more readily tolerated amino acids to expedite liver cell resynthesis.[40, 41] Acidic drugs, such as phenylbutazone, sulfonamides, diphenylhydantoin, thiopental and salicylates, will have reduced plasma protein binding, resulting in relatively high unbound levels in the blood.[42] Reduction of dosage of acidic drugs should thus be considered in the presence of liver disease. Increased drug "sensitivity" in the presence of liver disease may also reflect the competition of bilirubin for albumin-binding sites of some drugs.[43, 44]

The liver is the major organ responsible for the biotransformation of drugs, and liver disease can retard the transformation of many but not all drugs. Longer half-lives have been demonstrated in patients with chronic liver disease for drugs such as meprobamate, chloramphenicol, rifampin, isoniazid, amobarbital, lidocaine, digoxin and hexobarbital.[45]

It is not possible to predict which drugs will have delayed excretion or detoxification in patients with liver disease. The drug-metabolizing capacity of the liver does not correlate with common liver function tests or measurements of cytochrome P-450 enzymatic activity, since the significance of the latter determination is dependent on knowing liver volume as well. In addition, some patients with liver disease who are or have been on enzyme-inducing drugs, such as phenobarbital, may be capable of adequately handling the detoxification of drugs that would not be possible without the enzyme induction. Withdrawal of the inducer would then lead to toxic levels of the drug. In the presence of phenobarbital, for example, warfarin (Coumadin) dosage is increased because of an enzyme-induced increase in detoxification. On removal of phenobarbital, if the same dosage of warfarin is continued, generalized bleeding may result.

HEPATOTOXIC DRUGS

When impaired liver function and marginal ability to handle the detoxification of drugs exist, use of known hepatotoxic agents should be avoided when possible. Hepatotoxins are either themselves cytotoxic or are by-products of biotransformation of nontoxic substances.[46] Still other hepatotoxins produce cholestatic jaundice, which mimics obstruction of the biliary tree. A third group of hepatotoxic drugs that infrequently produce liver damage probably induce changes because of host hypersensitivity, either on an allergic or genetic basis.

DIRECT HEPATOTOXINS. — Direct hepatotoxins are those agents that produce characteristic lesions within the liver. The severity of the lesions is dose-related and can be produced experimentally. Chloroform, carbon tetrachloride, inorganic phosphorus and mushroom toxins are examples of direct hepatotoxins. The toxins cause generalized disruption of all hepatic cellular elements and zonal necrosis. The time between exposure to direct hepatotoxins and the appearance of symptoms of liver damage is quite short, and mortality is high. Fortunately, chlorinated hydrocarbons are now rarely used clinically.

INDIRECT CYTOTOXIC HEPATOTOXINS. — Indirect cytotoxic hepatotoxins may interfere with normal liver function by competitive inhibition of essential metabolites or interruption of specific metabolic pathways.[47] The degree of liver damage they produce is dose-dependent; histologic changes may develop within a day or two. High doses of tetracycline cause vacuolization of liver cells that contain small lipid droplets. Tetracycline is known to interfere with protein synthesis, and perhaps interference with lipoprotein synthesis prevents the mobilization of lipids from the liver. Liver damage has been observed in biopsy sections from patients on oral tetracycline and is more likely to occur in the presence of renal disease or during the last trimester of pregnancy.[48] Of 7 life-threatening reactions attributed to tetracycline collected by the Boston Collaborative Drug Surveillance Program, 2 occurred in patients who were cirrhotics. Three other patients evidenced renal, heart or pulmonary insufficiency.[49] Nausea, vomiting, diarrhea and anorexia were frequent side effects in these patients, and all had elevated blood urea nitrogen levels, which attest to the antianabolic effect and increased nitrogen turnover associated with tetracycline therapy.[50] Ethanol produces a fatty liver through both decreased oxidation and increased synthesis of fatty acids. In postoperative patients who still have high blood levels of alcohol, increased sensitivity to many drugs, including sedatives and analgesics, may be due to the binding of alcohol to the microsomal hemoproteins of the cytochrome P-450 enzyme system, effectively impeding drug biotransformation.[51]

Other commonly used cytotoxic drugs producing liver damage belong to the cancer chemotherapy group, including methotrexate, L-asparaginase, puromycin and cycloheximide. Cytotoxic drugs produce a clinical picture similar to that in viral hepatitis, characterized by jaundice, elevated transaminase and alkaline phosphatase levels, nausea and lassitude. If damage increases, ascites, spontaneous bleeding, coma and death may occur.

INDIRECT CHOLESTATIC HEPATOTOXINS. — Indirect hepatotoxins that cause minimal parenchymal damage but do cause obstructed bile flow have been classified as cholestatic hepatotoxins. Hepatic dysfunction is dose-related and begins by impairment of BSP excretion within a few days of beginning drug administration. Transaminase levels may be slightly elevated and, if portal inflammation occurs, alkaline phosphatase levels may be significantly elevated. Hepatocanicular obstruction sufficient to produce jaundice is not frequently seen during use of drugs causing cholestatic obstruction.

Many commonly used drugs have produced this type of liver injury. Methyltestosterone, norethandrolone and other C-17 alkylated drugs, including estrogen and progesterone derivatives, have been implicated. Patients on oral contraceptive steroids show a relatively high incidence of mild hepatic dysfunction.[47] Elevated serum cholesterol levels are frequently found in patients on anabolic steroids, oral contraceptives, corticosteroids and phenothiazines.[52] If drug therapy is continued, jaundice may supervene in patients with a genetic susceptibility.[53]

Gallbladder dyes and certain antibacterial rifamycin drugs produce a hepatic cholestatic type of injury characterized by unconjugated hyperbilirubinemia. Gallbladder dyes that contain iodine usually undergo conjugation with glucuronic acid in the liver, then are concentrated and stored in the gallbladder before elimination in the bile. These iodized fatty acids, because of their interference with the clearance of bilirubin, should be used with caution in the presence of liver disease. Rifampin, a semisynthetic derivative of rifamycin B, is widely used in the treatment of pulmonary tuberculosis; however, jaundice is a notable problem, which, in the presence of preexisting liver disease or with concomitant administration of other known hepatotoxic drugs, may lead to the hepatorenal syndrome and death. The biliary excretion of rifampin competes with gallbladder dyes, and when excretion is further hampered, either through overdosage or the presence of preexisting disease, nausea, vomiting and increasing lethargy herald the onset of severe hepatic damage. Novobiocin also can interfere with bilirubin conjugation, especially in neonates, which will lead to unconjugated hyperbilirubinemia. Because of this toxic effect and relatively narrow antibacterial spectrum, its clinical use is now discouraged.

Other drugs known to produce intrahepatic cholestasis include para-aminosalicylic acid (PAS), androgens and the phenothiazines.

HEPATOTOXINS WITH MANIFESTATIONS OF ALLERGY OR HYPERSENSITIVITY. — In some individuals hepatic injury develops unpredictably, infrequently and with signs suggestive of a hypersensitivity to the drug. When "sensitization" occurs, following exposure for a period of 1–4 weeks, these patients develop hepatic dysfunction on reexposure to the drug. Fever, rash and eosinophilia frequently occur. Liver biopsy may reveal eosinophilic granulomas. Drugs that produce hepatic disease in which drug allergy may play a role are Dilantin, propylthiouracil, sulfonamides, erythromycin, nitrofurantoin, aspirin, chlorpromazine, organic arsenicals, methyldopa and halothane.[47]

Still other drugs, while capable of infrequently producing hepatic dysfunction, fail to cause eosinophilia, fever, rash and other effects that characterize an allergic or hypersensitivity response. Isoniazid (INH) is such a drug, and the hepatic injury is due to an idiosyncratic metabolism of the drug.

Diagnosis of Postoperative Drug-Induced Hepatotoxicity

The postoperative patient has just experienced an event that may have affected liver function in many ways other than through drug additions, withdrawals or manipulations of dosage. As much as 20% of patients in a general surgical practice may be jaundiced, and 7% have abnormal liver function following surgery.[54] Hepatic blood flow may have been altered by surgical manipulation, and oxygen delivery may have been compromised by a hypoxic event or reduced cardiac output. Reduced renal function may have blocked an alternate route of excretion of toxic metabolites affecting liver function. Changes in liver function as a result of these occurrences may cloud interpretation of hepatic damage due to drugs. Onset of signs and symptoms of liver damage, particularly in patients with underlying disease, may occur immediately following the insult. Excessive bleeding during surgery may represent failure of the acutely damaged liver to synthesize prothrombin and the coagulation factors V, VII, IX and X. Bleeding may be aggravated by transfusion with factor-deficient stored citrated blood. Cirrhotic patients with portal hypertension may have inadequate vitamin K absorption, thrombocytopenia and elevated circulating fibrinolysins that aggravate intraoperative or postoperative bleeding. Short of a frank bleeding diathesis, intraoperative hepatic damage from shock will present postoperatively as increased BSP retention, increased serum bilirubin and prothrombin time and decreased urea formation leading to elevated blood urea nitrogen (BUN).[55] Prehepatic bilirubin levels will progressively increase following liver damage, since bilirubin is dependent on enzyme integrity for conjugation with glucoronic acid. While prehepatic bilirubin is frequently elevated following multiple transfusions, levels will rapidly fall as conjugated posthepatic bilirubin is formed and excreted through the biliary tract. Persistance of both forms of bilirubin suggest continued hepatic insufficiency and will lead to further hepatic damage.

Serum enzymes are especially helpful in detecting early changes in liver function. Serum glutamic-oxalacetic transaminase and serum glutamic-pyruvic transaminase (SGPT) rise rapidly following hepatic cell injury. Lactic dehydrogenase (LDH) is a glycolytic enzyme that catalyzes the reversible

tinely confirmed by analysis of oxygen and carbon dioxide blood gas tensions, and patients may receive oxygen therapy on an empirical basis. Unfortunately, oxygen therapy, while capable of elevating blood tension of oxygen, also produces undesirable and occasionally toxic effects.

EFFECTS OF OXYGEN INHALATION

The patient recovering from surgery and anesthesia and breathing spontaneously when given oxygen can be expected to experience a mild respiratory depression, reduction in heart rate and a 8–20% decrease in cardiac output. Three hours after exposure to 90% oxygen, impairment of mucus flow in the human trachea occurs, which may reduce the lungs' defenses against inhaled bacteria that are normally removed by ciliary action. Dogs breathing 100% oxygen for 6 hours develop diffuse tracheobronchitis with sloughing of ciliated epithelium. While 50% oxygen for 30 hours will produce tracheobronchitis in the dog, concentration as low as 40% will decrease mitochondrial respiration in cells from rat lungs.[63] Patients who inhale greater than 50% oxygen may develop sore throat, coughing, nasal congestion and a progressive decrease in vital capacity. If the $F_{I_{O_2}}$ is greater than 80%, these symptoms may appear within 12 hours.[64] High inspired oxygen tensions will eventually cause an inordinate increase in intrapulmonary shunting, yet restriction of the $F_{I_{O_2}}$ to "safe" levels in patients with significant shunting may produce arterial blood gas tensions well below 60 torr.[65]

WHAT IS "SAFE" OXYGEN THERAPY?

Most evidence suggests that inhalation of 100% oxygen for 24 hours does not lead to lung damage, and inspired tensions below 0.4–0.5 atmospheres are not associated with the development of pulmonary oxygen toxicity, even with prolonged exposures.[66, 67] While the accumulated data suggest that pure oxygen inhalation for more than 24 hours does produce pulmonary lesions, other factors associated with the treatment of critically ill patients may change the influence of exposure time and oxygen concentrations that are necessary to produce pulmonary lesions. While not recommended as a form of therapy, it has long been known, for example, that 15-minute interruptions of pure oxygen inhalation will markedly prolong survival in experimental animals.[68, 69]

Little is known about "safe" oxygen tensions in tissues other than the lungs and retinal vessels of premature infants. Most organs, with the exception of the kidney cortex, function with oxygen tensions ranging from 15 to 30 mm Hg. Utilizing a battery of micropolarographic electrodes, Kessler et al. have recently demonstrated that marked alterations in muscle blood flow and local oxygen supply can occur when oxygen concentrations below 21% or above 40% are inspired.[70] Changes in inspired oxygen tension have been found to alter regional blood flow in the liver as well.[71] Further investigation of the consequences of oxygen lack or excess on distribution of blood flow within organs and tissues hopefully will widen our understanding of what constitutes "safe" levels of oxygen tension in the blood.

O_2 THERAPY VIA NASAL CANNULA OR AEROSOL MASK

Patients recovering from major surgery often require supplemental oxygen, which is usually delivered under a plastic face mask or through nasal cannula. The relative merits of each delivery method have been well defined.[72, 73]

Blood oxygen tensions, however, drawn on postsurgical patients receiving this form of therapy cannot be expected to accurately reflect the degree of intrapulmonary shunting. Pain, sedation and surgical encroachments on the respiratory mechanism all serve to modify the depth and pattern of respiration, and these changes may alter the fraction of inspired oxygen. Factors of nasal patency and mask fit will also influence the fraction of the inspired oxygen. Figure 2 demonstrates the change in Pa_{O_2} of oxygen delivered by nasal cannula and aerosol mask in 9 recently extubated postsurgical patients requiring oxygen because of Pa_{O_2} values below 65 torr. Oxygen concentrations via mask and flow rates through the cannula were offered in a random order to each patient for 30-minute periods, and blood gases were drawn at the end of each period. Wide variations in Pa_{O_2} were observed among patients, and increases in Pa_{O_2} expected with incremental increases in Fi_{O_2} were seldom achieved. Control of the Fi_{O_2} in nonintubated patients is difficult, particularly when delivery flows of oxygen approach

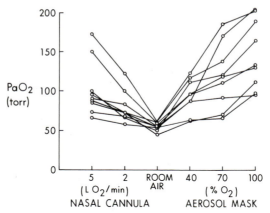

Fig 2. — Pa_{O_2} achieved by inhaling oxygen via nasal cannula or aerosol mask in 9 postoperative patients in need of supplemental oxygen. Aerosol generator when driven by 10 L/minute of 100% oxygen, delivered either 40 L/minute of 40% oxygen, 16 L/minute of 70% oxygen or 10 L/minute of 100% oxygen to the aerosol mask. Variations in nasal patency, minute and tidal volume, mask fit, gas flow and other factors account in part for wide variability in response and precludes meaningful assessment of changes in Pa_{O_2} during therapy.

the patients' inspiratory flow rate. Changes in Pa_{O_2} during oxygen therapy delivered by mask or cannula most frequently represent changes in the mechanics of delivery rather than changes in intrapulmonary shunting.

The nasal cannula offers some advantages over mask therapy in the postsurgical patient. A single nasal prong has proved as effective as a double nasal prong and can be used in patients with gastric tubes.[74] Oxygen therapy can be continued during eating, shaving and talking, and freedom of movement is improved when nasal cannulas are employed. Oxygen supplementation of the inspired air is equally effective with the mouth open or closed. With the mouth open, the nasopharynx is readily filled with oxygen and is depleted with the venturi effect of inspiration. When respiration is depressed, this venturi effect is less effective, and this may be partly responsible for the lack of evidence of CO_2 accumulation in patients with acute or chronic respiratory insufficiency for whom nasal prongs are used for supplemental oxygen.[73] Inspired oxygen tensions will tend to increase with increasing hypoventilation if oxygen is delivered via the aerosol mask, since air dilution at the mask is less likely.

Hypercarbia may result if ventilation has been dependent on a hypoxic drive. Such patients should receive supplemental O_2 via nasal prongs or high-flow venturi masks, the latter capable of delivering fixed, low concentrations of oxygen.[72] However, the excellent humidification of the inspired gases associated with aerosol mask therapy is lacking with both nasal cannula and venturi mask therapy. This may be an important consideration for many patients.

Effect of Cardiovascular Changes on Oxygen Delivery and Uptake

Arterial oxygen tensions (Pa_{O_2}) and oxygen delivery to the tissues are significantly affected by changes in cardiac output in patients with intrapulmonary shunting.[75] When high inspiratory oxygen tensions are required to maintain an adequate Pa_{O_2}, awareness of changes in cardiac output and/or tissue oxygen requirements can be obtained by serial analysis of mixed venous oxygen tension of blood from the superior vena cava, right atrium or pulmonary artery, simultaneously with arterial blood analysis.[76-78] Oxygen extraction may also be markedly increased by hyperthermia or shivering during hypothermia with little increase in cardiac output.[79] The ready availability of blood gas programs for desktop computers has made determinations of shunting and oxygen extraction a quick, accurate method for evaluating oxygen therapy.[80]

Perhaps the most commonly encountered "toxic" manifestation of hyperoxia, other than pulmonary damage, is respiratory depression and hypercarbia, which accrue when a patient who normally depends on a mild hypoxic drive for adequate alveolar ventilation is given excess oxygen. Preoperative blood gas analysis during air breathing for patients with chronic lung disease who may require postoperative ventilation control will delineate and expedite both the progress and goals of weaning in these patients.

Understandable hesitancy to reduce inspired oxygen tensions to "safe" levels ($<60\%$) may result from a fear of producing hypoxic tensions in patients with significant intrapulmonary shunting. This hesitancy may lead to prolonged inhalation of unnecessarily high inspired oxygen tensions, which may prolong weaning from respirators in some patients with chronic

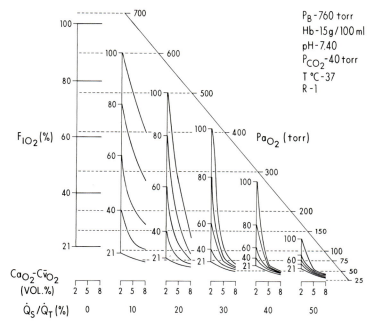

Fig 3. — Nomogram interrelating changes in $F_{I_{O_2}}$ with oxygen extraction ($C_{a_{O_2}}$ − $C_{\bar{v}_{O_2}}$), intrapulmonary shunting (Qs/Qt) and arterial oxygen tension ($P_{a_{O_2}}$). Raising the inspired oxygen concentration is less effective in raising the $P_{a_{O_2}}$ as Qs/Qt increases. Increases in cardiac output as reflected by reduction in $C_{a_{O_2}}$ − $C_{\bar{v}_{O_2}}$, however, will alone cause a significant improvement in $P_{a_{O_2}}$.

lung disease. Figure 3 demonstrates the effect of changes in $F_{I_{O_2}}$ and oxygen extraction on arterial oxygen tension, and is useful in understanding and managing this and other commonly encountered clinical problems.

For example, a patient with a $P_{a_{O_2}}$ of 105 while breathing 100% oxygen, and with a normal cardiac output and an oxygen extraction of 5 vol %, might experience a drop in the $P_{a_{O_2}}$ to approximately 70 torr when changed to a "safe" $F_{I_{O_2}}$ of 60 torr without a change in cardiac output or intrapulmonary shunting ($\dot{Q}_s/\dot{Q}_t$). The same patient, while still breathing 100% oxygen, might experience a reduction in $P_{a_{O_2}}$ to 65 torr, with no change in the $\dot{Q}_s/\dot{Q}_t$ of 30%, because of a reduction in cardiac output or an increase in oxygen extraction to 8 vol % due to shivering. The salutary effect on $P_{a_{O_2}}$ of maintaining or increasing cardiac output in the presence of large shunts is readily apparent, since a change in FI_{O_2} alone has less and less effect on Pa_{O_2} as amounts of shunted blood increase.

A Pa_{O_2} of 75 torr on 60% O_2 may suggest a shunt of 50% in a patient with high output septic shock but is also consistent with a shunt of 20% when oxygen extraction is increased or in the low output state. If the latter condition pertains, then the thrust of therapy should be to return the circulation to normal, and the arterial oxygen tension, in turn, will rise to 110 torr.

When cardiac output must increase to maintain oxygen delivery, the oxygen-carrying capacity of the blood should be maintained to minimize demands on the cardiovascular system, often already taxed by a surgical experience. To this end, maintenance of the hemoglobin at proper levels remains the cornerstone of proper oxygen therapy in patients with respiratory problems.

Problems of Parenteral Drug Therapy

Drugs may be given subcutaneously, intramuscularly, by intermittent or continuous intravenous injection or occasionally by absorption from the peritoneal cavity. Parenterally deposited lipid-soluble drugs readily diffuse through capillary endothelium, while larger lipid-insoluble molecules gain access through aqueous pores on the capillary surface. However, uptake from subcutaneous or intramuscular depots is dependent more on the amount of blood flow delivered to the area than on the ability of the drug to cross the capillary walls. Drug uptake can be expedited by local massage or heat or by mixing the drug with the enzyme hyaluronidase, which breaks down the hyaluronic acid in connective tissue and leads to increased drug distribution.[81] Uptake from SC or IM depots may be intentionally delayed by using aqueous or oil suspensions of poorly soluble salts of drugs. For example, insulin uptake may be delayed 4–6 hours by combining with protamine zinc. By increasing the size of a crystal of zinc insulin, which reduces surface area, uptake may be further delayed. Absorption of drugs, then, is affected by surface area, diluents and solubility of the drug in body fluids, but if vascularization is increased or tissue movement induced, uptake will increase.[82]

At times, drugs meant to be deposited SC or IM may induce arterial spasm, numbness, peripheral neuritis, local edema or hematoma formation. Arterial catheters are now commonly left in place to monitor blood pressure or blood gases of critically ill patients. When drugs such as a phenothiazine or thiopental are inadvertently given intra-arterially when the intravenous route was intended, arterial necrosis may occur, requiring digital or extremity amputation.[83] Irritants, such as solutions containing supplemental potassium or calcium salts or vasopressors, may induce increased permeability during intravenous infusions. The irritant effect of acidified solutions induces capillary transudation, while vasopressors constrict the vasa vasorum, which may permit leakage. If extravasation occurs, local necrosis and sloughing may result.[84, 85]

Once inadvertent arterial injection, venous extravasation or tissue injury has occurred during drug therapy, further reductions in local blood flow usually occur that will impede the uptake of drug from the site of deposition.

INADVERTENT ARTERIAL INJECTIONS

Arterial injections or suspected injections of sclerosing solutions are medical emergencies of the highest order. Pain, reflex vasoconstriction, stasis and edema rapidly follow injection. Efforts should be directed to maintaining the circulation and increasing drug uptake. If the brachial artery or its branches are involved, placement of a catheter for continuous brachial plexus, stellate ganglion or axillary block should be done. Systemic heparinization may prevent or delay the onset of arterial thrombosis that follows intimal damage and should be done as soon as prudent following establishment of local sympathetic blockade.[86] Should the use of heparin be temporarily contraindicated, dextran infusions may be tried. Experimental evidence exists that "dextran 70" and, to a lesser extent, "dextran 40" will inhibit thrombosis developing secondary to vascular injury.[87] Its effect is related to inhibition of platelet adhesiveness and release of platelet factor 3. An intravenous infusion of 7 mg/kg of 6% "dextran 70" followed by daily infusions of 3 ml/kg may be tried. Because of its lower molecular weight, however, dextran 40 is more likely to prevent or reverse cellular aggregation, which occurs in the microcirculation in low flow states. Systemic heparinization should be established as soon as possible with due regard to the synergistic effects of heparin and dextran on the coagulation mechanism. Anticoagulant therapy and sympathetic blockade should be continued for several days since a maximally dilated peripheral circulation may forestall further thrombosis, limit necrosis and aid in the healing process. Ancillary measures include narcotics, if pain is not completely controlled by sympathetic block, and slight elevation of the extremity to minimize stasis and induce venous return. Neither heat nor cold should be applied, and dressings, if necessary, should be nonocclusive.

Venous Extravasations

While the intravenous route for drug therapy is usually used for convenience or the establishment of stable blood levels, it is also used because many drugs are strongly acid or alkaline in solution. Subcutaneous deposition of these agents leads not only to tissue irritation or necrosis of tissue but to precipitation of the drug. Drug absorption from subcutaneous tissue is then dependent on simple diffusion. The osmotic pressure of the extracellular fluid must exceed that within the venous capillaries to maintain uptake of drug and its removal. Factors that induce hypotonicity of the extracellular fluid and favor collection of fluid near the area of extravasation will retard diffusion. Uptake of drug is then dependent on lymphatic drainage, which is more abundant in subcutaneous tissue than in the muscular areas. Lymphatics are a principal absorptive pathway for larger molecules and both warmth and activity will expedite absorption.[88]

Hyaluronidase historically was used as an effective expedient to subcutaneous diffusion of fluids, drugs and dyes for pediatric urography.[89] More recently it has been used to expedite the uptake of irritant drugs that have extravasated from veins.[90, 91] A combination of 150 units of hyaluronidase with 5–10 ml of 0.5–1% lidocaine may be injected into and around the periphery of the extravasated area. This serves to dilute the irritant, normalize extreme pH states of such drugs as thiopental or hydroxydione, and induce local vasodilation.[92] The greater interface of irritant drug with normal tissue induced by the hyaluronidase will expedite dilution and uptake of the drug.

Calcium chloride in 10% glucose, and calcium gluceptate are

capable, when extravasated, of producing a painful "subcutaneous burn," involving skin, fascia and underlying muscle.[93] Eschar formation and an indolent ulcer, resistant to early grafting, results. Heckler and McCraw have recently demonstrated experimentally the efficacy of clysis with NaCl plus hyaluronidase (150 units/1,000) in preventing full-thickness skin loss following extravasation of 10% calcium chloride. If clysis volume were 10 times the extravasated volume, the dilutional effect on the free calcium ion (Ca^{++}) was sufficient to prevent skin necrosis in all cases up to 1 hour following extravasation.[94]

Subcutaneous extravasation of continuous infusions of vasoconstrictors pose unique problems.[95] Levarterenol bitartrate (Levophed) and metaraminol (Aramine), used in the treatment of shock, and dopamine and epinephrine, frequently employed as cardiotonic drugs following open heart surgery, are examples of drugs that are capable of inducing local necrosis. Following extravasation, the local tissue becomes pale, indurated and cold. To overcome the intense local vasoconstriction, 5 mg of phentolamine (Regitine) in 10 ml of normal saline plus 150 units of hyaluronidase are injected throughout the affected area. According to McGinn et al., the hyaluronidase insures adequate penetration of the phentolamine into all affected areas.[96] Tissue slough was prevented in all of their patients so treated. Studies by Kirby et al. with local anesthetics and hyaluronidase, with and without epinephrine, indicate that although the accelerated absorption effect of hyaluronidase on local anesthetics is blocked in the presence of epinephrine, the spreading effect is actually enhanced.[97] The epinephrine presumably delays the uptake of hyaluronidase and allows it to produce maximal spreading.

Phentolamine appears to be required to prevent sloughing, however. Hyaluronidase and procaine alone have not prevented necrosis when injected into ischemic areas. Without locally induced vasodilatation, the hyaluronidase may serve only to disperse the vasopressor into a wider area.[98] When used with phentolamine, however, the hyaluronidase serves to distribute the vasodilator, to enlarge the absorbtive area for the offending drug and thereby effect its dilution. Its ability to reduce as well as prevent edema in traumatized tissue is well documented and may play a part in its use with phentolamine.[99]

Intravenous Drug Therapy

Many drugs, such as penicillins, in aqueous solutions can be given parenterally, and therapeutic blood levels may be temporarily exceeded without development of toxic symptoms. Wide fluctuations in antibiotic blood levels cannot only be well tolerated, but may have, in certain instances, therapeutic advantages.[100] Clinical studies indicate, for example, that isoniazid, streptomycin, rifampin or ethambutol, when given once every 3 days, is more efficacious in treating tuberculosis than a "time-concentration product" approach.[101] Most drugs commonly utilized in the early postoperative period, however, cannot be given in large intermittent doses without producing toxic symptoms. Antiarrhythmic agents and anticoagulants may be given as bolus loading doses followed by continuous infusions. Other agents, such as vasopressors or some antihypertensive drugs, which have a very short half-life, must be given by continuous infusions.

Dosages of some agents given by continuous infusions may be regulated by the establishment of the desired effect (reduction of blood pressure, abolition of arrhythmia, etc.) or limited by the development of toxic symptoms. In spite of the intactness of the hepatorenal system for drug metabolism and excretion, the rate of biotransformation of drugs may vary sixfold or more among individuals.

Lidocaine Infusion

Lidocaine is frequently given by continuous drip to control arrhythmias during or following cardiac surgery or myocardial infarction. Its dosage and specific effects are dependent on the efficiency of the biotransformation accomplished in the liver, and are unaffected by the presence or absence of renal function.[102] Oxidation of lidocaine is accomplished by the microsomal mixed function oxidases located in the hepatic endoplasmic reticulum. These enzymes convert lidocaine by dealkylation to monoethylglycine and xylidide. The latter compound, a toxin, is mainly dependent on the kidney for excretion.[103] Muscular twitching, diplopia, tinnitus and dizziness are reported during lidocaine administration, and some of these symptoms may be caused by unexcreted metabolic by-products of lidocaine metab-

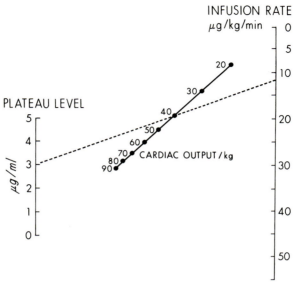

Fig 5. — Nomogram for determining the infusion rate of lidocaine necessary to attain the desired plateau concentration when cardiac output per kilogram body weight is known. Example: If the cardiac output is 40 ml/minute/kg body weight, a plateau concentration of 3 µg/ml would require an infusion rate of 12 µg/minute/kg body weight. (From Thomson, P. D., et al.[102])

centration of lidocaine when body weight and cardiac output are known.[102] It is based on the linear relationship of the rate of plasma clearance of lidocaine with cardiac output in patients with heart failure and in normal volunteers (Fig 5). If cardiac output measurements are not available, then lidocaine dosage should be reduced by half for patients with heart failure.[105, 108]

Serum lidocaine determinations should be done periodically in critically ill patients receiving lidocaine by infusion. Administration of lidocaine "to effect," without monitoring serum levels, is risky since the therapeutic range so often overlaps the toxic range. Ideally, the first determination should be done within a few hours of starting therapy before toxic or steady-state levels are achieved. The latter time is at least 6–8 hours, or 4 times the elimination half-life of lidocaine in normal subjects. The onset of toxic symptoms may be delayed several days in patients with a prolonged elimination time who may also have associated renal problems affecting clearance of toxic metabolites of lidocaine. Free-floating anxiety and personality changes, so often seen in acute stress situations, may actually reflect developing toxic levels.[109] If diazepam is mistakenly given for treatment, it will further mask the rising titer by increasing the threshold for convulsions.[110, 111]

PROPRANOLOL, PROCAINAMIDE, QUINIDINE AND DIGOXIN

The elimination half-life of lidocaine is approximately 1.5 hours. The half-lives of propranolol, procainamide, quinidine and digoxin are, respectively, 2–3 hours, 3.1 hours, 6.3 hours and 1.5 days. All four agents are rapidly absorbed when taken by mouth, yet their bioavailability may be markedly altered by postoperative changes in absorption for the gut and by the first-pass effect (presystemic hepatic extraction) on plasma concentration. Up to 70% of an oral dose of lidocaine, 80% of propranolol and 50% of an oral dose of procainamide can be metabolized in the first pass through the liver. While dosage regimes usually account for this loss in bioavailability, such surgical procedures as porta caval anastomoses or the presence of chronic or induced liver disease can markedly decrease the rate of metabolism and lead to toxic plasma concentrations.[112] Reductions in cardiac output and liver blood flow induced by propranolol not only will alter biotransformation of other drugs but will interfere with its own metabolism.[106] Digoxin is unaffected by the first-pass effect of hepatic disease, but both malabsorption from the gut and nuances in renal function, commonly encountered in the postoperative period, can complicate postoperative maintenance therapy or require use of the intravenous route.[113]

Dosage regimens and problems of clinical management and therapeutic assessment of these and other antiarrhythmics are beyond the scope of this report and can be found elsewhere.[102, 105-107, 109, 113] Let it be said, however, that drug monitoring serum levels of antiarrhythmics and other selected drugs is a rapidly developing clinical discipline. The sharing of problems of drug management with clinical pharmacokineticists can offer the surgical patient further protection against drug responses that may represent inappropriate drug dosage but which are mistakenly attributed to hypersensitivity, refractoriness or idiosyncracy.

Drug Monitoring

Knowledge of the uptake, distribution, metabolism and elimination of a drug is insufficient at times to predict individual response. Between the dose and its effect lie a multitude of factors that can alter the amount of drug reaching the site of action. Dosage of many drugs, such as antihypertensives or muscle relaxants, are monitored by the effect they produce, while other drugs are monitored by tests relevant to the effect desired. Prothrombin time determinations, for example, reflect the relative state of blood coagulability during heparin or Coumadin therapy. Other drugs, however, cannot always be monitored safely by dose manipulation without producing toxic effects. With still other drugs, toxicity may not be immediately evident, such as ototoxicity with certain antibiotics or retinal vessel damage due to excessive oxygen. For these and other drugs that produce clinically hidden toxic effects, measurement and interpretation of drug serum levels has sharpened considerably the physicians' ability to administer drugs safely as well as effectively.[102, 107, 114-117] Digoxin, theophylline, diphenylhydantoin, phenobarbital and lidocaine are notable examples of drugs now frequently monitored by measurement of plasma levels.

There is a more precise correlation between serum drug levels and drug effect compared to a drug dosage-to-effect sequence, because plasma levels reflect preconditioning by many biologic variables affecting dosage that are not detectable until a dose-response sequence has been completed.

Among these are: 1. Bioavailability, that is, the amount of drug reaching the general circulation and the rate at which it reaches the circulation, may vary greatly among patients, among different manufacturers' output of the same drug product (for example, digoxin) and from altered uptake due to surgery, malabsorption or altered circulation.[102, 105, 118]

2. Drug plasma levels also reflect changes in patient (or nursing) compliance, a not-infrequent cause of altered response to drugs. The greater the number of drugs taken and the more unpalatable the drug or its side effects, the more likely is patient noncompliance.

3. Plasma levels reflect unusual changes from predicted half-life, compartment size, protein binding and volume distribution of drugs due to concurrent disease. Antibiotics,[100, 119, 120] antiar-

rhythmics,[106, 121] anticonvulsants,[116, 117, 122] muscle relaxants,[22] antihypertensives,[123] bronchodilators[124, 125] and narcotics[126, 127] are a few classes of drugs whose serum levels are so affected.

4. The rate of hepatic clearance varies among drugs with changes in hepatic circulation and cirrhosis. Plasma drug levels are particularly helpful in establishing dosage for drugs with a high rate of hepatic clearance (first-pass effect) and for which the therapeutic-toxic range is small. Drugs with a large first-pass effect include lidocaine, propranolol, meperidine, methadone, reserpine, atropine, phenothiazines, L-dopa, $\propto$-methyldopa, estrogens and aspirin. In small doses, propranolol is almost completely extracted by the liver, with only small quantities escaping into the general circulation. With increasing dosage, both saturation of the propranolol binding sites and induced reductions in hepatic blood flow will lead to alarming increases in amounts of propranolol reaching the systemic circulation. Serum levels of such a drug reflect more precisely the amount of drug capable of reaching the target organ than do the effects of dose manipulation.

Problems of Monitoring Drug Levels

While techniques for measurement of drugs and, in some cases, their active metabolites have steadily improved, the correlation of serum levels and clinical effects have often been disappointing. Some drugs produce active metabolites, with longer half-lives than the parent drug. Lack of knowledge of the intensity of the metabolites' clinical effect as well as the inability of some laboratories to measure serum concentrations of metabolites, is responsible for some disappointing clinical studies.

A satisfactory therapeutic blood level may become insufficient for a patient as the disease process continues. This has long been observed clinically in patients with progressive heart disease treated with digitalis.

Measurement of drug blood levels must and has come under the scrutiny of those concerned with the alarming increase in the cost of health care delivery. Any reduction in morbidity derived from the measurements should be reflected in a decrease in overall patient care costs. Such studies are now underway. Blood level measurements of some drugs have played such a decided role in optimizing safe therapy, however, that their monitoring probably will continue as a necessary cost of treatment. Such drugs are digoxin, theophylline, oxygen, diphenylhydantoin and certain antiarrhythmics.

Perhaps the greatest problem in the clinical monitoring of drug levels lies in practicing physicians' general lack of knowledge of basic pharmacokinetics.[128, 129] Medical school curricula have only recently reflected some concern as to the relevancy of clinical pharmacology. Education of practicing physicians has principally been through consultations about drug problem cases with clinical pharmacologists in hospitals fortunate enough to have them.[116] Often the education of physicians rests with pharmacists trained in clinical pharmacokinetics and associated with hospital laboratories.[130, 131]

The flowering of this exciting new discipline will occur when practicing physicians, recognizing that clinical progress in this area may be passing them by, will turn to the clinical pharmacologist and recognize him as a valuable member of the ward rounds team.

REFERENCES

1. Huff, B. B. (ed.): *Physicians' Desk Reference* (Oradell, N. J.: Medical Economics Company, 1976).
2. Snyder, B. D.: Physostigmine: Antidote for anticholinergic poisoning, Minn. Med. 58:456, 1975.
3. Miller, R. R., and Greenblatt, D. J. (eds.): *Drug Effects in Hospitalized Patients* (New York: John Wiley & Sons, Inc., 1976).
4. Robinson, J. S.: Psychological effects of intensive care: Report of a personal experience, Anaesthetist 24:416, 1975.
5. Wilson, L. M.: Intensive care delirium, the effects of outside deprivation in a windowless unit, Arch. Intern. Med. 130:225, 1972.
6. Greene, L. T.: Physostigmine treatment of anticholinergic drug depression in postoperative patients, Anesth. Analg. (Cleve.) 50:222, 1971.
7. Sawyers, J. L., and Schenker, S.: How to handle the alcohol withdrawal state in surgical patients, Resident & Staff Physician 100:165, Feb. 1976.
8. Miller, L. C., and Heller, W. M.: Physical and Chemical Considerations in the Choice of Drug Products, in Modell, W. (ed.): *Drugs of Choice 1976-77* (St. Louis: The C. V. Mosby Company, 1976).
9. Fanning, G. L., and Colgan, F. J.: Diffusion hypoxia following nitrous oxide anesthesia, Anesth. Analg. (Cleve.) 50:86, 1971.
10. Stoelting, R. K., and Eger, E. I., II: Effect of ventilation and recovery from anesthesia: An in vivo and analog analysis before and after equilibrium, Anesthesiology 30:290, 1969.
11. Bastron, R. D., and Deutsch, S.: *Anesthesia and the Kidney* (New York: Grune and Stratton, 1976).

12. Habif, D. V., Papper, E. M., Fitzpatrick, H. F., Lawrence, P., Smythe, C. M., and Bradley, S. E.: The renal and hepatic blood flow, glomerular filtration rate and urinary output of electrolytes during cyclopropane, ether and thiopental anesthesia, operation and the immediate postoperative period, Surgery 30:241, 1951.

13. Mazze, R. I., Schwartz, F. D., Slocum, H. C., and Barry, K. G.: Renal function during anesthesia and surgery: The effects of halothane anesthesia, Anesthesiology 24:279, 1963.

14. Cousins, M. J., Greenstein, L. R., Hitt, A. B., and Mazze, R. I.: Metabolism and renal effects of enflurane in man, Anesthesiology 44:44, 1976.

15. Moran, W. H., Jr.: CPPB and vasopressin secretion, Anesthesiology 34:501, 1971.

16. Loughridge, L.: Anesthesia and the Kidneys, in Scurr, C. and Feldman, S. (eds.): Scientific Foundations of Anesthesia (Chicago: Year Book Medical Publishers, Inc., 1974).

17. Smith, J. W.: Digitalis toxicity: Epidemiology and clinical use of serum concentration measurements, Am. J. Med. 58:470, 1975.

18. Loehning, R. W., and Mazze, R. I.: Possible nephrotoxicity from enflurane in a patient with severe renal disease, Anesthesiology 40:203, 1974.

19. Brown, B. R., Jr.: Biotransformation of Anesthetics: Clinical Implications Explored, Clinical Trends in Anesthesiology, Vol. 6, no. 2 (New York: Science and Medicine Publishing Co., Inc., 1976).

20. De Wardner, H. E., Miles, B. E., Lee, G. De J., Churchill-Davidson, H. C., Wylie, W. D., and Sharpey-Schafer, E. P.: Circulatory effects of hemorrhage during prolonged light anesthesia in man, Clin. Sci. 12:175, 1953.

21. Churchill-Davidson, H. C., Way, W. L., and DeJong, R. H.: The muscle relaxants and renal excretion, Anesthesiology 28:540, 1967.

22. McLeod, K., Watson, J. J., and Rawlins, M. D.: Pharmacokinetics of pancuronium in patients with normal and impaired renal function, Br. J. Anaesth. 48:341, 1976.

23. Hillary, F. D., Renan, A. D., and Taylor, P.: Narcotic analgesics in anuric patients, Anesthesiology 43:745, 1975.

24. Bedfor, R. F., and Wollman, H.: Postoperative respiratory effects of morphine and halothane anesthesia: A study in patients undergoing cardiac surgery, Anesthesiology 43:1, 1975.

25. Berkowitz, B. A., Ngai, S. H., Yang, J. C., Hempstead, J., and Spector, S.: The disposition of morphine in surgical patients, Clin. Pharmacol. Ther. 17:629, 1975.

26. Stanski, P. R., Greenblatt, D. J., Lappas, D. B., Koch-Weser, J., and Lowenstein, E.: Kinetics of high-dose, intravenous morphine in cardiac surgery patients, Clin. Pharmacol. Ther. 19:752, 1976.

27. Clark, R. S. J., Doggart, J. R., and Lavery, T.: Changes in liver function after different types of surgery, Br. J. Anaesth. 48:119, 1976.

28. Biebuyck, J. F.: Anesthesia and hepatic metabolism: Current concepts of carbohydrate homeostasis, Anesthesiology 39:188, 1973.

29. Biebuyck, J. F., Lund, P., and Drebs, H. A.: The effects of halothane (2-bromo-2-chloro-1,1,1-trifluoroethane) on glycolysis and biosynthetic processes of the isolated perfused rat liver, Biochem. J. 128:711, 1972.

68. Barach, A. L., Eckman, M., Oppenheimer, E. T., Rumsey, C., Jr., and Soroka, M.: Observations on methods of increasing resistance to oxygen poisoning and studies of accompanying physiological effects, Am. J. Physiol. 142:462, 1944.
69. Wright, R. A., Weiss, H. S., Hiott, E. P., and Rustagi, J. S.: Risk or mortality in interrupted exposure to 100% O_2: Role of air vs. lowered PO_2, Am. J. Physiol. 210:1015, 1966.
70. Kessler, M., Hoper, J., and Krumme, B. A.: Monitoring of tissue perfusion and cellular function, Anesthesiology 45:184, 1976.
71. Krumme, B. A., Strehlan, R., Schonleben, K., and Kessler, M.: Redistribution of microcirculation—a new principle of regulation, Pfluegers Arch. 359:R35, 1975.
72. Shapiro, B. A., Harrison, R. A., and Trout, C. A.: *Clinical Application of Respiratory Care* (Chicago: Year Book Medical Publishers, Inc., 1975).
73. Cherniack, R. M., and Hakimpour, K.: The rational use of oxygen in respiratory insufficiency, J.A.M.A. 199:146, 1967.
74. Petty, T. L., Nett, L. M., and Lakshminarayan, S.: A single nasal prong for continuous oxygen therapy, Resp. Care 18:421, 1973.
75. Colgan, F. J., and Mahoney, P. D.: The effects of major surgery on cardiac output and shunting, Anesthesiology 31:213, 1969.
76. Stanley, T. H., and Isern-Amaral, J.: Periodic analysis of mixed venous oxygen tension to monitor the adequacy of perfusion during and after cardiopulmonary bypass, Can. Anaesth. Soc. J. 21:454, 1974.
77. Barratt-Boyes, B. G., and Wood, E. H.: The oxygen saturation of blood in the venae cavae, right-heart chambers and pulmonary vessels of healthy subjects, J. Lab. Clin. Med. 50:93, 1957.
78. Colgan, F. J., Nichols, F. A., and DeWeese, J. A.: Positive end expiratory pressure, oxygen transport and the low output state, Anesth. Analg. (Cleve.) 53:538, 1974.
79. Prys-Roberts, C.: The metabolic regulation of circulatory transport, in Scurr, C., and Feldman, S. (eds.): *Scientific Foundations of Anaesthesia* (London: William Heinemann Medical Books Ltd., 1970).
80. Ruiz, B. C., Tucker, W. K., and Kirby, R. R.: A program for calculation of intrapulmonary shunts, blood-gas and acid-base values with a programmable calculator, Anesthesiology 42:88, 1975.
81. La Du, B. N., Mandel, H. G., and Way, E. L. (eds.): *Fundamentals of Drug Metabolism and Drug Disposition* (Baltimore: The Williams & Wilkins Company, 1972).
82. Ballard, B. E., and Nelson, E.: Absorption of implanted solid drug, J. Pharm. Sci. 51:915, 1962.
83. Stone, H. H., and Donnelly, C. C.: The accidental intra-arterial injection of thiopental, Anesthesiology 22:995, 1961.
84. Brescoe, C. F., and Taylor, P. A.: Morbidity following intravenous injections, Anaesthesia 29:290, 1974.
85. Davies, D. D.: Local complications of thiopentone injection, Br. J. Anaesth. 38:530, 1966.
86. Kinmonth, J. B., and Shepherd, R. C.: Accidental injection of thiopentone into arteries, Br. J. Anaesth. 2:914, 1959.

87. Coon, W. W.: Drugs affecting the coagulation of blood, in Modell, W. (ed.): *Drugs of Choice 1976–77* (St. Louis: The C. V. Mosby Company, 1976).
88. Lowenthal, W.: Bioavailability, in Martin, E. W. (ed.): *Dispensing of Medication* (Easton, Pa: Mack Publishing Co., 1971).
89. Burket, L. C., and Gyorgy, P.: Clinical observations of the use of hyaluronidase, Ann. NY Acad. Sci. 52:1171, 1950.
90. Davis, H. S.: *Complications of Surgery and Their Management* (Philadelphia: W. B. Saunders Company, 1967).
91. Pashchuk, A.: Use of hyaluronidase in the complex measures for the prevention of necrotic inflammation in extravenous administration of calcium chloride, Klin. Khir. 5:1969.
92. Scurr, C. F.: Accidents with injections, Br. Med. J. 1:1350, 1956.
93. Yosowitz, P., Ekland, D. A., Shaw, R. C., and Parsons, R. W.: Peripheral intravenous infiltration necrosis, Ann. Surg. 182:553, 1975.
94. Heckler, F. R., and McCraw, J. B.: Calcium-related cutaneous necrosis, Surg. Forum 27:553, 1976.
95. Alexander, C. S., Sako, Y., and Mikulio, E.: Pedal gangrene associated with the use of dopamine, N. Engl. J. Med. 293:591, 1975.
96. McGinn, J. T., Schulger, J., and DiGregorio, N. J.: Prevention of levarterenol sloughs, NY State J. Med. 56:1950, 1956.
97. Kirby, C. K., Eckenhoff, J. E., and Looby, J. P.: The use of hyaluronidase with local anesthetic agents in surgery and dentistry, Ann. NY Acad. Sci. 52:1166, 1950.
98. Pelner, L., Waldman, S., and Rhoades, M. G.: The problem of levarterenol (Levophed) extravasation: An experimental study, Am. J. Med. Sci. 236:755, 1958.
99. Bennett, J. E., Zook, E. G., Ashbell, T. S., and Hugo, N. E.: The spreading enzymes and localized edema: A study of wringer crush injury in the rabbit, J. Trauma 10:240, 1970.
100. Kunis, C. M.: Blood level measurements and antimicrobial agents, Clin. Pharmacol. Ther. 16:251, 1974.
101. Jusko, W. J.: Pharmacokinetic management of antibiotic therapy, in Levy, G. (ed.): *Clinical Pharmacokinetics, a Symposium* (American Pharmaceutical Association, Academy of Pharmaceutical Sciences, Oct. 1974).
102. Thomson, P. D., Melmon, K. L., Richardson, J. A., Cohn, K., Steinbrunn, W., Cudihee, R., and Rowland, M.: Lidocaine pharmacokinetics in advanced heart failure, liver disease and renal failure in humans, Ann. Intern. Med. 78:499, 1973.
103. Ritchie, J. M., and Cohen, P. J.: Local anesthetics, in Goodman, L. S., and Gilman, A. (eds.): *The Pharmacological Basis of Therapeutics* (5th ed.; New York: Macmillan Publishing Co. Inc., 1975).
104. Boyes, R. N., Scott, D. B., Jebson, P. J., Godman, M. J., and Julian, D. G.: Pharmacokinetics of lidocaine in man, Clin. Pharmacol. Ther. 12:105, 1971.
105. Harrison, D. C., Stenson, R. E., and Constantine, R. T.: The Relationship of Blood Levels, Infusion Rates and Metabolism of Lidocaine to its Anti-Arrhythmic Action, in Sandoe, E., Flensted-Jensen, E., and Olesen, K. H.

monary reaction to remote infection. Complement seems to be
an important component in several studies, but nearly complete
depletion of complement in cats had little effect on the subsequent course after injection of endotoxin.[48] Bradykinin and serotonin are discussed more fully in the section "Vasoactive
Materials." The lung is active in regulating the homeostasis of
both substances, along with many other vasoactive mediators. A
pathologic effect on the lung itself implies a prior impairment of
the metabolic activity of the lung or overwhelming of the pertinent metabolic machinery. This is not impossible or even unlikely, and the hypothesis remains an attractive one but is still
unsubstantiated.

Platelets, polymorphonuclear leukocytes, fibrin and fibrin
degradation products are discussed in the section "Thromboembolism, Microembolism and Disseminated Intravascular Coagulation (DIC)." There is abundant evidence linking all of these
substances to pulmonary damage. The ultrastructural evidence
is perhaps strongest for polymorphonuclear leukocytes,[42, 45, 49, 50]
which are of primary importance in clearing blood-borne bacteria,[51] and there is evidence linking them to structural damage to
the lungs of primates given low doses of endotoxins repeatedly.[41]
Release of lysosomes was noted in this study, which is unlike the
response to phagocytosis of inert material. As noted in the later
section, however, recent clinical studies indicate that DIC,
platelets or polymorphonuclear leukocytes may not be essential
to the development of the clinical syndrome in infected patients.
Finally, there is evidence of an unidentified blood-borne factor in
infected animals that increases pulmonary capillary permeability and is inactivated by protease inhibitors.[52] In summary, it
currently appears possible that all of the substances mentioned
can participate in the genesis of pulmonary insufficiency after
remote sepsis, and that some changes may occur even without
any of them. The characteristic pattern is one of damage to the
pulmonary capillary endothelium with increased leakage of
fluids and protein.[53] This is compatible with the observed clinical changes. The temporal sequence suggests that the lung can
withstand these multiple challenges initially, but that its defenses (and perhaps defense of the systemic circulation) break
down as the onslaught continues. Clearly the best thing the
physician can do for the patient's lungs in these circumstances is
to control the remote infection. Abundant and still accumulat-

ing clinical evidence indicates that this may be the factor that determines survival in these patients.

Pulmonary Infection

There are three large "external" surfaces of the body: skin, intestine and airways. Of these, only the lower airway must remain sterile in order to function properly. In addition, the lungs as the main filter for blood-borne material bear the main brunt of bacteremic episodes. The pulmonary defense mechanisms are fairly complex and probably still incompletely defined.[54] The key elements appear to be the pulmonary alveolar macrophages, very metabolically active and efficient phagocytic cells.[54, 55] The ability of the lungs to clear and kill inhaled bacteria is adversely effected by serious injury,[56] hemorrhage,[57, 57a] aspiration,[58] hypoxia,[55] cigarette smoke and high concentrations of oxygen, among other things.[54] In addition, the lungs probably are affected by the suppression of systemic antibacterial defenses that results from anesthesia and operation.[59] There may be differences among various types of bacteria in the ability to survive in the lower airway, with *Pseudomonas* particularly difficult to sterilize.[60]

The bacterial challenge to the lower airway is increased in surgical patients by such factors as intubation, retained secretions, aspiration and dry gases (especially anesthetic gases). An interesting phenomenon is the conversion of the oropharyngeal flora of sick hospitalized patients to a predominantly gram-negative pattern.[61-65a] The reasons for this well-documented change are not clear; antibiotics probably intensify[61, 64, 65] but are not necessary for the change.[62, 65a] Hospital personnel do not share in this conversion.[66] This conversion undoubtedly facilitates contamination of the lower airway by gram-negative organisms and may signal more subtle impairments of defense mechanisms. Gram-negative pneumonia occurs primarily in patients who have first had the upper airway colonized by gram-negative bacteria.[67]

Most available evidence indicates that the gram-negative bacteria that colonize the lungs of sick postoperative patients arise from the patients themselves,[68, 69] although there are contrary data[70] and opinions. There are significant hazards in the environment, however, including nursing personnel and respiratory equipment.[71-74] Certain types of equipment may, in fact, spread contamination through nursing units.[75] Rigid adherence to technique will prevent cross-contamination in intensive care units, but it will do nothing for the colonizations and infections arising from endogenous sources. Once gram-negative tracheitis or pneumonia is established, dissemination throughout the entire lower airway may occur via ventilatory equipment. Use of elongated inspiratory-expiratory tubing (increased dead space) may be particularly harmful in redisseminating *Pseudomonas*.[73, 74] There are better ways of controlling CO_2 levels than by increasing dead space.

The topical characteristics of secondary gram-negative pneumonia in sick hospitalized patients are so striking that "topical" use of antimicrobial agents has been tried.[76-78a] The analogy to topical infection of burn wounds has a certain legitimacy. There seems little doubt that adding the proper antibiotic (usually an aminoglycoside) to a nebulization device in the ventilatory equipment will delay the appearance of gram-negative organisms in the airway, and may well improve the results of treatment with systemic antibiotics. The main problem is that with prolonged use on an individual patient or with routine use on all patients, resistant organisms appear that assume increasingly aggressive characteristics and that may rapidly colonize all patients admitted to the unit. More selective and intermittent use of nebulized antibiotics seems to avoid this problem, and may be a useful maneuver in very highly susceptible patients. Further controlled trials seem worthwhile. Another interesting approach is active immunization against *Pseudomonas,* which needs further evaluation.[79]

Gram-negative pneumonia can arise from bacteremic inoculation of the lungs. Experimentally, blood-borne polymorphonuclear leukocytes seem to be the key element of defense.[51] Bacteremic gram-negative pneumonias occur primarily in patients with significantly impaired antimicrobial defenses and carry a high mortality.[80] There have been no studies on the effect that brief, intermittent bacteremias, as might occur in the patient with multiple indwelling catheters, may have on the ability of the lungs to handle an inhaled bacterial challenge.

The diagnosis of gram-negative pneumonia can be difficult in a patient already ill with pulmonary complications. Fever, leukocytosis, pulmonary infiltrates and hypoxemia may be due to other causes. Proper interpretation of tracheal cultures in such a patient is very difficult.[80a] Most such patients will soon show gram-negative organisms in the tracheal aspirate, especially if intubated. Untimely use of antibiotics will probably do more harm than good. No one has established firm criteria for an accurate diagnosis of significant bronchopulmonary infection in this setting. One interesting study related serum antibody titers to the occurrence of gram-negative pneumonia; patients with colonization without pneumonia showed no change in titers.[81] This is not yet a practical diagnostic test. Distinguishing colonization from bronchopneumonia is a practical problem that is faced almost daily in every active intensive care unit but is very difficult to solve.

Superimposed pulmonary infection, usually gram-negative and most often *Pseudomonas,* is often the terminal event in those who die of postoperative or posttraumatic pulmonary insufficiency.[82] It is rarely the primary problem, but the superimposition of further loss of pulmonary function and an added septic burden prove insurmountable. Few patients who die of acute respiratory distress after operation or injury die with sterile lower airways. Pulmonary sepsis is a complication of complications, occurring in damaged lungs in a compromised host. All aspects of the problem need further investigation.

Hemorrhage

The relationship between hemorrhage and pulmonary insufficiency was reviewed by the author in 1972.[83] Briefly, the degree to which hemorrhage induces deterioration of pulmonary structure and function is not at all clear. Clinical evidence supporting such a relationship is rather thin, as pulmonary insufficiency is not a common event after hemorrhage alone or after the hypovolemic shock of cholera.[2] Experimental efforts to establish significant pulmonary insufficiency after hemorrhage alone have been almost universally unsuccessful. Morphologic changes of varying degrees have been reported, mostly in dogs. Compliance and shunt usually improve during hemorrhage, with decrease in pulmonary blood volume and extravascular lung water. Following treatment, there have been varying, usually unimpressive, decreases in compliance and little, if any, impairment in oxygenation. Few studies have extended into the postresuscitative period, few have treated the animals in a manner similar to clinical practice and few have systematically compared different treatment regimens. Those treatments that most effectively support survival may be associated with the least alteration in pulmonary structure and function.

One of the simplest explanations for any damage that does occur to the lungs as a result of hemorrhage would be hypoperfusion. The lungs are rather unique, however, in being able to tolerate total ischemia for several hours with surprisingly little detrimental effect, provided alveolar ventilation is maintained.[84-91] Even static inflation with nitrogen is largely protective. Atelectatic lung tolerates ischemia rather poorly.[87] Williams et al. reported that pulmonary arterial occlusion for one hour was well tolerated in otherwise normal animals, but very detrimental in animals with severe hypoxemia, indicating the potential role of systemic factors (or of overperfusion).[91]

Since our last review in 1972,[83] investigation into the relationship between hemorrhage and pulmonary function has continued. Several studies (including some in primates[96-98]) have again documented little functional change during or after hemorrhage.[92-95a] Several investigators continue to report significant structural alterations in the lungs of dogs after hemorrhage, but with little data on functional changes[99, 100a] or with minimal changes.[100a] Meyers et al.[101] and Garvey et al.[102] attempted to identify variables that might explain the discrepancies among observed changes in dogs after hemorrhage. Neither group succeeded and, even here, Meyers was unable to detect any notable changes, whereas Garvey reported "moderate or severe lesions" in half the animals but could not relate these to any of the several variables studied. Thus the unexplained discrepancies persist unabated, but with little documentation of functional impairment even by those describing marked structural changes. Hepatic inflow occlusion will increase pulmonary damage during hemorrhage in dogs.[102a]

Several groups have documented mild increases in lung water content when a salt solution was used instead of or in addition to shed blood.[103, 104] Moss et al. reported the paradoxical finding that interstitial edema and sodium content increase during hemorrhage in large primates and decrease after treatment with saline.[105] This is contrary to most reported findings on lung water content during and after hemorrhage and treatment.[83] A somewhat similar pattern was reported in cats,[106] but the method used labeled albumin and the assumption that all albumin in the lung is in plasma, which is clearly incorrect. Holcroft et al.[107, 107a] confirmed a finding by Moss that large primates resuscitated from hemorrhage with human albumin tend to sequester some of this colloid in the lungs. Gaisford et al.[108] reported the opposite in rhesus monkeys; that is, more interstitial edema and disruption occurred after treatment with salt water alone than with albumin. Thus, even when primates are used, contradictory results continue to be reported when the effect of hemorrhage on pulmonary function is investigated.

Anemia was proposed as a factor predisposing toward the development of postresuscitative pulmonary changes,[109] but the study was improperly controlled: the control dogs should have been bled and reinfused at the same interval before study as were the anemic dogs. Significant intrapulmonary trapping of platelets in dogs during and after hemorrhage was confirmed,[110] as was the previously well-described effect of acidosis in increasing pulmonary vascular resistance.[111, 112] Inspired CO_2 concentration was found to significantly effect pulmonary compliance during hemorrhage in dogs.[113] Steroids,[99] serotonin antagonists[100] and sodium bicarbonate[112] were reported to prevent the development of structural lesions in canine lungs after hemorrhage, but, as noted, some investigators cannot produce these lesions at all. Steroids had little effect in primates,[96] but the changes were minimal in controls.

An increased incidence of iron-laden macrophages was found in the tracheobronchial secretions of patients after hemorrhagic shock, confirmed by similar findings on studies in rats.[114] The significance of this is not clear. Border and associates described the use of alveolar-arterial N_2 differences to better define ventilation-perfusion mismatching in ill patients.[115]

The permeability of the pulmonary capillary membrane has become an area of active interest because of the many indications of increased permeability in patients with acute respiratory distress and because of the devastating effects of such a change. While there is abundant evidence to support such changes in patients with sepsis there are at best mixed results after hemorrhage. Studies in sheep[116] and dogs[117] failed to demonstrate increased permeability to protein in treated or untreated hemorrhagic shock, but other studies in dogs found evidence of a greatly increased leak.[118] Anderson and De Vries studied the pulmonary lymphatic drainage in dogs and found they could produce either result after hemorrhage.[119] The critical variable was the microvascular driving pressure. Perhaps this could explain the surprising and contradictory data on the effects of infused albumin on primate lungs after hemorrhage. Berman reported marked changes in permeability after extensive transfusion in rats, but this will be discussed in the section "Massive Transfusion."

The earlier findings of Henry *et al.*[120] that hemorrhagic shock in dogs led to alterations in the metabolic patterns of pulmonary tissue have been confirmed in rats using oxygen consumption with and without added glucose.[121] Other studies of pulmonary cellular function after hemorrhage were less impressive.[122] This is a very interesting line of investigation that should be pursued further: what are the temporal sequences, how does treatment alter these changes, how do the changes after hemorrhage compare with those after similar periods of ischemia without systemic hypotension?

The evidence relating hemorrhage to pulmonary dysfunction has not changed appreciably in recent years. With several contradictory results remaining unexplained, it appears that severe hemorrhage does induce some deterioration of pulmonary structure and function but that it is not marked (the functional changes are rather small) and is not progressive. The details of treatment may have more to do with subsequent functional changes than the hemorrhage itself. How much this degree of damage facilitates the development of other pulmonary complications remains an unanswered question, and is worth more investigative effort than is now evident.

There are some aspects of severe hemorrhage in man that alter pulmonary function, but they are not widely discussed. Many, perhaps most, patients with repeated hematemesis aspirate significant amounts of blood, especially if obtunded, or kept supine, or have tubes traversing the esophagus. This is a prominent cause of posthemorrhagic pulmonary dysfunction, sometimes labeled "shock lung." Blood is a very irritative agent when aspirated; if the patient is supine, the distribution will appear diffuse on radiographs taken in the anteroposterior plane. Hemorrhagic shock in the elderly, whatever the cause, is more likely to damage the left ventricle because of the increasing incidence of coronary arteriosclerosis with age. Known preexisting coronary disease or diffuse arteriosclerosis of course makes this more likely. Thus, patients with ruptured abdominal aortic aneurysms show a high incidence of left ventricular dysfunction after operation.[123] Measurement of pulmonary arterial wedge pressures help define this population, as the central venous pressure may initially be deceptively normal. Measurement of myocardial-specific creatine phosphokinase (CPK) isoenzymes is also a major diagnostic help. This is another group in which previously unexplained diffuse pulmonary consolidation following hemorrhage is now identifiable and can be treated more precisely. Based on experience with patients after myocardial infarctions, some form of mechanical assistance to the left ventricle, such as intra-aortic balloon pumping, might help some of these patients through hazardous postoperative periods.

Fluid Overload

The great wave of interest in the effects of hemodilutional resuscitation on pulmonary function now seems to be subsiding. Several excellent recent reviews of pulmonary edema are available, which indicate the complexity of the mechanisms for maintaining an appropriate content and distribution of fluids in the lungs, the effects of alterations in plasma oncotic pressure and in capillary hydrostatic pressure, and the impact of alterations in pulmonary capillary permeability.[124-127] Bredenberg's review of the effects of fluid overloading with salt solutions on pulmonary function is recommended.[128]

With some disagreement on details, it is clear that overloading the circulation produces pulmonary edema by elevating capillary hydrostatic pressure. This form of edema is associated with a prominent leak of protein along with fluid. Dilution of plasma-specific osmotic pressure allows edema to form at lower hydrostatic pressures. Such edema usually begins in the pulmonary interstitial space, but can extend to alveolar flooding with increased capillary permeability. Fatal pulmonary edema can be produced by extensive infusions of salt water in animals with normal central venous pressures; clinical examples of the same phenomenon have been too common. The earliest practical way of detecting interstitial edema is probably through changes in compliance,[129, 130] although there is some debate even on this point.[131] Interstitial pulmonary edema clearly need not cause shunting,[83, 132] but if alveolar flooding occurs, then shunting is inevitable. Even before alveolar flooding develops, the effects of interstitial edema on the closing of terminal airways could conceivably lead to atelectasis and shunting.[133]

The fact that excessive retention of salt and water results in pulmonary edema is neither new nor surprising. An important component of the clinical situation may be the ability of the patient to excrete the excess quantities of salt and water after resuscitation.[134, 135] This is reinforced by the common observation of improved oxygenation following diuresis, with or without supplemental albumin.[136, 137] The role of the concentration of albumin in the plasma in the genesis of acute respiratory failure remains in some dispute. Some of the contradictory work on the effect of albumin in the resuscitation of animals from hemorrhage was reviewed in the preceding section. Most clinical observations indicate that pulmonary insufficiency occurs in patients with lower concentrations of albumin,[34, 134, 135, 137-141] but this does not prove cause and effect, as many of the conditions associated with acute pulmonary insufficiency are also associated with hypoalbuminemia. The prospective study by Skillman et al.[142] is noteworthy in spite of its limitations, and is the best semicontrolled clinical study yet published in this area. Earlier studies by the Naval Surgical Research team showed little difference in postresuscitative concentrations of albumin in the plasma, whether combat casualties were given supplemental albumin or only simple salt solutions, but these studies did not deal with pulmonary function directly.[143]

There may be different considerations when pulmonary insufficiency is already established. There is abundant evidence for increased pulmonary capillary permeability in many such patients, including grossly increased permeability to albumin.[144] If such is the case, increasing the concentration of albumin in the plasma would have little effect on the exchange of fluids across the pulmonary capillary membrane. There is already good evidence of the inefficacy of administering albumin to patients while there is an increased capillary permeability to other materials of like size.[145] It is possible, however, that even in this situation there are relatively normal areas in the lungs that are, in fact, keeping the patient alive and should be protected from unnecessary flooding.

There is a general impression that with greater awareness of the limitations and dangers of resuscitation with salt water there has been much more judicious use of that substance, greater use of diuretics when the circulation has stabilized and before pulmonary problems develop, and a lower incidence of pulmonary insufficiency after resuscitation from major injury. This is all but impossible to prove, but it may well be that one form of posttraumatic, postoperative pulmonary insufficiency is now being more effectively prevented. The role of albumin in reversing established pulmonary insufficiency remains uncertain, but in general the use of albumin represents a logical approach unless there is a massive increase in pulmonary capillary permeability. Obviously, more clinical studies are needed on this very practical question.

There is an aspect to the treatment of severe hemorrhage in man that has received little attention. The traditional wisdom has been that a greater than normal blood volume is required for adequate resuscitation from severe hypotension. Measurements of blood volume in apparently well-resuscitated, stable patients following severe hemorrhage almost always reveal less than the predicted normal blood volumes for at least the first day, with (often) greater than normal blood volumes by the third day. This pattern has been consistent in studies on severely injured combat casualties,[146-148] even when central venous pressure was included as a guide for fluid replacement.[149] Reports on postoperative civilian patients have often been obscured by the inclusion of patients with sepsis, who usually require and develop blood volumes greater than normal. When data on hemorrhage alone can be extracted, however, a pattern similar to that reported in combat casualties is apparent,[150] again even when central venous pressure is included as a criterion for adequate replacement of blood loss.[151-153]

This pattern suggests that there may be a fixed contraction of the capacitance system (great veins) following severe blood loss.[154, 155] The classic study on the relationship of blood volume to central venous pressure showed no evidence of such a phenomenon, but was performed on normal volunteers in the supine position bled less than 15% of expected blood volume.[156] The study on combat casualties by Simmons et al. looked especially at this possibility.[149] They found that the degree of "undertransfusion," despite clinical stability and normal central venous pressure, was directly related to the amount of blood lost at injury. Of great interest is the fact that pulmonary edema developed in 4 of these casualties at a time when measured blood volumes were at predicted normal values or less. It appears that the pulmonary artery may also participate in the loss of vascular compliance that occurs in the response to stress.[157]

The earlier results showing less than expected blood volumes after resuscitation were ascribed to clinical error. It may be that persistent contraction of the capacitance and pulmonary arterial systems make the severely hemorrhaged patient much more susceptible to overtransfusion by removing a very useful volume buffering device. This possibility seems worthy of investigation.

Thromboembolism, Microembolism and Disseminated Intravascular Coagulation (DIC)

In recent years a great expansion of our knowledge of the incidence and natural history of deep venous thrombosis in the legs following major operations has resulted from studies using radiolabeled fibrinogen.[158-162] Similar data on pulmonary embolism have not accrued, but since deep venous thrombosis in the legs is the commonest event leading to postoperative, posttraumatic pulmonary embolism, the information obtained has been pertinent.

Factors predisposing toward deep venous thrombosis are those commonly associated with pulmonary embolism: congestive heart failure, certain malignancies, severe trauma, prolonged bed rest, obesity and a prior history of deep venous disease or of pulmonary embolism. Surprisingly, fully 50% of newly formed clots begin forming during the operation itself; most of the rest begin within a few days after. Most postoperative deep venous clots are asymptomatic; nearly half the patients with signs and symptoms suggesting thrombophlebitis in the calf do not have venous clots. In most circumstances, low doses of heparin are effective in preventing postoperative deep venous thrombosis except when clot is already present before operation.[163-165] Various mechanical maneuvers may also be effective.[162, 166] The usual compression stockings are probably not effective. With preexisting clots, fully anticoagulating doses of heparin are required. Continuous intravenous administration of heparin seems to be safer and at least as effective as the older practice of intermittent doses.[167] Heparin itself can cause thrombocytopenia in a significant percentage of patients.[168, 169]

Pulmonary emboli in man lyse spontaneously at a significant but somewhat unpredictable rate.[170, 171] Heparin prevents recurrent embolization, but may do little to alter the rate of resolution of existing emboli. The newer fibrinolysins derived from bacterial or human sources significantly hasten the resolution of pulmonary emboli and of peripheral deep venous clots.[172] They carry a significant risk of hemorrhage in early postoperative or posttraumatic patients, however, and also when used concurrently with heparin. These products may soon be approved for clinical use in the United States. Various mechanical devices inserted into the inferior vena cava transvenously appear to be effective in preventing recurrent embolization in high-risk patients who are unacceptable for heparin treatment or when heparin treatment has failed.[173, 174] The rate of complications of insertion decrease sharply with experience.

Pulmonary embolization is much more common in posttraumatic patients than is clinically apparent.[8,175-178] The degree is often fairly small, but occasionally inapparent recurrent embolization contributes significantly to pulmonary dysfunction in sick surgical patients. The clinical picture of hypoxemia, bilateral pulmonary infiltrates and fever can mimic many other causes. The diagnosis can be difficult to establish. In spite of heightened awareness, plain roentgenograms of the chest remain rather inaccurate.[179] Scintiscanning is often of little diagnostic value in such patients. Pulmonary arteriography is necessary to establish the diagnosis. The treatment involves either anticoagulation with heparin or interruption of the inferior vena cava.

Microembolization, especially of leukocytes and platelets, has received a great deal of attention in the past 20 years as a possible mechanism for pulmonary dysfunction in patients with sepsis or injury. A considerable amount of experimental work has yielded often contradictory results, but certain findings are fairly consistent. Platelets and serotonin sequester in the lungs after soft tissue injury, hemorrhage, endotoxemia or bacteremia. The primary functional effect seems to be bronchoconstriction, probably related to local release of serotonin. There is often little effect on oxygenation. When studied, white cells often sequester in the lungs along with platelets, especially after en-

sive hyperinflation of the lungs during general anesthesia prevents a significant and progressive fall in arterial oxygenation
that would otherwise occur, especially with tidal volumes less
than 8 ml/kg body weight. This probably represents a tendency
to closure of terminal airways and perhaps concomitant or subsequent alveolar collapse, especially if highly absorbable gas is
"trapped" behind the closed airways. There are marked changes
in compliance during general anesthesia, but much of this is due
to the lower functional residual capacity that occurs with recumbency and relaxation.

These effects persist into the early postoperative period, but
only for a matter of hours. The occurrence and degree of postoperative pulmonary impairment is dominated by such factors as
location of incision, obesity, duration of operation, preexisting
pulmonary disease and perhaps even "personality." The postoperative changes in pulmonary function have been reviewed by
Latimer et al.[194]

The influence of the incision on postoperative pulmonary
impairment dramatically demonstrates the importance of pain
and splinting. Churchill in 1927 first demonstrated the differential effect of upper abdominal incisions on pulmonary function
(vital capacity).[195] Many observations utilizing a variety of measurements have since reaffirmed the detrimental effects of incisions near the diaphragm. In some instances, upper laparoto-
mies were more detrimental than thoracotomies. Most studies
show decreases in vital capacity, functional residual capacity,
compliance and arterial oxygen tension, a restrictive pattern in
timed expiratory studies and a shift toward frequent shallow
breathing with an absence of deep breaths. All of these changes
are greatest with upper abdominal incisions and least or absent
with peripheral incisions.

There is general agreement (but not unanimity) that a number of variables clearly increase the risk of postoperative pulmonary complications. Preexisting pulmonary disease is one of
the most significant, leading to at least a twofold to threefold
increase in postoperative pulmonary complications. Even seemingly minor upper respiratory infections have been found to
greatly increase risk. Smoking is similarly a high-risk factor,
and much of these data are included in the group of patients
classified as having preoperative pulmonary disease. Obesity
seems to be a moderate risk factor. The location of the incision

has already been discussed. The type of incision (especially horizontal versus vertical) has been found both significant and not significant, but one of the best-controlled studies showed less respiratory impairment in massively obese patients explored through transverse as opposed to vertical abdominal incisions.[196] Age is a debatable risk factor, as much of the increased difficulty can be attributed to associated diseases rather than to age itself. The duration of operation is probably important, at least for prolonged (more than 3–4 hours) procedures. Sex is probably not significant; the several studies that showed more impairment in men usually did not correct for smoking. Surprisingly, the type of agent used for anesthesia showed little or no effect, and the incidence of delayed postoperative pulmonary complications was no less after regional than after general inhalation anesthesia. There may be differences relating to individual anesthesiologists, however, so technique probably is somewhat significant. A number of more recent studies further confirm this pattern of findings,[196-201] and have added the first demonstration of the importance of personality traits in the patients,[202] something well known to practicing surgeons.

The overall incidence of postoperative pulmonary complications varies widely in different series. The differences in criteria, selection of patients, and operative procedure are so great that any attempt to demonstrate an altered incidence related to treatment must be carefully controlled. A number of practices or devices designed to promote deep breathing postoperatively have been successful.[203-206] "Intermittent positive pressure breathing" as commonly dispensed is not one of these,[204, 206, 207] and should be specifically singled out because it is so commonly used, yet is at best worthless, always very wasteful of money, and at worst harmful (sepsis, meteorism, failure to adequately handle pulmonary problems). Some of the most effective maneuvers include careful use of narcotics,[208, 209] regional anesthesia for relief of postoperative pain,[210, 211] and preoperative chest physical therapy.[212, 213] The latter is particularly effective in patients with preexisting pulmonary disease, but requires several days to achieve full effectiveness.

Various other factors may contribute to pulmonary impairment during or after operation. Anesthetic gases as commonly used are almost totally dry. This is demonstrably harmful and probably accounts for some of the harmful effects of prolonged anesthesia.[214, 214a] Recumbency produces an instantaneous decrease in functional residual capacity.[208, 215] This can be minimized with tourniquets on the limbs,[208] so some must be due to shifting blood centrally and not all to elevating the diaphragm. Several studies indicated a modest fall in arterial oxygenation with prolonged bed rest,[216, 217] but a recent study found no change in normal volunteers after 48 hours' recumbency.[218] There has been little study of the changes in lung volumes and arterial oxygenation after changes in position in patients with recent upper abdominal incisions.

The pattern of findings confirmed in many studies over a 40-year period are rather clear and consistent. There are changes in pulmonary function induced by anesthesia and by narcotic drugs, but even more marked and prolonged changes result from operative wounds. These changes suggest that diaphragmatic motion is hindered by pain, with an altered pattern of breathing, changes in various lung volumes and a restrictive functional pattern all leading to airway closure and alveolar collapse. Some clearly defined factors make this more likely to happen, and various maneuvers can minimize the occurrence, extent and duration of these changes. These changes unquestionably contribute in a major way to the development of more severe forms of pulmonary insufficiency, at least by allowing certain complications to occur more easily, if not contributing directly to whatever causes the severe impairment.

Aspiration

The true incidence of aspiration pneumonitis is almost impossible to define. The mortality after clinically diagnosed aspiration remains surprisingly high, mostly because of the type of patients who aspirate. A number of recent reviews are available.[219-224]

"Silent" regurgitation occurs rather predictably in patients under general anesthesia. A number of sizable studies have documented its occurrence and have identified several factors leading to a higher risk of aspiration: operations on the abdomen or oropharynx, the presence of nasogastric tubes (doubles the incidence), tracheostomy and perhaps the anesthetic agent. Much of this aspiration produces little in the way of clinical disease and probably represents primarily an increased bacterial challenge to the lower airway.

Aspiration is a more complex disease than it appears. The threats to function and survival are most likely drowning, chemical damage, bacterial contamination and mechanical obstruction of the airway. Failure to distinguish between these various components makes some clinical reports and experimental studies difficult to evaluate. Drowning is straightforward, it obviously requires a grossly distended stomach, and hence is associated with improper intragastric feeding by tube, forced oral intake or severe ileus. The treatment is immediate suctioning of the airway, intubation and mechanical ventilatory support, and safely emptying the stomach to prevent recurrence. It is much more likely to happen in obtunded or unconscious patients.

Chemical damage is usually the result of low pH of the aspirate, and is probably a combined acid-peptic lesion. There is experimental evidence that a threshold pH exists, in the range of 2 to 3, above which little chemical damage occurs. It is difficult to determine how frequently this form of aspiration occurs. Much experimental work and some clinical series seem to assume that this is the dominant or sole form of clinical aspiration, but it is difficult to imagine large volumes of highly acid gastric contents except in gastric hypersecretors, who clearly constitute a small minority of those who aspirate. In the absence of better data, it seems likely that this form of aspiration has received far more attention than it deserves. If there is a rule for using steroids in patients who have aspirated, it is to use steroids only for this highly acid form, and even then there is some contrary evidence.[225, 226] The incidence of late infection is not clear, but can only be increased by using steroids. If significant aspiration is thought to have occurred, and especially if impairment of oxygenation has been documented, early use of mechanical ventilatory assistance will probably be beneficial.[225-226a]

Most sizable aspirations that occur clinically involve either recently ingested food or obstructed intestinal contents; occasionally purulent material is involved. The problem here is double: removing mechanically obstructing material and controlling bacterial contamination. If particles are observed in the mouth or returned in the tracheal aspirate, bronchoscopic exam-

ination and removal of remaining particles should be undertaken quickly. With the fiberoptic devices now available, bronchoscopy in the recovery room, intensive care unit or emergency
room is feasible and can be performed while the patient is receiving mechanical ventilatory support. Removal of particles is
more cumbersome, but the initial examination can demonstrate
the extent of the problem and the need for rigid bronchoscopy.
Bacterial contamination is especially prominent with aspiration
of obstructed intestinal contents. With either food or obstructed
contents, late infection is probably the leading cause of death.
The bacterial flora is very broad and nonspecific following aspiration and the use of antibiotics prophylactically is of uncertain
value.[227-231] Aspiration by hospitalized patients tends to result in
more gram-negative and staphylococcal infections, but anaero-
bic organisms predominate in out-of-hospital aspiration. If purulent material is aspirated, it seems incumbent to provide early antibiotic coverage; if the aspirate is foul-smelling, antian-
aerobic prophylaxis is probably advantageous. The role of early
ventilatory support in this group of patients is not as well established. These forms of aspiration need more experimental study.
It may be neater to use fluids of defined composition and pH, but
that is not what many patients are aspirating.

Aspiration of blood produces a particularly intense inflammatory response. This is usually seen with endobronchial bleeding,
which is fortunately not usually great or prolonged after accidental or violent trauma, even with direct injury to the lungs.
More commonly, since the subsidence of tuberculosis, aspiration
of blood occurs with upper gastrointestinal hemorrhage. The
supine position, drug- or disease-induced stupor and nasogastric
tubes all greatly increase the chance for aspiration in the patient who is vomiting or regurgitating blood. Repeated hematemesis is probably usually associated with significant aspiration
of blood, and this accounts for much of the pulmonary impairment in such patients. Effective therapy for aspiration of blood
is largely preventive.

The available data indicate that aspiration is underestimated
in incidence and extent and that the favorite form among investigators (acid aspiration) is not the main problem clinically.
Early use of positive pressure ventilation seems very beneficial
in some forms, the role of prophylactic antibiotics is not settled
and steroids are of limited, if any, value.

Vasoactive Materials

The lungs receive the entire cardiac output. All venous blood passes through the pulmonary capillary bed before reaching the systemic circulation, coming in contact with a hugh endothelial surface area. Normally 60–100 ml of blood is in contact with a surface area of up to 70 m². This is a unique situation, and it is not surprising that the lungs have been found to be metabolically and hormonally very active. This is still an area of active investigation, but a certain pattern of biologic activity is already evident. A number of recent reviews have summarized the field.[232-235]

The lungs are of prime importance in determining the activity of many circulating vasoactive substances. The vasoactive amines are selectively inactivated: acetylcholine, 5-hydroxytryptamine (5-HT) and norepinephrine are variably inactivated on single passages. About 65% of an injected dose of 5-HT is taken up by the normal human lungs on single passage. About 25% of norepinephrine is inactivated on single passage. Acetylcholine is so rapidly inactivated in the blood that the potential for inactivation in the lung is probably rarely used. In contrast to the lungs' activity on norepinephrine, epinephrine, dopamine and isoproterenol are not altered. Histamine is also unchanged, although some may be taken up and stored. Among the peptides, angiotensin I is almost completely converted to angiotensin II, bradykinin is 95–99% inactivated, and there is evidence of activity against gastrin and insulin. The prostaglandins are selectively inactivated: the E and F compounds may be altered up to 80% at low concentrations in the venous plasma, while the A compounds are unchanged.[236] There are major differences among species in activity toward the various groups of prostaglandins, however, and it is not clear what occurs in human lungs. It is also possible that some of the metabolic conversion of the prostaglandins yields compounds that are still biologically active. The adenine nucleotides are rapidly inactivated by ATPase and 5'-nucleotidase. For some of these processes, specific enzymes have been identified on or are suspected to be on the lumenal surface of the endothelial cells. For the prostaglandins, there is probably a transport mechanism that determines specificity. The structural alterations occur within the endothelial cells. Norepinephrine and 5-HT are also selectively transported

showed a lower incidence of hypoxemia in the patients for whom filters were used, more control patients had wounds of the chest and abdomen, which are associated with a higher incidence of hypoxemia (see also section on "Anesthesia and Operation"). Under this circumstance, even though the mortality was much higher in controls (8/16 versus 3/13), the most fervent advocates could hardly attribute such efficacy to fine filtration. The weight of available evidence fails to support the hypothesis that these microaggregates are clinically significant. Nevertheless, it is unlikely that they do any good, so until better clinical studies are available we continue to use fine filters in patients in whom more than one half of a blood volume is likely to be transfused. Under no circumstances, however, should the "need" for fine filters be allowed to impede the transfusion of blood into rapidly bleeding patients. Potential delay represents the real disadvantage of the extra filters; this delay is caused not so much by flow rates through the filters as by the extra steps necessary to set up and transfuse multiple units of blood.

The relationship of DIC to pulmonary failure is discussed elsewhere. A hemolytic transfusion reaction is a classic cause of DIC. More subtly, stored blood undergoes partial activation of various clotting factors and release of some cellular thromboplastic debris. The recipient of extensive transfusion is usually hypoperfused and may have extensive tissue damage. DIC is therefore more likely to occur and may be further facilitated by the stored blood. This is at present only speculative. Many if not most of the clotting disorders documented in massively transfused patients suggest DIC as the underlying etiology,[243] and pulmonary dysfunction is very common in patients exhibiting clinically impaired hemostasis after injury or operation.

There are now several documented instances of human pulmonary edema with an immunologic basis resulting from single blood transfusions. These have been reviewed recently.[244] Reactions to IgA, leukocyte, platelet and red cell antigens have all been implicated. There is usually other evidence of an acute immunologic reaction. Prior exposure to allogeneic tissue has almost always been noted (multiple pregnancies or transfusions). Obviously, the more blood transfused, the more likely the occurrence of such a reaction, although it is almost certainly a rare if usually misdiagnosed event.

A more unusual immunologic phenomenon is the graft-versus-host reaction. Lymphocytes remain viable in liquid stored blood[245] and can persist and perhaps proliferate in an immunosuppressed transfused recipient.[246-249] A variety of effects are possible, including pulmonary problems. This disease occurs only in severely immunologically crippled recipients. It can be prevented by irradiating the blood or by removing the leukocytes before transfusion.[250]

Stored blood contains a variety of vasoactive materials. Serotonin and bradykinin are present in increased amounts,[251] as are a variety of unidentified altered plasma proteins. There is indirect evidence of biologic activity in stressed animals,[252, 253] but the effects of these materials during extensive transfusion in patients is unknown. (See the section on "Vasoactive Materials.")

Berman *et al.*,[254] in an interesting series of experiments, found evidence of increased capillary permeability (total albumin content) in hemorrhaged and transfused rats that was largely but not completely related to the presence of buffy coat, was partially preventable by filtration, was perhaps related to storage in plastic and was related to duration of storage. These observations raise a number of possibilities; however, using a more severe hemorrhagic challenge we found practically no increase in total lung water in rats at a similar period following transfusion with whole blood while there were significant increases in lung water with nonblood fluids.[83] The differences are difficult to explain, but it would have been preferable if Berman and co-workers had included a marker for whole blood in their experiments so that total albumin content could have been at least partially partitioned into intravascular and extravascular components.

Perhaps the most common cause of pulmonary insufficiency after extensive transfusion is left ventricular failure. This is most likely to occur in the elderly or in those with coronary arterial disease. It is likely that the left ventricle is damaged during periods of hypotension, so that the margin between hypovolemia and overtransfusion becomes hazardously small. Measurements of pulmonary capillary wedge pressures lead to correct diagnoses more frequently than when central venous pressure is the guide for heart failure. Aspiration of bloody vomitus is another clinically common occurrence in the setting of massive transfusion. When postresuscitative pulmonary insufficiency seems unexplained, samples of tracheal fluid may reveal this occurrence.

With uncomplicated hemorrhage and even extensive transfusion, the incidence of pulmonary insufficiency remains rather low (see section on "Systemic Infection"). Much of the pulmonary insufficiency that does occur has a well-recognized cause. There may be subtle forms of pulmonary damage during transfusion, but more work is needed to establish their incidence and importance.

Oxygen Toxicity

This is now a well-recognized hazard of the treatment of hypoxemia. Many excellent reviews are available.[255-258] Briefly, the changes induced by high inspired concentrations of oxygen are dependent on both time of exposure and concentration of inspired oxygen, with changes occurring rather rapidly when 100% oxygen is inspired. These changes can be fatal. Animals with hypoxemia may be somewhat less susceptible, but this has been challenged.[260] The control settings on older style ventilators are often very inaccurate for determining the percentage of oxygen supplied to the patient; periodic check of inspired oxygen concentration should be made with specially designed and calibrated instruments.

It is ironic that the lung is so resistant to hypoxia and so sensitive to hyperoxia. Evidence still accumulating indicates how destructive hyperoxia is to the metabolic processes of the lung. Most clinicians are now well aware of this problem and include it in considering the day-to-day management of patients in respiratory failure. When more than 50% inspired oxygen is required to maintain arterial oxygenation, other maneuvers must be considered (diuresis, positive end-expiratory pressure, bronchoscopy, etc.), depending on the circumstances. An arterial oxygen tension above 70 mm Hg adds little in the way of arterial oxygen content and the added risk of high oxygen concentrations in the lungs is clearly not worth it. The practice of measuring arterial blood oxygen tension after breathing 100% oxygen for 20 minutes is rather popular. There is evidence that in sick surgical patients the intrapulmonary shunt can increase during this period.[261, 262] Even though some of this is due to redistribution of blood flow, which reverses when the inspired oxygen concentration is lowered, some of it seems to be due to atelectasis. Since this maneuver adds no unique information, and in fact usually requires an additional analysis of arterial blood to confirm proper long-range setting of the ventilator, its continued wide use does not seem wise.

Fat Embolism

Fat embolism is a less common and usually overlooked cause of ventilatory failure in injured patients.[263, 264] It can mimic other forms quite closely. The clinical onset is usually 1 to several days after injury. The presentation is one of progressively worsening hypoxemia, perhaps with disproportionate deterioration of mental status. The roentgenographic picture is that of generalized bilateral fluffy infiltrates progressing to nearly complete opacification. Death occurs from hypoxemia, and at autopsy the lungs are very heavy and congested. Microscopically, there is hemorrhagic infiltration and consolidation with small skip areas of nearly normal architecture. Fat is not seen unless stained for, and may be mostly gone by the time the patient dies. Other factors such as aspiration, bacterial pneumonitis, thromboembolism, oxygen toxicity and fluid overloading may be superimposed, but fat embolism alone can cause death from ventilatory insufficiency.

The diagnosis of fat embolism is rather nonspecific. Fat occurs in the sputum and urine of normal or minimally injured patients who are not clinically ill, and it may be absent in patients with severe fat embolism. Changes in circulating lipase appear not to correlate with the disease at all, and circulating lipids change in a nonspecific manner. Typical changes in the retina and characteristic petechiae suggest but do not establish the diagnosis. A significantly elevated alveolar-arterial gradient for oxygen is present in nearly all clinically significant instances. The nonspecific roentgenographic changes already described usually lag behind the changes in oxygenation of the blood.

The clinical incidence of fat embolism is hard to estimate because of the difficulty of establishing a firm diagnosis and the degree to which it mimics other pulmonary problems that occur in injured patients. It is almost never diagnosed in institutions where the disease is rarely thought of, and it is diagnosed frequently where someone has an active interest in it. The true incidence is probably not greater than 10–20% of adult patients with major long-bone fractures. The term "incidence" needs some definition, because embolic fat can be found in the lungs of most patients with long-bone fractures, or indeed after all major orthopedic procedures. It is likely that there is a continuum that extends from the subclinical event — never detected unless death occurs early from some other cause and a specific search is made for it — all the way to massive, fatal embolization of fat and marrow to the lungs, brain, heart and kidneys, with steadily decreasing incidence toward the fatal end of the spectrum. More importantly, with modern ventilatory management, the mortality should be less than 10% in those patients with a firm clinical diagnosis. It is important to realize that sudden, dramatic improvement is quite common. This can easily convince the uninformed that some "specific" drug or remedy has been marvelously effective. Controlled trials are mandatory to evaluate such drugs.

The nature and especially the cause of posttraumatic fat embolism have been the subject of an unfortunate degree of controversy and confusion, unfortunate because there is, in fact, little evidence to support the exotic interpretations of the disease that have been popular in recent years. There is a substantial body of reasonably confirmed clinical and experimental observations regarding this disease, and it is well to emphasize what is known. By far the most common clinical occurrences are in patients with major fractures, especially of the femur, tibia and axial skeleton. The more fractures and the larger the bones involved, the greater the incidence of fat embolism. No other diseases, including those associated with lipemia, bear such a relationship. Almost all nonfracture settings in which fat embolism has occurred with some regularity involve direct mechanical disruption of depot fat or bone marrow: sickle cell crisis, caisson disease and fatty liver. The low incidence of fat embolism in children is noteworthy, as the incidence rises sharply in conditions in which the normally cellular marrow is replaced with fat. All of this is compelling evidence in favor of the "classic" theory of fat embolism, namely that direct mechanical injury results in entrance of depot fat into the venous circulation with embolization to the lungs.

Less extensive but reasonably firm data from animals and

man indicate that embolization of fat continues from the injured parts for several days after injury, and that motion of the injured parts increases and prolongs this continued embolization. Embolization of bone marrow proper seems to occur primarily at the time of injury.

Fat embolism is manifested as a pulmonary disorder, with extensive pulmonary embolism found in almost all patients with systemic embolization. The apparently pure neurologic manifestations are usually accompanied by clinically unsuspected but severe hypoxemia. The life-threatening functional disorder is loss of functioning alveoli and extensive "shunting" (venous blood traversing the lungs without oxygenation). Retention of CO_2 is relatively easily avoided until the situation is terminal.

The histologic and perhaps the functional changes are very time-dependent and somewhat organ-dependent. Fat embolism in the lungs is initially bland but is later associated with hemorrhagic consolidation as the neutral fat disappears. In organs with less lipase activity, especially renal glomeruli, the fat remains with little tissue reaction or destruction until removed by mechanically traversing the endothelium and basement membrane into the lumen of the nephron or until swept back into the venous circulation to be trapped in the lungs. These observations suggest that more than simple mechanical embolization is involved in the lungs. Local breakdown with release of unbound fatty acids would be destructive to the regional pulmonary capillaries, leading to all the observed structural, clinical and functional changes. This interpretation is compatible with a wide array of observed events but lacks direct confirmation.

Other theories of the pathogenesis of fat embolism involve release of the fat from its normally bound forms in the circulating blood as a nonspecific response to injury or stress. The strong association with bony injury is unexplained by these theories, as is the unimpressive incidence in sick patients with hyperlipemia. The only documented instances of "desuspension" of fat from circulating blood involve cardiopulmonary bypass and collecting blood under a strong vacuum, both obviously ex vivo types of situations. Various theories involving circulating fatty acids seem popular in the United States, judging by the use of bolus injections of fatty acids as experimental models of "fat embolism." Fatty acids are mobilized in times of stress to several

Miscellaneous

Intracranial injury is often accompanied by pulmonary edema.[265-267] The effect is probably produced by massive shifts of blood volume centrally following peripheral vasoconstriction.[268-272] Many changes in experimental models can be prevented or reversed with sympathetic blockade. It is possible that direct neurally induced changes in pulmonary vascular compliance also contribute.[157] Fibrin in parts of the central nervous system may also induce similar changes.[273] A nonrandomized clinical study suggests that steroids may be effective in reducing the pulmonary dysfunction that follows head injury;[274] it is not clear whether this is due to effects on intracranial pressure, pulmonary vasculature or renal fluid balance. The well-known relationship between cerebral injury and pulmonary edema has recently been extended to implicate the cerebral hypoxia that accompanies hemorrhage as a cause of posttraumatic respiratory failure.[275] As noted in the section on "Hemorrhage," the relationship between blood loss and pulmonary dysfunction is tenuous at best. Efforts by other groups to produce pulmonary changes on the basis of cerebral hypoxia have been unsuccessful.[276]

Pulmonary insufficiency seems to be a particularly prominent complication of acute pancreatitis.[277-279] This must be viewed with some caution, as pancreatitis results in upper abdominal peritonitis, which is likely to significantly impair pulmonary function, whatever the cause. There is some experimental evidence, however, that there is additional damage to the pulmonary vasculature in acute pancreatitis, presumably due to vasoactive material released from the pancreas or surrounding tissue.[280-282]

Severely burned patients often have pulmonary complications that occasionally are the primary cause of death.[283-285] The early complications are related to direct injury by noxious gases. There is little that can be done for this condition except for nonspecific ventilatory assistance, although at least one report claims benefit from early use of steroids.[286] The later complications are related to sepsis. Older patients are prone to left ventricular failure because of the initially large fluid shifts and the sustained high cardiac outputs that accompany the large unhealed wounds. Some of the ventilatory patterns after major burns can be adversely affected by treatment; mafenide (Sulfamylon) is an inhibitor of carbonic anhydrase and increases the work of maintaining CO_2 balance.[287] Simultaneous ventilation-perfusion lung scans may allow earlier definition of the extent of inhalation injury.[288] Fiberoptic bronchoscopy allows direct serial observation of the tracheobronchial tree.[289] Hopefully, therapeutic improvements will also be developed.

Burk *et al.* have proposed that excessive beta-adrenergic stimulation is responsible for some degree of posttraumatic pulmonary insufficiency.[290-292] Since catecholamines represent a significant response to injury, one must be suspicious of another theory of autodestruction. Other studies with epinephrine produced practically no pulmonary changes.[293]

Patients with severe liver disease manifest both sustained hyperventilation and hypoxia.[294, 295] Both changes are largely unexplained. It is not known whether acute hepatic impairment, as frequently occurs after severe hemorrhage or with prolonged intraperitoneal sepsis, contributes to acute pulmonary insufficiency by the same mechanisms. There is some clinical evidence that sustained hypocarbia in patients with acute pulmonary insufficiency impairs oxygenation, but these studies were performed with 100% oxygen as the inspired gas.[296]

Severe metabolic alkalosis clearly depresses ventilation and presumably can lead to the complications of sustained hypoventilation.[297-299] This condition seems to be increasing in frequency as sicker patients survive longer with prolonged nasogastric suctioning. It may be necessary to use hydrochloric acid parenterally in such patients, especially if attempting to discontinue mechanical ventilatory assistance.

Protein-calorie malnutrition accompanies or precedes ventilatory failure in many patients. Such malnutrition may impair a variety of antimicrobial defenses and may lead to wasting of ventilatory muscles, especially when they are placed at prolonged rest by mechanical ventilatory assistance. More recently in otherwise normal subjects a calorie-electrolyte regimen simulating the usual pattern of parenteral fluids resulted in significant depression of hypoxic ventilatory drive after only 10 days.[300] Nutrition may well be an important, occasionally critical element in recovery from ventilatory failure.

Pulmonary edema is a common complication of acute uremia. There is abundant evidence that the lungs share in a wide-

spread increase in capillary permeability and that a large component of the pulmonary insufficiency is due to this increased
capillary permeability.[301-304] This, plus the tendency to hypervo-
lemia and the decreased resistance to infection, makes the patient in posttraumatic or postoperative acute renal failure prone
to develop significant pulmonary insufficiency.

Closing Comments on Treatment

Despite the multiplicity of causes of postoperative, posttraumatic pulmonary insufficiency and the specific aspects of treatment that relate to each, the central core of treating such
patients is the same. Just as the lung is rather repetitive and
nonspecific in its response to various noxious stimuli, the therapeutic response is essentially repetitive and nonspecific. Significant advances have been made in the past few years in the treatment of acute respiratory failure. These cannot be reviewed in
detail here, and are well known to those clinically active in this
area. The reviews by Pontoppidan et al.[3] and by Shoemaker[305]
are concise yet informative. Several advances, however, must at
least be mentioned. Positive end-expiratory pressure has
unquestionably greatly improved the care of such patients, at
least by allowing use of lower concentrations of inspired oxygen
and probably by preventing the development of further atelectasis and perhaps by hastening the resolution of already existing atelectasis. Some believe it has prophylactic value,[306] but
such is difficult to prove. Guidelines for most effective and safest
use are still evolving. Intermittent mandatory ventilation has
made the "weaning" process significantly safer, especially in
patients with wasting of the respiratory motor mechanisms.[307]
Measurement of pulmonary capillary wedge pressure in special
care units has improved the accuracy of managing fluid loads in
difficult situations and of detecting subclinical left heart failure,
as noted previously. Conversely, there may also be patients in
falsely apparent heart failure whose management is also improved.[308] New ventilators allow flexibility, individualization
and a degree of control not previously possible. This can make a
significant difference in "borderline" patients. Current clinical
investigations are now extending into important related areas,
such as circulatory-respiratory interactions,[309] the increased
metabolic demands in septic states[310] and the role of the in-

creased work of breathing in clinical outcome.[311] As might be expected, steroids have been advocated for this condition; as usual, the clinical reports are uncontrolled.[312, 313] Many believe that the mortality from respiratory failure after operation or injury is decreasing.[33] This probably reflects better preventive measures, earlier detection and the improvements in methods of management already cited. We are certainly not dealing with a progressively healthier population of patients. One of the more encouraging aspects of this condition is the remarkably complete functional recovery that is so common; late disability is distinctly the exception in survivors.[314-317] This has encouraged such heroic therapeutic measures as the use of extracorporeal membrane oxygenators for prolonged periods. Perhaps because of the criteria used to select patients, the results have been disappointing; but, as noted, the results with "standard" treatment may well be improving.

REFERENCES

1. Moore, F. D., Lyons, J. H., Pierce, E. C., Morgan, A. P., Drinker, P. A., MacArthur, J. D., and Dammin, G. J.: *Post-Traumatic Pulmonary Insufficiency* (Philadelphia: W. B. Saunders Company, 1969).
2. Collins, J. A.: The causes of progressive pulmonary insufficiency in surgical patients, J. Surg. Res. 9:685, 1969.
3. Pontoppidan, H., Geffin, B., and Lowenstein, E.: *Acute Respiratory Failure in the Adult* (Boston: Little, Brown and Company, 1973).
4. Blaisdell, F. W., and Schlobohm, R. M.: The respiratory distress syndrome: a review, Surgery 74:251, 1973.
5. Webb, W. R. (ed.): Symposium on pulmonary problems in surgery, Surg. Clin. North Am. 54:941, 1974.
6. Campbell, G. S.: Respiratory failure in surgical patients, Curr. Probl. Surg. 13:1, 1976.
7. Teplitz, C.: The core pathobiology and integrated medical science of adult acute respiratory insufficiency. Surg. Clin. North Am. 56:909, 1976.
8. Blaisdell, F. W.: Pathophysiology of the respiratory distress syndrome, Arch. Surg. 108:44, 1974.
9. Swensson, S. A.: Artificial respiration in severe abdominal disease, Arch. Dis. Child. 37:149, 1962.
10. Burke, J. F., Pontoppidan, H., and Welch, C. E.: High output respiratory failure. An important cause of death ascribed to peritonitis or ileus, Ann. Surg. 158:581, 1963.
11. Clowes, G. H., Vucinic, M., and Weidner, M. G.: Circulatory and metabolic alterations associated with survival or death in peritonitis, Ann. Surg. 163:866, 1966.
12. Rosoff, L., Weil, M., Bradley, E. C., and Berne, C. J.: Hemodynamic and

metabolic changes associated with bacterial peritonitis, Am. J. Surg. 114:180, 1967.

13. Siegel, J. H., Greenspan, M., and Del Guercio, L. R.: Abnormal vascular tone, defective oxygen transport and myocardial failure in human septic shock, Ann. Surg. 165:504, 1967.

14. Clowes, G. H., Zuschneid, W., Turner, M., Blackburn, G., Rubin, J., Toala, P., and Green, G.: Observations on the pathogenesis of the pneumonitis associated with severe infections in other parts of the body, Ann. Surg. 167:630, 1968.

15. Border, J. R., Tibbetts, J. C., and Schenck, W. G.: Hypoxic hyperventilation and acute respiratory failure in the severely stressed patient: massive pulmonary arteriovenous shunts, Surgery 64:710, 1968.

16. McLean, A. P., Duff, J. H., and MacLean, L. D.: Lung lesions associated with septic shock, J. Trauma 8:891, 1968.

17. Bredenberg, C. E., James, P. M., Collins, J. A., Anderson, R. W., Martin, A. M., and Hardaway, R. M.: Respiratory failure in shock, Ann. Surg. 169:392, 1969.

18. Simmons, R. L., Heisterkamp, C. A., Collins, J. A., Bredenberg, C. E., Mills, D. E., and Martin, A. M.: Respiratory insufficiency in combat casualties. IV Hypoxemia during convalescence, Ann. Surg. 170:53, 1969.

19. Skillman, J. J., Bushnell, L. S., and Hedley-Whyte, J.: Peritonitis and respiratory failure after abdominal operations, Ann. Surg. 170:122, 1969.

20. Wilson, R. F., Kafi, A., Asuncion, Z., and Walt, A. J.: Clinical respiratory failure after shock or trauma, Arch. Surg. 98:539, 1969.

21. Lowery, B. D., Cloutier, C. T., and Carey, L. C.: Blood gas determinations in the severely wounded in hemorrhagic shock, Arch. Surg. 99:330, 1969.

22. Clowes, G. H., Farrington, G. H., Zuschneid, W., Cossette, G. R., and Sarovis, C.: Circulating factors in the etiology of pulmonary insufficiency and right heart failure accompanying severe sepsis (peritonitis), Ann. Surg. 171:663, 1970.

23. Moseley, R. V., and Doty, D. B.: Hypoxemia during the first twelve hours after battle injury, Surgery 67:765, 1970.

24. Proctor, H. J., Ballantine, T. V., and Broussard, N. D.: An analysis of pulmonary function following non-thoracic trauma, with recommendations for therapy, Ann. Surg. 172:180, 1970.

25. Hirsch, E. F., Fletcher, R., and Lucas, S.: Hemodynamic and respiratory changes associated with sepsis following combat trauma, Ann. Surg. 174:211, 1971.

26. Lavin, I., Weil, M. H., Shubin, H., and Sherwin, R.: Pulmonary failure associated with clinical shock states, J. Trauma 11:22, 1971.

27. McLaughlin, J. S.: Physiologic consideration of hypoxemia in shock and trauma, Ann. Surg. 173:667, 1971.

28. Horovitz, J. H., Carrico, C. J., and Shires, G. T.: Pulmonary response to major injury, Arch. Surg. 108:349, 1974.

29. Fulton, R. L., and Jones, C. E.: The cause of post-traumatic pulmonary insufficiency in man, Surg. Gynecol. Obstet. 140:179, 1975.

30. Milligan, G. F., MacDonald, J. A., Mellon, A., and Ledingham, I. McA.:

Pulmonary and hematologic disturbances during septic shock, Surg. Gynecol. Obstet. 138:43, 1974.

31. Vito, L., Dennis, R. C., Weisel, R. D., and Hechtman, H. B.: Sepsis presenting as acute respiratory insufficiency, Surg. Gynecol. Obstet. 138: 896, 1974.

32. Schulz, V., Schnabel, K. H., and Schmidt, W.: Untersuchungen zum pulmonaren Gasaustausch in der akuten Schockphase und nach Ubergang in eine Schocklunge, Klin. Wochenschr. 52:624, 1974.

33. Walker, L., and Eiseman, B.: The changing pattern of post-traumatic respiratory distress syndrome, Ann. Surg. 181:693, 1975.

34. Finley, R. J., Holliday, R. L., Lefcoe, M., and Duff, J. H.: Pulmonary edema in patients with sepsis, Surg. Gynecol. Obstet. 140:851, 1975.

35. Clowes, G. H., Hirsch, E., Williams, L., Kwasnik, E., O'Donnell, T. F., Cuevas, P., Sani, V. K., Moradi, I., Farizan, M., Sarovis, C., Stone, M., and Kuffler, J.: Septic lung and shock lung in man, Ann. Surg. 181:681, 1975.

36. McClusky, B.: The stressed lung in severe non-thoracic sepsis, Aust. N. Z. J. Surg. 44:102, 1974.

37. Clowes, G. H.: Pulmonary abnormalities in sepsis, Surg. Clin. North Am. 54:993, 1974.

38. Buckberg, G., Cohn, J., and Darling, C.: Escherichia coli bacteremic shock in conscious baboons, Ann. Surg. 173:122, 1971.

39. Pool, J. L., Owen, S. E., Meyers, F. K., Coalson, J. J., Holmes, D. D., Guenter, C. A., and Hinshaw, L. B.: Response of the subhuman primate in gram-negative septicemia induced by live Escherichia coli, Surg. Gynecol. Obstet. 132:469, 1971.

40. Pingleton, W. W., Coalson, J. J., Hinshaw, L. B., and Guenter, C. A.: Effects of steroid treatment on development of shock lung: hemodynamic, respiratory, and morphologic studies, Lab. Invest. 27:445, 1972.

41. Balis, J. V., Gerber, L. I., Rappaport, E. S., and Neville, W. E.: Mechanism of blood-vascular reactions of the primate lung to acute endotoxemia, Exp. Mol. Pathol. 21:123, 1974.

42. Wittels, E. H., Coalson, J. J., Welch, M. H., and Guenter, C. A.: Pulmonary intravascular leukocyte sequestration: a potential mechanism of lung injury, Am. Rev. Respir. Dis. 109:502, 1974.

43. Hinshaw, L. B., Kuida, H., Gilbert, R. P., and Visscher, M. B.: Influence of perfusate characteristics on pulmonary vascular response to endotoxin, Am. J. Physiol. 191:293, 1957.

44. Kuida, H., Hinshaw, L. B., Gilbert, R. P., and Visscher, M. B.: Effect of gram-negative endotoxin on pulmonary circulation. Am. J. Physiol. 192:335, 1958.

45. Kux, M., Coalson, J., Massion, W. H., and Guenter, C. A.: Pulmonary effects of E. coli endotoxin: role of leukocytes and platelets, Ann. Surg. 175:26, 1972.

46. Centora, I., Saad, B., Goodale, R. L., Motsay, G. W., and Borner, J. W.: Further studies of endotoxin and alveolocapillary permeability: effect of steroid pre-treatment and complement depletion, Ann. Surg. 179:372, 1974.

47. Bessa, S. M., Dalmasso, A. P., and Goodale, R. L.: Studies on the mecha-

nism of endotoxin induced increase of alveolocapillary permeability, Proc. Soc. Exp. Biol. Med. 147:701, 1974.

48. Kitzmiller, J. L., Lucas, W. E., and Yelonosky, P. F.: The role of complement in feline endotoxin shock, Am. J. Obstet. Gynecol. 112:414, 1972.

49. Cochrane, C. G., and Aiken, B.: Polymorphonuclear leukocytes in immunologic reactions: the destruction of vascular basement membrane in vivo and in vitro, J. Exp. Med. 124:733, 1966.

50. Janoff, A., and Zelig, J. D.: Vascular injury and in vitro lysis of basement membrane by neutral protease of human leukocytes, Science 161:702, 1968.

51. Harrow, E. M., Jakab, G. J., Brody, A. R., and Green, G. M.: The pulmonary response to a bacteremic challenge, Am. Rev. Respir. Dis. 112:7, 1975.

52. Voss, H. J., MacNicol, M. D., Saravis, C. A., Altug, K., and Clowes, G. H.: The pathogenesis of pneumonitis in sepsis, Surg. Forum 22:27, 1971.

53. Brigham, K. L., Woolverton, W. C., Blake, L. H., and Staub, N. C.: Increased sheep lung permeability caused by Pseudomonas bacteremia, J. Clin. Invest. 54:792, 1974.

54. Newhouse, M., Sanchis, J., and Bienenstock, J.: Lung defense mechanisms, N. Engl. J. Med. 295:990, 1045, 1976.

55. Cohen, A. B., and Cline, M. J.: Human alveolar macrophage isolation, cultivation and morphological and functional characteristics, J. Clin. Invest. 50:1390, 1971.

56. Dressler, D. P., and Skornik, W. A.: Pulmonary bacterial susceptibility in the burned rat, Ann. Surg. 180:221, 1974.

57. Roth, R. R., Mullane, J. F., Huber, G. L., Phelps, T. D., and Wilfong, R. G.: Blood loss and factors affecting pulmonary antibacterial defenses, J. Surg. Res. 17:36, 1974.

57a. Esrig, B. C., and Fulton, F. L.: Sepsis, resuscitated hemorrhagic shock and "shock lung": an experimental correlation, Ann. Surg. 182:218, 1975.

58. Mullane, J. F., Huber, G. L., Popvic, N. A., Wilfong, R. G., Bielke, S. R., O'Connel, D. M., and La Force, F. M.: Aspiration of blood and pulmonary host defense mechanisms, Ann. Surg. 180:236, 1974.

59. Slade, M. S., Simmons, R. L., Yunis, E., and Greenburg, L. J.: Immunodepression after major surgery in normal patients, Surgery 78:363, 1975.

60. Southern, P. M., Mays, B. B., Pierce, A. K., and Sanford, J. P.: Pulmonary clearance of Pseudomonas aeruginosa, J. Lab. Clin. Med. 76:548, 1970.

61. Redman, L. R., and Lockey, E.: Colonization of the upper respiratory tract, Anaesthesia 22:220, 1967.

62. Johanson, W. G., Pierce, A. K., and Sanford, J. P.: Changing pharyngeal bacterial flora of hospitalized patients, N. Engl. J. Med. 281:1137, 1969.

63. Glover, J. L., and Jolly, L.: Gram negative colonization of the respiratory tract in post-operative patients, Am. J. Med. Sci. 261:24, 1971.

64. Bryant, L. R., Trinkle, J. K., Mobin-Uddin, K., Baker, J., and Griffen, W. D.: Bacterial colonization profile with tracheal intubation and mechanical ventilation, Arch. Surg. 104:647, 1972.

65. Schlenker, J. D., and Hubay, C. A.: Colonization of the respiratory tract and postoperative pulmonary infections, Arch. Surg. 107:313, 1973.

65a. Rose, H. D., and Babcock, J. B.: Colonization of intensive care unit patients with gram-negative bacilli, Am. J. Epidemiol. 101:495, 1975.

66. Rahal, J. J., Meade, R. H., Bump, C. M., and Reinauer, A. J.: Upper respiratory tract carriage of gram-negative enteric bacilli by hospital personnel, J.A.M.A. 214:754, 1970.

67. Johanson, W. G., Pierce, A. K., Sanford, J. P., and Thomas, G. D.: Nosocomial respiratory infections with gram-negative bacilli: the significance of colonization of the respiratory tract. Ann. Intern. Med. 77:701, 1972.

68. Smith, H. B., and Tuffnell, P. G.: Pseudomonas aeruginosa in respiratory illness: endogenous or exogenous? Can. Anaesth. Soc. J. 17:516, 1970.

69. Michel-Briand, Y., Michel-Briand, C., Vieu, J. F., and Le Bras, Y.: Infections pulmonaires graves à Pseudomonas aeruginosa dans un service de réanimation, à propos de dix cas: études épidémiologiques et déspistage systématique chez 623 malades, Presse Med. 79:2103, 1971.

70. Khanan, T., Branthwaite, M. A., English, I. C., and Preutis, J. J.: The control of pulmonary sepsis in intensive therapy units, Anaesthesia 28: 17, 1973.

71. Pierce, A. K., Sanford, J. P., Thomas, G. D., and Leonard, J. S.: Long-term evaluation of decontamination of inhalation-therapy equipment and the occurrence of necrotizing pneumonia, N. Engl. J. Med. 282:528, 1970.

72. Grieble, H. G., Colton, F. R., Bird, T. J., Toigo, A., and Griffith, L. G.: Fine-particle humidifiers: source of Pseudomonas aeruginosa infections in a respiratory-disease unit, N. Engl. J. Med. 282:531, 1970.

73. Babington, P. C., Baker, A. B., and Johnston, H. H.: Retrograde spread of organisms from ventilator to patient via the expiratory limb, Lancet 1:61, 1971.

74. Harris, T. H., Ramon, T. K., Richards, W. J., Covert, S. V., Blake, J. A., and Accurso, J.: An evaluation of bacteriologic contamination of ventilator humidifying systems, Chest 63:922, 1973.

74a. Perea, E. J., Criado, A., Moreno, M., and Avello, F.: Mechanical ventilators as vehicles of infection, Acta Anaesthesiol. Scand. 19:180, 1975.

75. Dyer, E. D., and Peterson, D. E.: How far do bacteria travel from the exhalation valve of IPPB equipment? Anesth. Analg. (Cleve.) 51:516, 1972.

76. Greenfield, S., Teres, D., Bushnell, L. S., Hedley-Whyte, J., and Feingold, D. S.: Prevention of gram-negative bacillary pneumonia using aerosol polymixin as prophylaxis. I. Effect on colonization pattern of the upper respiratory tract of seriously ill patients, J. Clin. Invest. 52:2935, 1973.

77. Klick, J. M., du Moulin, G. C., Hedley-Whyte, J., Teres, D., Bushnell, L. S., and Feingold, D. S.: Prevention of gram-negative bacillary pneumonia using aerosol polymixin as prophylaxis. II. Effect on the incidence of pneumonia in seriously ill patients, J. Clin. Invest. 55:514, 1975.

78. Feeley, T. W., du Moulin, G. C., Hedley-Whyte, J., Bushnell, L. S., Gil-

bert, J. P., and Feingold, D. S.: Aerosol polymyxin and pneumonia in seriously ill patients, N. Engl. J. Med. 293:471, 1975.

78a. Klastersky, J., Hensgens, C., Noterman, J., Mouawad, E., and Meunier-Carpentier, F.: Endotracheal antibiotics for the prevention of tracheobronchial infections in tracheotomized unconscious patients: a comparative study of gentamycin and aminosidin-polymyxin B combination, Chest 68:302, 1975.

79. Polk, H. C., Borden, S., and Aldrete, J. A.: Prevention of Pseudomonas respiratory infection in a surgical intensive care unit, Ann. Surg. 177:607, 1973.

80. Iannini, P. B., Claffey, T., and Quintiliani, R.: Bacteremic Pseudomonas pneumonia, J.A.M.A. 230:558, 1974.

80a. Polk, H. C.: Quantitative tracheal cultures in surgical patients requiring mechanical ventilatory assistance, Surgery 78:485, 1975.

81. Espinoza, H., Palmer, D. L., Kisch, A. L., Olrich, J., Eberle, B., and Reed, W. P.: Clinical and immunological response to bacteria isolated from tracheal secretions following tracheostomy, J. Thorac. Cardiovasc. Surg. 68:432, 1974.

82. Ashbaugh, D. G., and Petty, T. L.: Sepsis complicating the acute respiratory distress syndrome, Surg. Gynecol. Obstet. 135:865, 1972.

83. Collins, J. A., Braitberg, A., and Butcher, H. R.: Changes in lung and body weight and lung water content in rats treated for hemorrhage with various fluids, Surgery 73:401, 1973.

84. Blades, B., Beattie, E. J., Hill, R. P., and Thistlethwaite, R.: Ischemia of the lung, Ann. Surg. 136:56, 1952.

85. Hankinson, H. W., and Edwards, F. R.: The effect of pulmonary ischaemia on lung function, Thorax 14:122, 1959.

86. Blumenstock, D. A., Hechtman, H. B., and Collins, J. A.: Preservation of the canine lung, J. Thorac. Cardiovasc. Surg. 44:771, 1962.

87. Edmunds, L. H., and Hohn, J. C.: Effect of atelectasis on lung changes after pulmonary arterial ligation, J. Appl. Physiol. 25:115, 1968.

88. Veith, F. J., and Richards, K.: Lung transplantation with simultaneous contralateral pulmonary artery ligation, Surg. Gynecol. Obstet. 129:768, 1969.

89. Kondo, Y., Turner, M. D., Cockrell, J. V., and Hardy, J. D.: Ischemic tolerance of the canine autotransplanted lung, Surgery 76:447, 1974.

90. Fonkalsrud, E., Sanchez, M., Higashijima, I., Gyepes, M., and Arima, E.: Evaluation of pulmonary function in the ischemic expanded canine lung, Surg. Gynecol. Obstet. 142:573, 1976.

91. Williams, W. G., Manley, R. W., and Drew, C.: Pulmonary circulatory arrest, Thorax 20:523, 1965.

92. Katsuya, H., Ohtsu, H., Inoue, K., Isa, T., and Morioka, T.: Effects of acute hemorrhage and rapid infusion of colloid solution on the pulmonary shunt ratio, Anesth. Analg. (Cleve.) 52:355, 1973.

93. Steenblock, U., Mannhart, H., and Wolff, G.: Effect of hemorrhagic shock on intrapulmonary right to left shunt and dead space, Respiration 33:133, 1976.

94. Kallos, T., Wyche, M. Q., and Marshall, B. E.: Effects of hemorrhagic

shock on pulmonary diffusion and capillary blood volume of the dog, J. Trauma 13:218, 1973.

95. Bo, G., and Hauge, A.: A two-phased change in dynamic lung compliance during hemorrhagic hypotension, Acta Physiol. Scand. 87:448, 1973.

95a. Silberschmid, M., Szczepanski, K. P., and Lund, C.: Hemorrhagic shock in dogs without major pulmonary changes, Eur. Surg. Res. 7:10, 1975.

96. Pingleton, W. W., Coalson, J. J., Hinshaw, L. B., and Guenter, C. A.: Effects of steroid pre-treatment on development of shock lung: hemodynamic, respiration, and morphologic studies, Lab. Invest. 27:445, 1972.

97. Herman, C. M., Moquin, R. B., and Horwitz, D. L.: Coagulation changes of hemorrhagic shock in baboons, Ann. Surg. 175:197, 1972.

98. Siegel, D. C., Cochin, A., and Moss, G. S.: The ventilatory response to hemorrhagic shock and resuscitation, Surgery 72:451, 1972.

99. Kasujima, K., Wax, S. D., and Webb, W. R.: Effects of methylprednisolone on pulmonary microcirculation, Surg. Gynecol. Obstet. 139:1, 1974.

100. Kasujima, K., Ozdemir, I. A., Webb, W. R., Wax, S. D., and Parker, F. B.: Role of serotonin and serotonin antagonists on pulmonary hemodynamics and microcirculation in hemorrhagic shock, J. Thorac. Cardiovasc. Surg. 67:908, 1974.

100a. Connell, R. S., Swank, R. L., and Webb, M. C.: The development of pulmonary ultrastructural lesions during hemorrhagic shock, J. Trauma 15:116, 1975.

100b. Tiefenbrun, J., Dikman, S., and Shoemaker, W. C.: The correlation of sequential changes in the distribution of pulmonary blood flow in hemorrhagic shock with histopathologic anatomy, Surgery 78:618, 1975.

101. Meyers, J. R., Meyer, J. S., and Baue, A. E.: Does hemorrhagic shock damage the lungs? J. Trauma 13:509, 1973.

102. Garvey, J. W., Hagstrom, J. W., and Veith, F. J.: Pathologic pulmonary changes in hemorrhagic shock, Ann. Surg. 181:870, 1975.

102a. Porcelli, R., Foster, W. M., Bergofsky, E. H., Bicker, A., Kaur, R., Demeny, M., and Reich, T.: Pulmonary circulatory changes in pathogenesis of shock lung, Am. J. Med. Sci. 268:250, 1974.

103. Magilligan, D. J., Oleksyn, T. W., Schwartz, S. I., and Yu, P. N.: Pulmonary intravascular and extravascular volumes in hemorrhagic shock and fluid replacement, Surgery 72:780, 1972.

104. Fulton, R. L., and Fischer, R. P.: Pulmonary changes due to hemorrhagic shock: resuscitation with isotonic and hypertonic saline, Surgery 75:881, 1974.

105. Moss, G. S., Das Gupta, T. K., Newsom, B., and Nyhus, L. M.: The effect of saline solution resuscitation on pulmonary sodium and water distribution, Surg. Gynecol. Obstet. 136:934, 1973.

106. Aarseth, P., and Bo, G.: Blood and extravascular water in cat lungs during changes in total blood volume, Acta Physiol. Scand. 85:343, 1972.

107. Holcroft, J. W., and Trunkey, D. D.: Extravascular lung water following hemorrhagic shock in the baboon: comparison between resuscitation with Ringer's lactate and plasmanate, Ann. Surg. 180:408, 1974.

107a. Holcroft, J. W., Trunkey, D. D., and Lim, R. C.: Further analysis of lung water in baboons resuscitated from hemorrhagic shock, J. Surg. Res. 20: 291, 1976.

108. Gaisford, W. D., Pandey, N., and Jensen, C. G.: Pulmonary changes in treated hemorrhagic shock. II. Ringer's lactate solution versus colloid infusion, Am. J. Surg. 124:738, 1972.

109. Moss, G., and Stern, A. A.: Shock lung—anemia as a predisposing factor, Am. J. Surg. 126:419, 1973.

110. Ljungqvist, V. E., and Schwartz, S. I.: Pulmonary platelet trapping during shock and pulmonary embolism, J. Surg. Res. 18:559, 1975.

111. Shubrooks, S. J., Schneider, B., Dubin, H., and Turino, G. M.: Acidosis and pulmonary hemodynamics in hemorrhagic shock, Am. J. Physiol. 225:225, 1973.

112. Kim, S. I., and Shoemaker, W. C.: Role of the acidosis in the development of increased pulmonary vascular resistance and shock lung in experimental hemorrhagic shock, Surgery 73:723, 1973.

113. Patterson, R. W., and Sullivan, S. F.: The interrelationship between lung compliance and airway carbon dioxide concentration during hemorrhagic shock, J. Trauma 13:238, 1973.

114. Friedman-Mor, Z., Chalon, J., Katy, J. S., Gorstein, F., Turndorf, H., and Orkin, L. R.: Tracheobronchial and pulmonary cytologic changes in shock, J. Trauma 16:58, 1976.

115. Markello, R., Schuder, R., and Border, J.: Arterial-alveolar N_2 differences documenting ventilation-perfusion mismatching following trauma, J. Trauma 14:423, 1974.

116. Demling, R. H., Selinger, S. L., Bland, R. D., and Staub, N. S.: Effect of acute hemorrhagic shock on pulmonary microvascular fluid filtration and protein permeability in sheep, Surgery 77:512, 1975.

117. Horovitz, J. H., and Carrico, C. J.: Lung colloid permeability in hemorrhagic shock, Surg. Forum. 23:6, 1972.

118. Northrup, W. F., and Humphrey, E. W.: Relationship of pulmonary capillary protein flux to irreversible hypotension following hemorrhagic shock and reinfusion, Surg. Forum 26:13, 1975.

119. Anderson, R. W., and De Vries, W. C.: Transvascular fluid and protein dynamics in the lung following hemorrhagic shock, J. Surg. Res. 20:281, 1976.

120. Henry, J. N., McArdle, A. H., Buonous, G., Hampson, L. G., Scott, H. J., and Gurd, F. N.: The effect of experimental hemorrhagic shock on pulmonary alveolar surfactant, J. Trauma 7:691, 1967.

121. Rohatgi, P., Tauber, I., and Massaro, D.: Hemorrhagic hypotension and the lung: in vitro respiration, Am. Rev. Respir. Dis. 113:763, 1976.

122. Sayeed, M. M., Chaudry, I. H., and Baue, A. E.: Na+-K+ transport and adenosine nucleotides in the lung in hemorrhagic shock. Surgery 77: 395, 1975.

123. Hechtman, H. E.: Unpublished data.

124. Fishman, A. P., and Hecht, H. H. (eds.): *The Pulmonary Circulation and Interstitial Space* (Chicago: University of Chicago Press, 1969).

125. Fishman, A. P.: Pulmonary edema: the water-exchanging function

of the lung, Circulation 46:390, 1972.
126. Robin, E. D., Cross, C. E., and Zelis, R.: Pulmonary edema, N. Engl. J. Med. 288:239, 246, 292, 1973.
127. Staub, N. C.: Pulmonary edema, Physiol. Rev. 54:678, 1974.
128. Bredenberg, C. E.: Acute respiratory distress, Surg. Clin. North Am. 54: 1043, 1974.
129. Terzi, R. G., and Peters, R. M.: The effect of large fluid loads on lung mechanics and work, Ann. Thorac. Surg. 6:16, 1968.
130. Gump, F. E., Zikria, B. A., and Mashima, Y.: The effect of interstitial edema on pulmonary function in the dog, J. Trauma 12:764, 1972.
131. Bo, G., Hauge, A., Nicolaysen, G., and Waaler, B. J.: Does interstitial lung edema cause changes in lung compliance? N. Engl. J. Med. 289: 218, 1973.
132. Hechtman, H. E., Weisel, R. D., Vito, L., Ali, J., and Berger, R. L.: The independence of pulmonary shunting and pulmonary edema, Surgery 74:300, 1973.
133. Harken, A. H., and O'Connor, N. E.: The influence of clinically undetectable pulmonary edema on small airway closure in the dog, Ann. Surg. 184:183, 1976.
134. Gump, F. E., Kinney, J. M., Iles, M., and Long, C. G.: Duration and significance of large fluid loads administered for circulatory support, J. Trauma 10:431, 1970.
135. Abrams, J. S., Diane, R. S., and Davis, J. H.: Adverse effects of salt and water retention on pulmonary function in patients with multiple trauma, J. Trauma 13:788, 1973.
136. Fleming, W. H., and Bowen, J. C.: The use of diuretics in the treatment of early wet lung syndrome, Ann. Surg. 175:505, 1972.
137. Skillman, J. J., Parikh, B. M., and Tanenbaum, B. J.: Pulmonary arteriovenous admixture: improvement with albumin and diuresis, Am. J. Surg. 119:440, 1970.
138. Skillman, J. J., Bushnell, L. S., and Hedley-Whyte, J.: Peritonitis and respiratory failure after abdominal operations, Ann. Surg. 170:122, 1969.
139. Gutierrez, V. S., Berman, I. R., Soloway, H. B., and Hamit, H. F.: Relationship of hypoproteinemia and prolonged mechanical ventilation to the development of pulmonary insufficiency in shock, Ann. Surg. 171: 385, 1970.
140. Giordano, J. M., Joseph, W. L., Klingemaier, C. H., and Adkins, P. C.: The management of interstitial pulmonary edema. Significance of hypoproteinemia, J. Thorac. Cardiovasc. Surg. 64:739, 1972.
141. Lundsgaard-Hansen, P.: Oncotic deficit and albumin treatment, Proc. Workshop on Albumin, DHEW Publ. No. 76-295:242, 1976.
142. Skillman, J. J., Restall, D. S., and Salzman, E. W.: Randomized trial of albumin vs. electrolyte solutions during abdominal aortic operations, Surgery 78:291, 1975.
143. Cloutier, C. T., Lowery, B. D., and Carey, L. C.: The effect of hemodilutional resuscitation on serum protein levels in humans in hemorrhagic shock, J. Trauma 9:514, 1969.

144. Gump, F. E., Mashima, Y., Ferenczy, A., and Kinney, J. M.: Pre- and postmortem studies of lung fluids and electrolytes, J. Trauma 11:474, 1971.

145. Pruitt, B. A., Mason, A. D., and Moncrief, J. A.: Hemodynamic changes in the early postburn patient: the influence of fluid administration and of a vasodilator (hydralazine), J. Trauma 11:36, 1971.

146. Prentice, T. C., Olney, J. M., Artz, C. P., and Howard, J. M.: Studies of blood volume and transfusion therapy in the Korean battle casualty, Surg. Gynecol. Obstet. 99:542, 1954.

147. Doty, D. B., Hulfnagel, H. V., and Moseley, R. V.: The distribution of body fluids following hemorrhage and resuscitation in combat casualties, Surg. Gynecol. Obstet. 130:453, 1970.

148. Doty, D. B., Moseley, R. V., and Simmons, R. L.: Sequential changes in blood volume after injury and transfusion, Surg. Gynecol. Obstet. 130:801, 1970.

149. Simmons, R. L., Heisterkamp, C. A., and Doty, D. B.: Postresuscitative blood volumes in combat casualties, Surg. Gynecol. Obstet. 128:1193, 1969.

150. Williams, J. A., Grable, E., Frank, H. A., and Fine, J.: Blood loss and plasma volume shifts during and following major surgical operations, Ann. Surg. 156:648, 1962.

151. Brisman, R., Parks, L. C., and Benson, D. W.: Pitfalls in the clinical use of central venous pressure, Arch. Surg. 95:902, 1967.

152. Wilson, R. F., Sarver, E., and Birks, R.: Central venous pressure and blood volume determinations in clinical shock, Surg. Gynecol. Obstet. 132:631, 1971.

153. Northfield, T. C., and Smith, T.: Physiologic significance of central venous pressure in patients with hemorrhage, Surg. Gynecol. Obstet. 135:267, 1972.

154. Alexander, R. S.: Venomotor tone in hemorrhage and shock, Circ. Res. 3:181, 1955.

155. Cleland, J., Pluth, J. R., Tauxe, W. N., and Kirklin, J. W.: Blood volumes and body fluid compartment changes soon after closed and open intracardiac surgery, J. Thorac. Cardiovasc. Surg. 52:698, 1966.

156. Gauer, D. H., Henry, J. P., and Sieker, H. O.: Changes in central venous pressure after moderate hemorrhage and transfusion in man, Circ. Res. 4:79, 1956.

157. Szidon, J. P., and Fishman, A. P.: Participation of pulmonary circulation in the defense reaction, Am. J. Physiol. 220:364, 1971.

158. Flanc, C., Kakkar, V. V., and Clarke, M. B.: The detection of venous thrombosis of the legs using ^{125}I labelled fibrinogen, Br. J. Surg. 55:742, 1968.

159. Negus, P., Pinto, D. J., Le Quesne, L. P., Brown, N., and Chapman, M.: [125]I labelled fibrinogen in the diagnosis of deep vein thrombosis and its correlation with phlebography, Br. J. Surg. 55:835, 1968.

160. Kakkar, V. V., Howe, C. T., Flanc, C.: Natural history of post-operative deep vein thrombosis, Lancet 2:230, 1969.

161. Kakkar, V. V., Howe, C. T., Nicolaides, A. N., Renney, J. T., and Clarke,

M. B.: Deep vein thrombosis — is there a "high risk" group? Am. J. Surg. 120:527, 1970.

162. Skillman, J. J.: Postoperative deep vein thrombosis and pulmonary embolism: a selective review and personal viewpoint, Surgery 75:114, 1974.

163. Nicolaides, A. N., Dupont, P. A., Desai, S., Lewis, J. D., Douglas, J. N., Dodsworth, H., Fourides, G., Luck, R. J., and Jamieson, C. W.: Small doses of subcutaneous sodium heparin in preventing deep venous thrombosis after major surgery, Lancet 2:890, 1972.

164. Clagett, G. P., and Salzman, E. W.: Prevention of venous thromboembolism in surgical patients, N. Engl. J. Med. 290:93, 1974.

165. Kakkar, V. V.: Prevention of fatal postoperative pulmonary embolism by low doses of heparin: an international multicentre trial, Lancet 2:45, 1975.

166. Colton, L. T., and Roberts, V. C.: The prevention of deep vein thrombosis, with particular reference to mechanical methods of prevention, Surgery 81:228, 1977.

167. Salzman, E. W., Deykin, D., Shapiro, R. M., and Rosenberg, R.: Management of heparin therapy: controlled prospective trial, N. Engl. J. Med. 292:1046, 1975.

168. Natelson, E., Lynch, E., Alfrey, C., Gross, J.: Heparin-induced thrombocytopenia; an unexpected response to treatment of consumption coagulopathy, Ann. Intern. Med. 71:1121, 1969.

169. Rhodes, G., Dixon, R., and Silver, D.: Heparin induced thrombocytopenia with thrombotic and hemorrhagic manifestations, Surg. Gynecol. Obstet. 136:409, 1973.

170. Fred, H. L., Axelrod, M. A., Lewis, J. M., and Alexander, J. K.: Rapid resolution of pulmonary thromboemboli in man, J.A.M.A. 196:1137, 1966.

171. Dalen, J. E., Banas, J. S., Brooks, H. L., Evans, G. L., Paraskos, J. A., and Dexter, L.: Resolution rate of acute pulmonary embolism in man, N. Engl. J. Med. 280:1194, 1969.

172. Fratantoni, J. C., Ness, P., and Simon, T. L.: Thrombolytic therapy: current status, N. Engl. J. Med. 293:1073, 1975.

173. Mobin-Uddin, K., Collard, G. M., Bolooki, H., Robinson, R., Michie, D., and Jude, J. R.: Transvenous caval interruption with umbrella filter, N. Engl. J. Med. 286:55, 1972.

174. Greenfield, L. J., McCurdy, J. R., Brown, P. P., and Elkins, R. C.: A new intracaval filter permitting continued flow and resolution of emboli, Surgery 73:599, 1973.

175. Eeles, G. H., and Sevitt, S.: Microthrombosis in injured and burned patients, J. Pathol. Bact. 93:275, 1967.

176. Moseley, R. V., and Doty, D. B.: Death associated with multiple pulmonary emboli soon after battle injury, Ann. Surg. 171:336, 1970.

177. Lindquist, O., Rammer, L., and Saldeen, T.: Pulmonary insufficiency, microembolism and fibrinolysis inhibition in a post-traumatic autopsy material, Acta Chir. Scand. 138:545, 1972.

178. Remmele, W., and Goebel, U.: Zur pathologischen Anatomie des Kreis-

laufschocks beim Menschen. V. Pathomorphologie der Schocklunge, Klin. Wochenschr. 51:25, 1973.

179. Janson, R., Thelen, M., Rommelsheim, K., Louven, B., and Siege, P.: Synopsis von Thorax-und Obduktionsbefunden bei chirurgischen Intensivpflegepatienten, Fortschr. Geb. Röntgenstr. Nuklearmed. 124:427, 433, 1976.

180. Thomas, D., Stein, M., Tanabe, G., Rege, V., and Wessler, S.: Mechanism of bronchoconstriction produced by thromboemboli in dogs, Am. J. Physiol. 206:1207, 1964.

181. Stein, M., and Thomas, D. P.: Role of platelets in the acute pulmonary responses to endotoxin. J. Appl. Physiol. 23:47, 1967.

182. Olsson, P., Swedenborg, J., and Lindquist, O.: Effects of slow defibrinogenation on the canine lung, J. Trauma 14:325, 1974.

183. Kux, M., Coalson, J., Massion, W. H., and Guenter, C. A.: Pulmonary effects of E. coli endotoxin: role of leukocytes and platelets, Ann. Surg. 175:26, 1972.

184. White, M. K., Shepro, D., and Hechtman, H. B.: Pulmonary function and platelet-lung interaction, J. Appl. Physiol. 34:697, 703, 1973.

185. Douglas, M. E., Downs, J. B., Dannemiller, F. J., and Hodges, M. R.: Acute respiratory failure and intravascular coagulation, Surg. Gynecol. Obstet. 143:555, 560, 1976.

186. Hechtman, H. B., Lonegan, E. A., and Shepro, D.: Platelet and leukocyte lung interactions in patients with respiratory failure, Surgery. In press.

187. Hardaway, R. M.: Disseminated intravascular coagulation as a possible cause of acute respiratory failure, Surg. Gynecol. Obstet. 137:419, 1973.

188. Hoie, J., and Schenk, W. G.: Pulmonary hemodynamics and function in acute experimental disseminated intravascular coagulation, J. Trauma 13:887, 1973.

188a. Josephson, S., Swedenborg, J., and S. E.: Dahlgren, Delayed lung lesion in dogs after thrombin-induced disseminated intravascular coagulation, Acta Chir. Scand. 140:431, 1974.

189. Milligan, G. F., MacDonald, J. A., Millon, A., and Ledingham, I. McA.: Pulmonary and hematologic disturbances during septic shock, Surg. Gynecol. Obstet. 138:43, 1974.

190. Laterman, A., Manwaring, D., and Curreri, P. W.: The role of fibrinogen degradation products in the pathogenesis of the respiratory distress syndrome, Surgery. In press.

191. Robboy, S. J., Minna, J. D., Colman, R. W., Birndorf, N. I., and Lopas, H.: Pulmonary hemorrhage syndrome as a manifestation of disseminated intravascular coagulation: analysis of ten cases, Chest 63:718, 1973.

192. Marshall, B. E., and Wyche, M. Q.: Hypoxemia during and after anesthesia, Anesthesiology 37:178, 1972.

193. Weil, J. V., McCullough, R. E., Kline, J. S., and Sodal, I. E.: Diminished ventilatory response to hypoxia and hypercapnia after morphine in normal man. N. Engl. J. Med. 292:1103, 1975.

194. Latimer, R. G., Dickman, M., Day, W. C., Gunn, M. L., and Schmidt, C. D.: Ventilatory patterns and pulmonary complications after upper abdominal surgery determined by preoperative and postoperative com-

puterized spirometry and blood gas analysis, Am. J. Surg. 122:622, 1971.

195. Churchill, E. D., and McNeil, D.: The reduction in vital capacity following operation, Surg. Gynecol. Obstet. 44:483, 1927.

196. Vaughan, R. W., and Wise, L.: Choice of abdominal operative incision in the obese patient: a study using blood gas measurements, Ann. Surg. 181:829, 1975.

197. Pecora, D. V.: Predictability of effects of abdominal and thoracic surgery upon pulmonary function, Ann. Surg. 170:101, 1969.

198. Alexander, J. I., Horton, P. W., Millar, W. T., Parikh, R. K., and Spence, A. A.: The effect of upper abdominal surgery on the relationship of airway closing point to end tidal position, Clin. Sci. 43:137, 1972.

199. Zikria, B. A., Spencer, J. L., Kinney, J. M., and Broell, J. R.: Alterations in ventilatory function and breathing patterns following surgical trauma, Ann. Surg. 179:1, 1974.

200. Siler, J. N., Rosenberg, H., Mull, T. D., Kaplan, J. A., Bardin, H., and Marshall, B. E.: Hypoxemia after upper abdominal surgery: comparison of venous admixture and ventilation/perfusion inequality components, using a digital computer, Ann. Surg. 179:149, 1974.

201. Ali, J., Weisel, R. D., Layung, A. B., Kripke, B. J., and Hechtman, H. B.: Consequences of postoperative alterations in respiratory mechanics, Am. J. Surg. 128:376, 1974.

202. Dalrymple, D. G., Panbrook, G. D., and Steel, D. F.: Factors predisposing to postoperative pain and pulmonary complications, Br. J. Anaesth. 45:589, 1973.

203. Van de Water, J. M., Watring, W. G., Linton, L. A., Murphy, M., and Byron, R. L.: Prevention of postoperative pulmonary complications, Surg. Gynecol. Obstet. 135:229, 1972.

204. Bartlett, R. H., Gazzaniga, A. B., and Geraghty, T. R.: Respiratory maneuvers to prevent postoperative pulmonary complications, J.A.M.A. 224:1017, 1973.

205. Bartlett, R. H., Brennan, M. L., Gazzaniga, A. B., and Hanson, E. L.: Studies on the pathogenesis and prevention of postoperative pulmonary complications, Surg. Gynecol. Obstet. 137:925, 1973.

206. Meyers, J. R., Lembeck, L., O'Kane, H., and Baue, A. B.: Changes in functional residual capacity of the lung after operation, Arch. Surg. 110: 576, 1975.

207. Gold, M. I.: Is intermittent positive pressure breathing therapy (IPPRx) necessary in the surgical patient? Ann. Surg. 184:122, 1976.

208. Anscombe, A. R.: *Pulmonary Complications of Abdominal Surgery* (Chicago: Year Book Medical Publishers, Inc., 1957).

209. Bromage, R. R.: Spirometry in assessment of analgesia after abdominal surgery, Br. Med. J. 2:589, 1955.

210. Guis, J. A.: Paravertebral procaine block in the treatment of postoperative atelectasis, Surgery 8:832, 1940.

211. Spence, A. A., and Smith, G.: Postoperative analgesia and lung function: a comparison of morphine with extradural block, Br. J. Anaesth. 43:144, 1971.

212. Thoren, L.: Postoperative pulmonary complications: observations on

their prevention by means of physiotherapy, Acta Chir. Scand. 107:193, 1954.

213. Stein, M., and Lassara, E. L.: Preoperative pulmonary evaluation and therapy for surgery patients, J.A.M.A. 211:787, 1970.

214. Fonkalsrud, E. W., Sanchez, M., Higashyima, I., and Arima, E.: A comparative study of the effects of dry vs. humidified ventilation on canine lungs, Surgery 78:373, 1975.

214a. Weeks, D. B.: Humidification during anesthesia, NY State J. Med. 75: 1216, 1975.

215. Altschule, M. D.: The significance of changes in the lung volume and its subdivisions during and after abdominal operation, Anesthesiology 4: 385, 1943.

216. Berggren, S. M.: The oxygen deficit of arterial blood caused by non-ventilating parts of the lung, Acta Physiol. Scand. [Suppl.] 4:11, 1942.

217. Cardus, D.: O_2 alveolar-arterial tension difference after 10 days recumbency in man, J. Appl. Physiol. 23:934, 1967.

218. Trimble, C., Smith, D. E., Cook, T. I., and Trummer, M. J.: The effect of supine bed rest upon alveolar-arterial oxygen gradients and intrapulmonary shunting in normal man, J. Thorac. Cardiovasc. Surg. 63:873, 1972.

219. Blitt, C. D., Gutman, H. L., Cohen, D. D., Weisman, H., and Dillon, J. B.: "Silent" regurgitation and aspiration during general anesthesia, Anesth. Analg. (Cleve.) 49:707, 1970.

220. Lewis, R. T., Burgess, J. H., and Hampson, L. G.: Cardiorespiratory studies in critical illness: changes in aspiration pneumonitis, Arch. Surg. 103:335, 1971.

221. Cameron, J. L., and Zuidema, G. D.: Aspiration pneumonia: magnitude and frequency of the problem, J.A.M.A. 219:1194, 1972.

222. Cameron, J. L., Mitchell, W. H., and Zuidema, G. D.: Aspiration pneumonia: clinical outcome following documented aspiration, Arch. Surg. 106:49, 1973.

223. Turndorf, H., Rodis, I. D., and Clark, T. S.: "Silent" regurgitation during general anesthesia, Anesth. Analg. (Cleve.) 53:700, 1974.

224. Bartlett, J. G., and Gorbach, S. L.: The triple threat of aspiration pneumonia, Chest 68:560, 1975.

225. Chapman, R. L., Downs, J. B., Modell, J. H., and Hood, C. I.: The ineffectiveness of steroid therapy in treating aspiration of hydrochloric acid, Arch. Surg. 108:858, 1974.

226. Dudley, W. R., and Marshall, B. E.: Steroid treatment for acid-aspiration pneumonitis, Anesthesiology 40:136, 1974.

226a. Flint, L., Gosdin, G., and Carrico, C. J.: Evaluation of ventilatory therapy for acid aspiration, Surgery 78:492, 1975.

227. Cameron, J. L., Caldini, P., Toung, J. K., and Zuidema, G. D.: Aspiration pneumonia: physiologic data following experimental aspiration, Surgery 72:238, 1972.

228. Bartlett, J. G., Gorbach, S. L., and Finegold, S. M.: The bacteriology of aspiration pneumonia, Am. J. Med. 56:202, 1974.

229. Lorber, B., and Swenson, R. M.: Bacteriology of aspiration pneumonia, Ann. Intern. Med. 81:329, 1974.

230. Aldrete, J. A., Liem, S. T., and Carrow, D. J.: Pulmonary aerobic bacterial flora after aspiration pneumonitis, J. Trauma 15:1014, 1975.
231. Bartlett, J. G., and Gorbach, S. L.: Treatment of aspiration pneumonia and primary lung abscess, J.A.M.A. 234:935, 1975.
232. Gillis, C. N.: Metabolism of vasoactive hormones by lung, Anesthesiology 39:626, 1973.
233. Tierney, D. F.: Lung metabolism and biochemistry, Annu. Rev. Physiol. 36:209, 1974.
234. Fishman, A. P., and Pietra, G. P.: Handling of bioactive materials by the lung, N. Engl. J. Med. 291:884, 953, 1974.
235. Said, S. I.: Endocrine role of the lung in disease, Am. J. Med. 57:453, 1974.
236. Anderson, M. W., and Eling, T. E.: Prostaglandin removal and metabolism by isolated perfused rat lung, Prostaglandins 11:647, 1976.
237. O'Donnell, T. F., Clowes, G. H., Talamo, R. C., and Colman, R. W.: Kinin activation in the blood of patients with sepsis, Surg. Gynecol. Obstet. 143:539, 1976.
238. Moseley, R. V., and Doty, D. B.: Changes in the filtration characteristics of stored blood, Ann. Surg. 171:329, 1970.
239. Tobey, R. E., Koprina, C. J., Homer, I. D., Solis, R. T., Dickson, L. G., and Herman, C. M.: Pulmonary gas exchange following hemorrhagic shock and massive blood transfusion in the baboon, 179:316, 1974.
240. Bennett, S. H., and Geelhoed, G. W.: Filtration of stored and autotransfused blood in the prevention of "shock lung" in the canine and primate, Presented at 9th Annual Meeting, Assn. Acad. Surg., 1975.
241. McNamara, J. J.: International Forum: Does a relationship exist between massive blood transfusions and the adult respiratory distress syndrome? If so, what are the best preventive measures? Vox Sang. In press.
242. Reul, G. J., Greenburg, S. D., Lefrak, E. A., McCollum, W. B., Beall, A. C., and Jordan, G. L.: Prevention of post-traumatic pulmonary insufficiency: fine screen filtration of blood, Arch. Surg. 106:386, 1973.
243. Collins, J. A.: Massive blood transfusion, Clin. Haematol. 5:201, 1976.
244. Wolf, C. F., and Canale, V. C.: Fatal pulmonary hypersensitivity reaction to HL-A incompatible blood transfusion: report of a case and review of the literature, Transfusion 16:135, 1976.
245. McCullough, J., Benson, S. J., Yunis, E. J., and Quie, P. G.: Effect of blood-bank storage on leucocyte function, Lancet 2:1333, 1969.
246. Schechter, G. P., Soehnlen, F., and McFarland, W.: Lymphocyte response to blood transfusion in man, N. Engl. J. Med. 287:1169, 1972.
247. Beaulieu, R., Pirofsky, B., and Noonan, M.: Lymphocyte response to blood transfusion, N. Engl. J. Med. 288:853, 1973.
248. Parkman, R., Mosier, D., Umansky, I., Cochran, W., Carpenter, C. B., and Rosen, F. S.: Graft-versus-host disease after intrauterine and exchange transfusions for hemolytic disease of the newborn, N. Engl. J. Med. 290:359, 1974.
249. Schwartz, R. S.: Trojan-horse lymphocytes, N. Engl. J. Med. 290:397, 1974.
250. Groff, P., Torhorst, J., Speck, B., Nissur, C., Weber, W., Cornu, P., Ros-

sier, J., and Biland, L.: Die Graft-versus-Host-Krankheit, eine wenig bekamte Komplikation der Bluttransfusion, Schweiz. Med. Wochenschr. 106:634, 1976.

251. Strauss, H. W., Smith, R. B., Polimeni, P., Schenker, A. C., Schenker, V. J., and Stuckey, J. H.: Plasma serotonin levels in stored human blood, Angiology 18:535, 1967.

252. Rush, B. F., and Wilder, R. J.: Mortality and renal tubular necrosis in hemorrhagic shock in dogs: the effect of blood handling, Surg. Forum 14: 1, 1963.

253. Hardaway, R. M., Johnson, D. G., Houchin, D. N., Jenkins, E. B., Bucas, J. W., and Jackson, D. R.: The influence of extracorporeal handling of blood on hemorrhagic shock in dogs, Exp. Med. Surg. 23:28, 1965.

254. Berman, I. R., Iliescu, H., Ranson, J. H., and Eng, K.: Pulmonary capillary permeability – a transfusion lesion, J. Trauma 16:471, 1976.

255. Haugaard, N.: Cellular mechanisms of oxygen toxicity, Physiol. Rev. 48: 311, 1968.

256. Clark, J. M., and Lambertsen, C. J.: Pulmonary oxygen toxicity: a review, Pharmacol. Rev. 23:37, 1971.

257. Senior, R. M., Wessler, S., and Avioli, L. V.: Pulmonary oxygen toxicity, J.A.M.A. 217:1373, 1971.

258. Winter, P. M., and Smith, G.: The toxicity of oxygen, Anesthesiology 37: 210, 1972.

259. Winter, P. M., Gupta, R. K., Michalski, A. H., and Lanphier, E. H.: Modification of hyperbaric oxygen toxicity by experimental venous admixture, J. Appl. Physiol. 23:954, 1967.

260. Miller, W. W., Waldhausen, J. A., and Rashkind, W. J.: Comparison of oxygen poisoning of the lung in cyanotic and acyanotic dogs, N. Engl. J. Med. 282:943, 1970.

261. McAslan, T. C., Chiu, J. M., Turney, S. Z., and Cowley, R. A.: Influence of inhalation of 100% oxygen on intrapulmonary shunt in severely traumatized patients, J. Trauma 13:811, 1973.

262. Suter, P. M., Fairley, H. B., and Schlobohm, R. M.: Shunt, lung volume and perfusion during short periods of ventilation with oxygen, Anesthesiology 43:617, 1975.

263. Sevitt, S.: Fat Embolism (London: Butterworth & Co., Ltd., 1962).

264. Beck, J. P., and Collins, J. A.: Theoretical and clinical aspects of posttraumatic fat embolism syndrome, American Academy of Orthopedic Surgery, Instructional Course Lectures 22:38, 1973.

265. Ducker, T. B.: Increased intra-cranial pressure and pulmonary edema. I. Clinical study of eleven patients, J. Neurosurg. 28:112, 1968.

266. Simmons, R. L., Martin, A. M., Heisterkamp, C. A., and Ducker, T. B.: Respiratory insufficiency in combat casualties, II. Pulmonary edema following head injury, Ann. Surg. 170:39, 1969.

267. Sugimoto, T., Katsurada, K., Yamada, R., Ogawa, M., Minami, T., and Onji, Y.: Posttraumatische Respiratorische Insuffizienz bei Kopfverletzten, Anaesthesist 23:263, 1974.

268. Ducker, T. B., Simmons, R. L., and Anderson, R. W.: Increased intracranial pressure and pulmonary edema III. The effect of increased intra-

cranial pressure on the cardiovascular hemodynamics of chimpanzees, J. Neurosurg. 29:475, 1968.

269. Berman, I. R., and Ducker, T. B.: Pulmonary, somatic and splanchnic circulatory responses to increased intracranial pressure, Ann. Surg. 169:210, 1969.

270. Beckman, D. L., Bean, J. W., and Baslock, D. R.: Sympathetic influence on lung compliance and surface forces in head injury, J. Appl. Physiol. 30:394, 1971.

271. Droste, P. L., and Beckman, D. L.: Pulmonary effects of prolonged sympathetic stimulation, Proc. Soc. Exp. Biol. Med. 146:352, 1974.

272. Chen, H. I., Sun, S. C., and Chai, C. Y.: Pulmonary edema and hemorrhage resulting from cerebral compression, Am. J. Physiol. 224:223, 1973.

273. Sarnoff, S. J., and Sarnoff, L. C.: Neurohemodynamics of pulmonary edema. II. The role of sympathetic pathways in the evaluation of pulmonary and systemic vascular pressures following the intracisternal injection of fibrin, Circulation 6:51, 1952.

274. Abrams, J. S., Deane, R. S., and Davis, J. H.: Pulmonary function in patients with multiple trauma and associated severe head injury, J. Trauma 16:543, 1976.

275. Moss, G., Staunton, C., and Stein, A. A.: The centrineurogenic etiology of the acute respiratory distress syndrome: universal, species independent phenomenon, Am. J. Surg. 126:37, 1973.

276. Kasajima, K., Wax, S. D., and Webb, W. W.: Cerebral hypotension and shock lung syndrome, J. Thorac. Cardiovasc. Surg. 67:969, 1974.

277. Kellum, J. M., De Meester, T. R., Elkins, R. C., and Zuidema, G. D.: Respiratory insufficiency secondary to acute pancreatitis, Ann. Surg. 175:657, 1972.

278. Ransom, J. H., Turner, J. W., Roses, D. F., Rifkind, K. M., and Spencer, F. C.: Respiratory complications in acute pancreatitis, Ann. Surg. 179:557, 1974.

279. Rovner, A. J., and Westcott, J. L.: Pulmonary edema and respiratory insufficiency in acute pancreatitis, Radiology 118:513, 1976.

280. Morgan, A. P., Jenny, M. E., and Haessler, H.: Phospholipids, acute pancreatitis, and the lungs: effect of lecithinase infusion on pulmonary surface activity in dogs, Ann. Surg. 167:329, 1968.

281. Halmagyi, D. F., Karis, J. H., Stenning, F. G., and Vorga, D.: Pulmonary hypertension in acute hemorrhagic pancreatitis, Surgery 76:637, 1974.

282. Warshaw, A. L., Lesser, P. B., Rie, M., and Cullen, D. J.: The pathogenesis of pulmonary edema in acute pancreatitis, Ann. Surg. 182:505, 1975.

283. Pruitt, B. A., Flemma, R. J., DiVincenti, F. C., Foley, F. D., and Mason, A. D.: Pulmonary complications in burn patients: 697 patients, J. Thorac. Cardiovasc. Surg. 59:7, 1970.

284. Pruitt, B. A., Erickson, D. R., and Morris, A.: Progressive pulmonary insufficiency and other pulmonary complications of thermal injury, J. Trauma 15:369, 1975.

285. Luce, E. A., Su, C. T., and Hoopes, J. E.: Alveolar-arterial oxygen gradient in the burn patient, J. Trauma 16:212, 1976.
286. Dressler, D. P., Skornik, W. A., and Kupersmith, S.: Corticosteroid treatment of experimental smoke inhalation, Ann. Surg. 183:46, 1976.
287. Petroff, P. A., Hander, E. W., and Mason, A. D.: Ventilatory patterns following burn injury and effect of Sulfamylon, J. Trauma 15:650, 1975.
288. Agee, R. N., Long, J. M., Hunt, J. L., Petroff, P. A., Lull, R. J., Mason, A. D., and Pruitt, B. A.: Use of ^{133}Xenon in the early diagnosis of inhalation injury, J. Trauma 16:218, 1976.
289. Hunt, J. L., Agee, R. N., and Pruitt, B. A.: Fiberoptic bronchoscopy in acute inhalation injury, J. Trauma 15:641, 1975.
290. Berk, J. L., Hagen, J. F., Koo, R., Beyer, W., Dochat, G. R., Rupright, M., and Nomoto, S.: Pulmonary insufficiency caused by epinephrine, Ann. Surg. 178:423, 1973.
291. Berk, J. L., Hagen, J. F., and Koo, R.: Effect of alpha and beta adrenergic blockade on epinephrine induced pulmonary insufficiency, Ann. Surg. 183:369, 1976.
292. Berk, J. L., Hagen, J. F., Koo, R., and Maly, G.: Pulmonary insufficiency produced by isoproterenol, Surg. Gynecol. Obstet. 143:725, 1976.
293. Aarseth, P., Karlsen, J., and Bo, G.: Effects of catecholamine infusions and hypoxia on pulmonary blood volume and extravascular lung water content in cats, Acta Physiol. Scand. 95:34, 1975.
294. Bashour, F. A., McConnell, T., and Miller, W. F.: Circulatory and respiratory changes in patients with Laennec's cirrhosis of the liver, Am. Heart J. 74:569, 1967.
295. Siegel, J. H., Goldwyn, R. M., Farrell, E. J., Gallin, P., and Friedman, H. P.: Hyperdynamic states and the physiologic determinants of survival in patients with cirrhosis and portal hypertension, Arch. Surg. 108: 282, 1974.
296. Trimble, C., Smith, D. E., Rosenthal, M. H., and Fosburg, R. G.: Pathophysiologic role of hypocarbia in post-traumatic pulmonary insufficiency, Am. J. Surg. 122:633, 1971.
297. Goldring, R. M., Cannon, P. J., Heinemann, H. O., and Fishman, A. P.: Respiratory adjustment to chronic metabolic alkalosis in man, J. Clin. Invest. 47:188, 1968.
298. Tuller, M. A., and Mehdi, F.: Compensatory hypoventilation and hypercapnia in primary metabolic alkalosis: report of 3 cases, Am. J. Med. 50: 281, 1971.
299. Steer, M. L., Cloeren, S. E., Bushnell, L. S., and Skillman, J. J.: Metabolic alkalosis and respiratory failure in critically ill patients, Surgery 72:408, 1972.
300. Dockel, R. C., Zwilbich, C. W., Scoggin, C. H., Kryger, M., and Wiel, J. V.: Clinical semi-starvation: depression of hypoxia ventilatory response, N. Engl. J. Med. 295:358, 1976.
301. Sova, J., and Jirásek, V.: Mechanism of pulmonary edema, Biochem. Clin. 4:263, 1964.
302. Gibson, D. G.: Haemodynamic factors in the development of acute pulmonary oedema in renal failure, Lancet 2:1217, 1966.

303. Merrill, J. P., and Hampers, C. L.: Uremia, N. Engl. J. Med. 282:953, 1014, 1970.
304. Lee, H. Y., and Stretton, T. B.: The lungs in renal failure, Thorax 30:46, 1975.
305. Shoemaker, W. C. (ed.): *The Lung in the Critically Ill Patient: Pathophysiology and Therapy of Acute Respiratory Failure* (Baltimore: Williams & Wilkins Company, 1976).
306. Schmidt, G. B., O'Neill, W. W., Kotb, K., Hwang, K. K., Bennett, E. J., and Bombeck, C. T.: Continuous positive airway pressure in the prophylaxis of the adult respiratory distress syndrome, Surg. Gynecol. Obstet. 143:615, 1976.
307. Downs, J. B., Perkins, H. M., Modell, J. H.: Intermittent mandatory ventilation: an evaluation, Arch. Surg. 109:519, 1974.
308. Civetta, J. M., and Gabel, J. C.: "Pseudocardiogenic" pulmonary edema, J. Trauma 15:143, 1975.
309. Siegel, J. H., Farrell, E. J., Miller, M., Goldwyn, R. M., and Friedman, H. P.: Cardiorespiratory interactions as determinants of survival and the need for respiratory support in human shock states, J. Trauma 13:602, 1973.
310. Halmagyi, D. F., and Kinney, J. M.: Metabolic rate in acute respiratory failure complicating sepsis, Surgery 77:492, 1975.
311. Proctor, H. J., and Woolson, R.: Prediction of respiratory muscle fatigue by measurements of the work of breathing, Surg. Gynecol. Obstet. 136:367, 1973.
312. James, P. M., and Myers, R. T.: Experience with steroids, albumin, and diuretics in progressive pulmonary insufficiency, South. Med. J. 65:945, 1972.
313. Sladen, A.: Methylprednisolone: pharmacologic doses in shock lung syndrome, J. Thorac. Cardiovasc. Surg. 71:800, 1976.
314. Downs, J. B., and Olsen, G. N.: Pulmonary function following adult respiratory distress syndrome, Chest 65:92, 1974.
315. Yernault, J. C., Englert, M., Sergysels, R., and DeCosta, A.: Pulmonary mechanics and diffusion after "shock lung," Thorax 30:252, 1975.
316. Lakshiminarayan, S., Stanford, R. E., and Petty, T. L.: Prognosis after recovery from adult respiratory distress syndrome, Am. Rev. Respir. Dis. 113:7, 1976.
317. Klein, J. J., van Haeringen, J. R., Sluiter, H. J., Holloway, R., and Peset, R.: Pulmonary function after recovery from the adult respiratory distress syndrome, Chest 69:350, 1976.

Abdominal Ultrasound in Surgical Patients

RAYMOND GRAMIAK and SETH A. BORG

Department of Radiology, Division of Ultrasound, University of Rochester School of Medicine and Dentistry, Rochester, New York

Ultrasound has become established as a useful technique that provides valuable information in abdominal disease processes. It evolved in the early 1950s from concepts developed in World War II for radar and sonar. Detailed description of these interesting developments is beyond the scope of this presentation, but publications by Howry[1] and Holmes and Howry[2] review this topic as well as those of early instrumentation and clinical imaging. This chapter is intended to present a brief overview of the physical and clinical aspects of abdominal imaging with ultrasound and will emphasize topics of interest to surgeons. The reader who may be stimulated to seek a more comprehensive description of technical concepts and clinical applications is referred to recent textbooks.[3, 4]

Physical Principles

The physical principles governing the generation and display of ultrasound, as well as the characteristics of the tissues that reflect the sound energy, control the production of images, influence their content and provide the diagnostic criteria used clinically.

Ultrasound is defined as that portion of the acoustic spectrum above the range of human perception, 20,000 cps (20 kHz). In

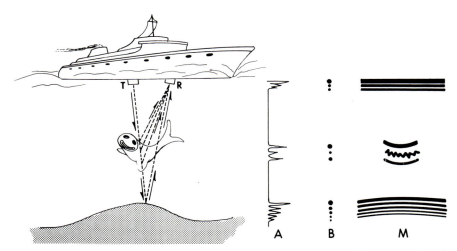

Fig 1.—Imaging modes in ultrasound. A sonar system illustrates the propagation of a single pulse of ultrasound from a transmitter *(T)* and reflections from a moving fish and the ocean bottom to a receiver *(R)*. A-mode display *(A)* features oscilloscopic baseline deflections whose amplitude varies with the intensity of the signal. In B-mode *(B)* the spikes are converted into dots whose brightness represents echo strength. When a recording medium is swept across these dots, motion derived from transit of the ship or from targets within the beam is presented as a variation in the position of reflectors as they change with time; this is designated M-mode *(M)*. The information contained in these modes is one-dimensional in nature.

clinical systems, ultrasound is generated by certain crystalline or ceramic materials that possess piezoelectric properties. These materials, when stressed by high-voltage pulses, can be made to vibrate at a high frequency, usually in the $1-3$ million cps range $(1-3$ MHz$)$. These vibrations can be formed into a beam and made to propagate into tissues, where they are reflected, refracted, scattered, absorbed and transmitted. Reflection is primarily used in ultrasonic imaging, while the other interactions mainly result in acoustic artifacts, though absorption with resultant shadowing produces information of diagnostic importance.

The pulse-echo principle, widely used in sonar and radar as well as in nondestructive testing of metals, is illustrated in Figure 1 and represents the basis on which all clinical ultrasound systems operate. A brief pulse of ultrasonic energy (usually $1-2$ μsec in duration) is emitted by a crystal housed in a suitable casing, the transducer. This energy is transmitted through tissue at a known speed until a reflecting interface is encountered. Reflections occur at those interfaces where the product of density multiplied by the speed of sound (acoustic impedance) changes. This physical factor is unique to ultrasound and allows detection of tissue properties that are invisible in radiologic examinations. Part of the energy is reflected from the surface of the structure, while the rest passes through and is, in turn, reflected from other deeper interfaces. The returning energy impinges on a receiving crystal or on the sending crystal, which operates as a sender-receiver. The mechanical energy deforms the piezoelectric element slightly and produces an electrical impulse that can be detected electronically. Since the speed of sound in tissue is known (1,540 m/second), the depth of the reflecting surface can be calculated from the time of flight between emission of the pulse and arrival of returning echoes. The pulses are repeated 1,000 times/second to provide sufficient information density for diagnosis.

The echo returns are usually displayed on an oscilloscope in one of three modes. A-mode displays the amplitude of returning echoes as a series of spikes in which depth is shown along the X-axis while echo strength is indicated by the amplitude of the deflection. In B-mode, the spikes that indicate reflector position are converted into a series of dots whose brightness represents echo strength. As reflectors move, their distance from the transducer changes. These movements can be recorded by sweeping a recording medium, such as light-sensitive film or paper, past the B-mode display to produce a motion record or M-mode. In all of these display modes, the information recorded is one-dimensional, and the anatomical relationship of adjacent structures is not shown.

To obtain anatomical relationships, a device is interposed between the transducer and the oscilloscope to determine position of the transducer in space, as well as the angle of the beam for spatially correct orientation of the B-mode (Fig 2). The device consists of a multijointed arm that derives positional signals, from which a small analog computer calculates the spatial coordinates of the ultrasonic beam. Individual lines are used to build up a composite image on an oscilloscope or video screen from which permanent records are obtained photographically.

The transducer is placed on the skin, and the beam is directed into the body in one of two fashions. Linear, arc or sector scans

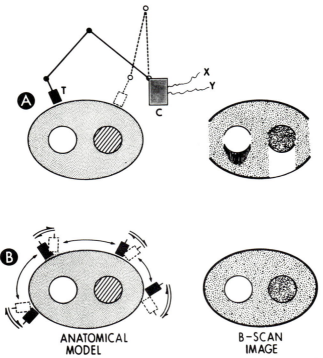

ANATOMICAL
MODEL

B-SCAN
IMAGE

Fig 2. – B-scanning principles and techniques. The depiction of spatially correct anatomical information requires positioning of ultrasonic B-mode echoes with the same angle and position as the transducer *(T)* used during recording. A small analog computer *(C)* calculates display coordinates *(X* and *Y)* for correct oscilloscopic presentation. A single transducer sweep **(A)** images structure margins incompletely *(right)*. Transmission through a fluid-filled cavity *(open circle)* is accentuated and results in increased echoes posteriorly. A solid mass *(crosshatched circle)* attenuates the beam and produces an acoustic shadow. Compound scanning **(B)** utilizes multiple transducer angles and sweeps, producing more complete anatomical information. However, the transmission characteristics of tissue are masked by the multiple transducer sweeps employed.

are produced by a rapid single transducer pass over the area of interest, usually during suspended respiration. This gives the best detail and clearly demonstrates changes in sound transmission through tissues. Some loss of information occurs, since certain reflectors may "drop out" if their position relative to the sender-receiver transducer is not perpendicular.

More complete rendition of anatomical information may be obtained by the technique of compound scanning (see Fig 2, B).

In this method, multiple transducer passes are used with a combination of sector scanning and selection of beam angles for ideal sonic illumination of all structures. More operator skill is required to visualize all areas of the image optimally, and alterations of instrument sensitivity in designated areas may also be necessary. Respiratory motion causes the image to be less sharp, and tissue transmission characteristics may be masked.

Tissue characteristics also influence the content of the record. Bone absorbs the sonic energy so that structures lying deep to these barriers cannot be imaged. Gas transmits sound so poorly that free or contained air also blocks the passage of the ultrasonic beam. Gaseous bowel distention may render abdominal examination impossible, but localized gas collections may usually be dealt with by altering patient position or by angling the scanning plane to "look" under the individual bowel loops. Calcifications produce strong echoes and well-defined shadowing to allow identification of stones and deposits of calcium. Fluids can be distinguished from solids by their ultrasonic appearance. A typical fluid-containing mass such as a cyst will show no internal echo sources and will transmit and possibly concentrate the ultrasonic energy beyond the confines of its margins. This results in the production of an intense ultrasonic "tail" behind cystic lesions, which represents a useful parameter for cyst identification. Solid tumors, on the other hand, contain internal echoes, especially as receiver sensitivity is increased. Tumors that contain collagen absorb much of the incident energy and therefore do not exhibit the same transmission potentiation of cysts, and frequently produce shadowing.

Examination Technique

The ultrasound technique requires direct access to the skin, so surgical dressings may have to be removed. A coupling gel is applied to exclude air and to enhance the transmission of sonic energy into the body. Therefore, open wounds present a problem, since it is usually not feasible to scan over them.

Patient preparation has been useful to minimize the gas normally present in the gastrointestinal tract. Ideally, we recommend 24 hours of clear liquids, nothing by mouth after midnight and ultrasound examination in the morning. A distended bladder is required for pelvic organ scanning, since it displaces bowel loops and provides a noninterfering pathway for the ultrasonic beam.

The ultrasonic records represent cross-sectional anatomical views that may be longitudinal, transverse or oblique. Atlases of cross-sectional anatomy provide anatomical relationships; however, the examiner must synthesize nonstandard oblique planes and three-dimensional relationships from multiple sequential cross sections. Anatomical demonstration, therefore, differs from the layer-to-layer approach familiar to surgeons.

Early ultrasonic equipment selected only those echoes whose intensity exceeded a specified threshold and presented them with a single brightness. These images, therefore, consisted only of strong echo sources and contained no graded-intensity information. Current equipment has the capability to display intensity in shades of gray and has greatly expanded the informational content of the image, which now shows the internal architecture of abdominal structures.

Ultrasonic diagnosis utilizes organ contour changes or displacements, altered or inappropriate echo intensities, changes induced by physiologic maneuvers such as the Valsalva and motion or fixation of structures. Correlation with clinical and radiologic findings is necessary for maximal information.

The current popularity of ultrasound in abdominal imaging stems directly from its unique physical properties. It appears to be totally safe at the low power levels required for clinical imaging. There have been no reports of early or late tissue damage from the nonionizing energy used. Soft tissue contrast is obtained as a result of the natural interaction of ultrasound with tissue so that patient invasion, x-ray exposure and contrast medium injection are avoided. When ultrasound is used with a full appreciation of its capabilities and limitations, valuable clinical and diagnostic data can be obtained easily, repeatedly, safely and relatively inexpensively.

It is convenient to review abdominal ultrasound imaging in the format of regional anatomy. Most often, clinical requests for information are organ oriented, but frequently it is necessary to examine an entire region to localize, identify and characterize suspected pathology. We have, therefore, divided the clinical discussion into regional anatomical areas; this satisfies the majority of clinical indications for study.

Clinical Ultrasonography of the Upper Abdomen

Transverse and longitudinal (sagittal) scans are obtained from the xiphoid to the level of the umbilicus at 2-cm intervals. When it is necessary to visualize a given structure more fully, the transducer may be oriented along oblique pathways.

LIVER

The liver can usually be studied to demonstrate its diaphragmatic aspect and the subhepatic margin with identification of individual lobes. Internally, parenchymal structures are represented as a fine stippling of echo sources, and larger ducts and vessels may be imaged as tubular branching or round sonolu-

Fig 3. – Hepatic metastases. **A,** longitudinal scan of the right lobe of a normal liver shows uniform hepatic architecture. **B,** a similar scan of a patient with pancreatic carcinoma contains many areas of high-intensity reflection from metastatic deposits. **C** is a transverse scan in which liver substance has been replaced by metastases whose low reflectance is best appreciated in the areas designated by arrows. k = kidney; s = spine.

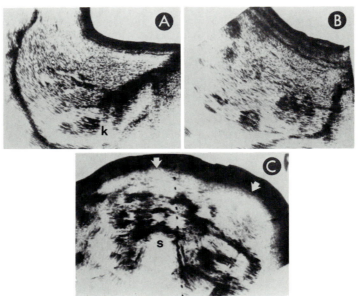

cent spaces. At the porta hepatis, large vessels entering the liver are seen as dense reflectors.

Diffuse disease processes, such as cirrhosis and extensive infiltrative metastases, alter the normal orderly appearance of the liver and change liver size. Cirrhosis may be detected by the high intensity of internal echoes, the presence of dilated intrahepatic portal radicles and splenomegaly resulting from portal hypertension.[5, 6]

Metastases, when focal and not diffusely replacing liver parenchyma, are identified as disparate echo sources, usually less dense than surrounding normal liver parenchyma. However, metastatic foci are occasionally seen as more intense reflectors than surrounding parenchyma, especially when highly vascularized, as are the metastases produced by colonic carcinoma or other adenocarcinomas (Fig 3, B). The response to irradiation or chemotherapy of metastatic liver disease can be followed by serial ultrasound examinations.[7]

In contradistinction to the usual focal metastasis, primary hepatic carcinoma is a source of accentuated echo pattern with indistinct margins that gradually blend with proximal normal parenchyma.[5]

Intrahepatic abscesses are well-marginated lesions containing no or few internal echo reflectors when viewed in the acute stage. The homogeneous echo-free depiction of the core of these abscesses results from the intrinsic lack of internal stroma. The image may resemble that of a simple cyst, but transmission of the beam will be reduced as the result of absorption by a homogeneously solid abscess. During the healing process, as organization occurs, internal echo patterns become evident, producing a complex pattern that may be difficult to differentiate from those of other solid space-occupying lesions (Fig 4).

Liver size is easily determined by ultrasound, and the location of the hepatic edge can be indelibly marked on the skin surface. Serial observations of the response to various therapies, such as portal decompression surgery, can be readily followed.[8] The potential also exists for quantitative hepatic volume determination from multiple cross-sectional scans.

Radionuclide liver scintiscans also provide information concerning liver size and parenchymal replacement. Isotope studies have been shown by Lomonaco et al. to be a more sensitive indicator of disease, but in their comparative study, ultrasound of-

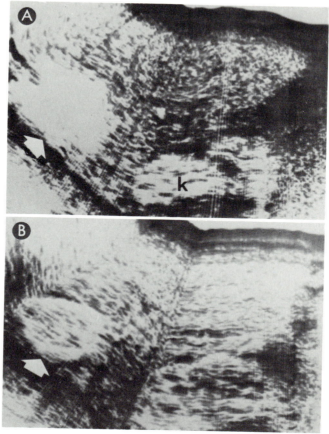

Fig 4. — Amebic abscess of the liver. The abscess cavity *(arrows)* lies posteriorly near the dome of the liver. In an early study **(A)** the cavity is echo-free but shows no potentiation of sonic energy behind it. Following medical therapy **(B)** the abscess has decreased significantly in size and presents evidence of organization, as indicated by its internal echo pattern. *k* = kidney.

fered fewer false positive diagnoses (15% vs 3%).[9] Definable space-occupying lesions are all depicted as foci of diminished activity by isotopic studies, but information concerning the internal architecture of lesions is lacking so that solid and fluid-filled lesions cannot be differentiated. Ultrasound, on the other hand, recognizes lesions of approximately the same size (1.5 – 2 cm) and not only confirms their presence but also details their internal composition. Therefore, the two examination modalities are complementary and are informationally additive.

GALLBLADDER

Oral cholecystography and intravenous cholangiography remain the most precise evaluative tools in the diagnosis of biliary tract disease. However, there are circumstances when such examinations are unrewarding. Hyperbilirubinemia, either as

Fig 5.—Cholelithiasis. In **A** the gallbladder is dilated, contains a single stone and shows dilatation of the cystic duct *(arrow)* as the result of an obstructing pancreatic carcinoma that is not included in this longitudinal section. **B,** mobility of the stone is demonstrated in a decubitus position. **C,** shadowing behind a stone is present in another patient studied transversely in the recumbent position.

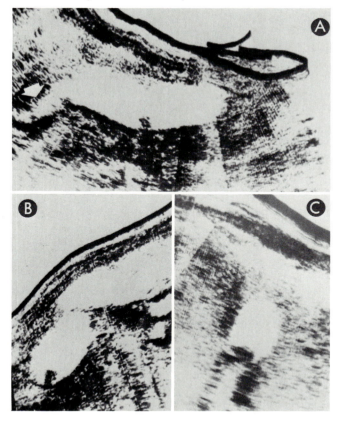

an absolute elevation or as an increasing index, often results in nonvisualization by either modality. Ultrasound, since it lacks dependence on gallbladder and liver function, offers an excellent opportunity to study the gallbladder.

The normal gallbladder is visualized as a well-defined structure lacking internal echo reflectors. With the patient fasting for 8–12 hours or on a fat-free diet for the same period, the normally distended gallbladder is easily located. Doust and

Fig 6. – Biliary tract obstruction. **A,** transverse section of the liver reveals a honeycombed appearance with several prominently dilated biliary ducts *(arrows).* A normalsized portal vein is shown crossing the midline and entering the liver. An enlarged gallbladder *(gb)* and distended proximal biliary radicles are viewed sagittally in **B.**

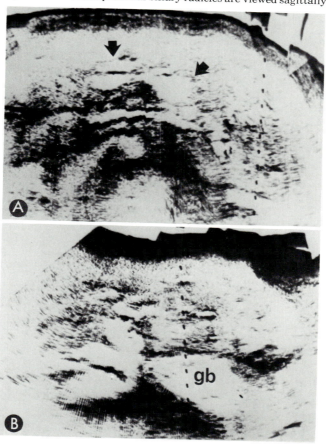

Maklad[10] were able to identify 92% of gallbladders, including both normal and pathologic organs.

Gallstones are shown as mobile intraluminal echo sources and must be sizable (greater than 0.5– 0.8 cm) if single;[11, 12] multiple stones are more easily imaged. Both calcified and uncalcified stones are strong reflectors of ultrasound, and shadowing distal to the stone is a common observation (Fig 5,C). A thickened gall-bladder wall can occasionally be seen.

Doust and Maklad were able to detect 80% of gallstones, while 72% were identified by Goldberg et al.[13] Radiographic accuracy in their study, combining plain and contrast radiography, was 89%.

Ultrasound offers a safe and rapid means of screening patients with painless jaundice to distinguish among hepatocellular dysfunction, obstruction due to calculus and obstruction due to carcinoma of the pancreas or bile ducts.

In hepatocellular jaundice, the gallbladder is either of normal size or is small, and the intrahepatic biliary ducts are not distended. The combination of these findings usually excludes obstruction as an etiology for the clinical jaundice. On the other hand, should common or hepatic duct obstruction be present, the intrahepatic biliary radicles will be distended with inspissated bile (Fig 6). Cystic duct stone impaction will lead to proximal cystic duct and gallbladder dilatation, and distal common duct calculus obstruction will dilate the entire system proximal to it. Pancreatic carcinoma, as a cause of common duct obstruction, will be manifest usually as a mass within the head of the pancreas.

It is recommended, therefore, that ultrasound be employed as the initial evaluative tool prior to examinations such as transhepatic cholangiography or endoscopic retrograde cholangiopancreatography. In many instances it may prove to be the only examination necessary prior to surgical intervention.

PANCREAS

The pancreas, one of the most elusive of all organs to visualize with any diagnostic modality, has been extensively studied with ultrasound. The results of this vigorous attempt[14-16] have led to a recognition of several of the pathologic states that occur within this complex glandular organ. Ultrasonic imaging of the pancreas is dependent on careful scanning techniques utilizing normal anatomical landmarks as reference areas. Identification of the superior mesenteric artery, for example, is extremely useful in locating the pancreas. This artery is seen either just posterior to the pancreas or as a vessel piercing it.

Since the pancreas is not encapsulated, it may be difficult to define its margins precisely. However, the gland itself is the source of a rather homogeneous, finely stippled echo pattern, which is normally of greater intensity than that of the liver. The contour of the pancreas, therefore, can be identified by the distribution of its characteristic echoes.

Fig 7. – Normal pancreas. **A,** midline longitudinal scan shows the pancreas *(arrow)* lying under the liver margin and anterior to the superior mesenteric artery, which branches from the aorta *(ao).* **B,** in a transverse scan the pancreas *(arrows)* is draped over the sonolucent oval image of the aorta and contains stippled echoes from its parenchyma.

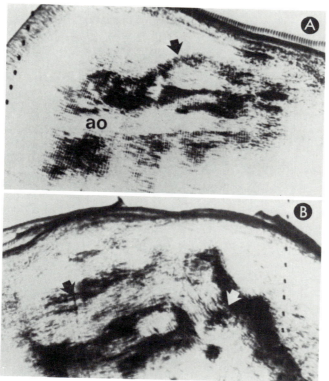

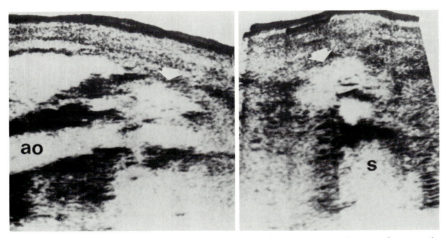

Fig 8. — Pancreatic edema. The arrows localize the pancreas in its usual preaortic position. The relatively high gain used in the transverse scan *(right)* emphasizes the sonolucent character of pancreatitis. *ao* = aorta; *s* = spine.

The normal pancreas has the appearance of an inverted U with a somewhat bulbous head and tail and a slender, tapered body. The pancreas is usually not transversely oriented, but lies rather in an oblique plane roughly paralleling the right costal margin (Fig 7).

In acute pancreatitis, the inflamed gland is enlarged and is considerably more sonolucent (echo-free) than normal. The usual internal reflectors become less prominent as a result of edema, which produces significant separation of the stromal content of the pancreas (Fig 8).

Pseudocysts of the pancreas can achieve rather impressive dimensions. Regardless of size, however, they are sonographically identified as sharply marginated sonolucent masses; they may contain solid or echo-dense components that represent floating cellular debris (Fig 9).[17]

Pancreatic carcinoma results in a mass of variable echo intensity, echo-dense in most instances, which distorts the pancreatic contour.[18] When the carcinoma lies in the head of the pancreas, distention of the gallbladder and intrahepatic ducts occurs and the inferior vena cava may show an impression on its anterior margin. Chronic inflammatory masses may mimic the findings of carcinoma and require histologic study (Fig 10).

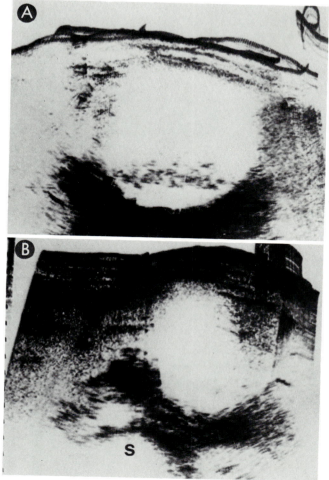

Fig 9. — Pancreatic pseudocyst. A huge sonolucent space lying to the right of the spine *(s)* is shown in longitudinal (**A**) and transverse (**B**) scans. Its fluid-filled nature is revealed by the marked increase of sound transmission posteriorly. Debris floating in the dependent portion of the pseudocyst is responsible for the echoes present within the cavity in **A**.

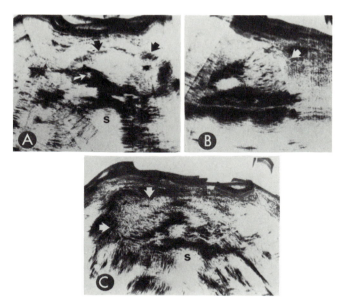

Fig 10. — Pancreatic masses. **A** and **B,** chronic inflammatory disease produced a mass in the head of the pancreas *(arrows).* A calcification is responsible for the strong echo source lying within the pancreas, under the arrow to the far right in **A.** The horizontal white arrow indicates the superior mesenteric artery in this transverse scan. **C,** a carcinoma of the tail of the pancreas *(arrows)* is shown in this transverse scan. *s* = spine.

Ultrasound has been shown to be a better screening tool than the myriad of radiologic, endoscopic and isotopic studies commonly employed. Superselective arteriography remains the best presurgical examination technique for diagnosis and planning of interventions. In many instances, confirmation of malignancy may be obtained with percutaneous needle aspiration biopsy of the pancreas[19] guided by ultrasound.

In addition to lesion detection, ultrasound can be employed as a staging modality by demonstrating the presence of hepatic or other local soft tissue metastases.

Spleen

The normal spleen is a sharply demarcated structure with a homogeneous, low-amplitude internal reflection pattern, usually lower in intensity than that of the liver. Stomach gas often blocks an anterior abdominal approach; however, the right lateral decubitus position usually makes the spleen more accessible to examination, as the spleen is interposed between the transducer and stomach gas.

Two different clinical questions can often be answered by ultrasound examination of the spleen. One is spleen size and volume, important in reticuloproliferative diseases as well as in hepatic disease (cirrhosis). Ninety-five percent of patients with liver disease were found by Koga and Morikawa[20] to have splenic enlargement. Serial ultrasound examination can be quite useful in monitoring the response to therapy.

The other clinical indication is splenic trauma. Seventy such patients were studied by Asher et al.[21] The results of 61 studies were verified as negative. There were 4 true positives, 4 false positives and 1 false negative result. These authors propose that the criteria for splenic injury include (1) splenic enlargement, (2) irregular contour, (3) change in contour with change in patient position, (4) progression in enlargement and (5) free peritoneal fluid.

It appears reasonable to conclude that patients whose hematologic indices remain stable following trauma and whose ultrasound studies give negative results probably do not have splenic disease requiring surgery.

Clinical Ultrasonography of the Pelvic Cavity

Structures lying within the pelvis that are amenable to ultrasound visualization include the urine-filled bladder, uterus, ovaries and prostate.

Patient bowel preparation is necessary to investigate this compartment since small-bowel and colonic gas will interfere with the study. Distention of the bladder is helpful for several reasons, and patients are requested to refrain from voiding for 4–6 hours preceding the examination.

BLADDER AND PROSTATE

Sonographically, the full bladder is the easiest organ to image.[22] Since it is essentially nothing more than a balloon filled with fluid, it is imaged as a well-defined structure lacking any normal internal reflectors. The walls are smooth and the con-

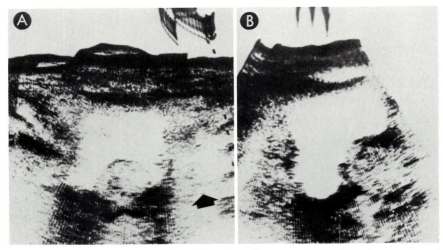

Fig 11.—Prostatic hypertrophy. The enlarged prostate domes into the sonolucent image of the bladder in transverse (**A**) and longitudinal (**B**) studies. A lymphomatous mass is also present *(arrow)* and deforms the contour of the bladder.

tour symmetrical. Pelvic masses extraneous to the bladder can be localized by their impression upon the bladder. Tumors or abscesses arising from adjacent structures, such as the colon, prostate (Fig 11), uterus or ovary, may erode through the bladder wall and be seen as an exophytic echo source within the normally echo-free bladder.

Similarly, ultrasound may prove quite useful in the staging of primary bladder cancer. Cystoscopy allows for direct visualization of tumor but cannot assess depth of penetration or direct tumor invasion beyond the bladder wall. Ultrasound can image not only the endoluminal component of tumor but also gross tumor extension outside the wall. Since the mode of therapy of bladder cancer is dependent on depth of penetration and extravesicular adhesion, ultrasound may yield considerable information regarding these enigmas.

In addition to tumor evaluation and staging, ultrasound offers a unique ability to visualize the bladder for suprapubic aspiration. Percussion of the bladder is useful, but ultrasound is precise and reliable. It is particularly useful in infants and small children where bladder volume may diminish precipitously and be unobserved.

The deep position of the prostate gland within the pelvis requires study through the distended bladder and a rather steep caudal transducer angulation.[23] The prime use of ultrasound is tumor staging in prostatic carcinoma, whereby extension of tumor into the bladder can be demonstrated.

UTERUS AND OVARIES

The gamut of indications for study of female reproductive organs ranges from identification of intrauterine devices to evaluation of uterine and ovarian masses. Frequently, it is the ultrasound examination that offers the first suggestion of the type and extent of neoplasm when a pelvic mass is present.

The uterus is a retrovesicular midline structure, pear-shaped, and containing a linear echo source arising from the coapted endometrial walls. Many intrauterine contraceptive[24] devices produce intense echo sources along the endometrial canal. When doubt exists regarding the location of such devices, ultrasound may be useful in demonstrating their intrauterine position.

Of the various causes of uterine enlargement, early pregnan-

Fig 12. – Uterus. The bladder *(bl)* forms a sonolucent window for imaging the uterus in longitudinal sections. **A,** myomas distort the uterine contour and produce typical internal echoes. **B,** an intrauterine contraceptive device is imaged as a strong reflector in the endometrial canal.

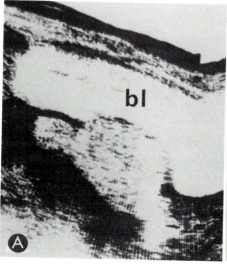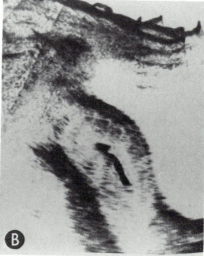

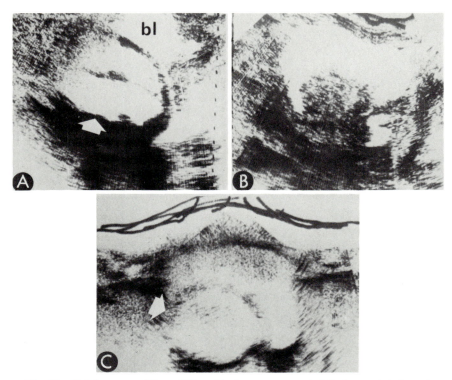

Fig 13. — Pelvic masses. Three different lesions are presented. In **A** a septated ovarian cystadenoma *(arrow)* lies behind the bladder *(bl)* and transmits sonic energy like a fluid-filled mass. In **B** the bladder contour is altered by an invading cystadenocarcinoma of the ovary, which results in an endoluminal exophytic mass. In **C** a pelvic abscess *(arrow)* displaces and deforms the bladder. **A** and **B** represent longitudinal scans, while **C** is a transverse section.

cy is best suited to ultrasonic evaluation.[25] The fluid-filled gestational sac is readily imaged along with the developing embryo. Leiomyomas and uterine carcinoma may enlarge and distort the contour of the uterus and produce echoes that indicate their solid nature (Fig 12). The presence of regional node enlargement may be useful in differentiating these ultrasonically similar conditions. Ovarian cysts and cystic teratomas are echo-free masses, though teratomas may contain either a nidus of dense echoes or multiple echo sources. Serous cystadenoma of the ovary is a multiseptated mass containing echo-free compart-

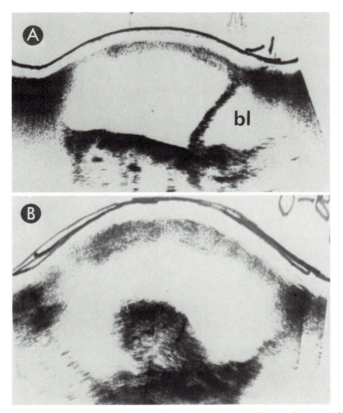

Fig 14.—Cystic lesions of the ovary. An enormous simple ovarian cyst is demonstrated in **A** in a longitudinal midline scan. **B,** a dense echo-producing mass in another large ovarian cyst identifies this lesion as a teratoma (transverse scan). *bl* = bladder.

ments not readily differentiated from serous cystadenocarcinoma (Figs 13 and 14).[26]

RENAL TRANSPLANTS

Ultrasound information gathered in patients with renal transplantation may be extremely useful.[27] Accurate measurement of renal size in the postoperative patient (following removal of surgical dressings) should be obtained as a baseline. Since the kidney is superficial and lies just beneath the skin, accurate measurement of size is possible. Serial evaluation or repeat study when indicated may help confirm early rejection when the kidney increases slightly or moderately in size. Urinoma or lymphocele is readily identified as an echo-free "cystic" mass, usually interposed between the transplanted kidney and the bladder. Because of the similarity in appearance, it is not possible to distinguish between them.

Clinical Ultrasonography of the Retroperitoneum

Aorta

The aorta is usually an easy structure to image with ultrasound, provided there is little interfering bowel gas.

Ideally, the entire course of the aorta from the level of the diaphragm to its bifurcation can be visualized.[28] In fact, several centimeters of each common iliac artery are usually also seen. Initial transverse scans of the upper abdomen will locate the course of the aorta, and subsequent sagittal transducer sweeps will depict its entire length. One-centimeter interval transverse sections characterize the aortic walls, whose outer transverse diameter should not exceed 25 mm.

Ectasia of the aorta is depicted as mild, diffuse enlargement frequently accompanied by tortuosity. Fusiform enlargement is not present and, characteristically, no intraluminal thrombus is seen (Fig 15).

Aneurysms of the aorta, whether fusiform or saccular, will be imaged as an area of divergent walls, variable in length. The length of such aneurysms can be measured and extension to the proximal iliac arteries evaluated. Involvement of the renal arteries is not easily perceived.

Birnholz[29] studied 22 patients with abdominal aortic aneurysms using ultrasound and isotope aortography. All aneurysms were visualized by ultrasound, and only 2 involved the renal arteries. Ultrasound measurement of transverse diameter was within 4 mm of actual size. Mulder, Winsberg et al.[30] performed ultrasound examinations on 115 patients with suspected aneurysm of the aorta. Fifty-four aneurysms were verified by arteriography, surgery or autopsy. In all cases, ultrasound gave the correct result.

Ultrasound also offers a unique visualization of the aortic

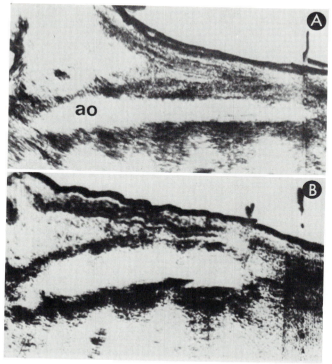

Fig 15. — Aortic ectasia. A normal aorta *(ao)* is presented in **A** for comparison with an ectatic aorta in **B**. Dilatation, lumen irregularity and strong echo sources arising in calcium deposits are characteristic.

walls, aortic lumen and periaortic tissue. Calcification of the walls, depicted by extremely dense curvilinear echoes, often accompanies aneurysmal dilatation. Of greater significance is visualization of intraluminal thrombus, extraluminal extravasation or dissection.

Thrombus is demonstrated as a "solid" tissue interposed between the aortic wall and the sonolucent lumen (Fig 16). Extraluminal extravasation produces a sonolucent space adjacent to the aorta. In the presence of dissection, the true and false lumens can be identified as sonolucent spaces separated by a thin moving echo source, the dissected intima.

Ultrasound aortography is thought by many, including Wheeler et al.,[31] to be of greater accuracy than clinical exami-

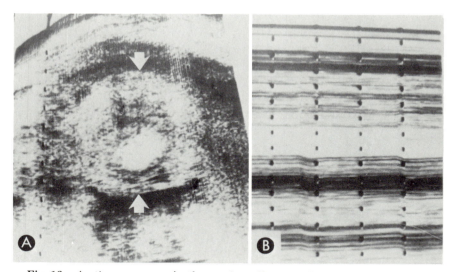

Fig 16.—Aortic aneurysm. **A,** the aortic walls are indicated by arrows and are separated from the sonolucent lumen by laminated thrombus. **B,** an M-mode recording made through the aneurysm at the plane of the arrows clearly reveals pulsatile movement of the luminal margins.

nation, plain radiography and contrast or isotope aortography. It provides accurate depiction of true aortic size, characterization of the aortic walls and assessment of aortic extravasation. Normal ultrasound aortography reliably excludes the presence of an abdominal aortic aneurysm.

INFERIOR VENA CAVA

After the aorta, the inferior vena cava is the most easily studied vascular abdominal structure. Its longitudinal path is usually within 4 cm of the midline, in the right hemiabdomen. This vessel is distinguished from the aorta by its gently diverging walls, its continuity with the right atrium and its significant change in caliber with the Valsalva maneuver.

Patients with hepatomegaly of unknown etiology may benefit from ultrasound venacavography. Unsuspected right heart disease results in engorgement of the vena cava so that dilatation occurs and no further enlargement can be produced by the Valsalva maneuver.[32]

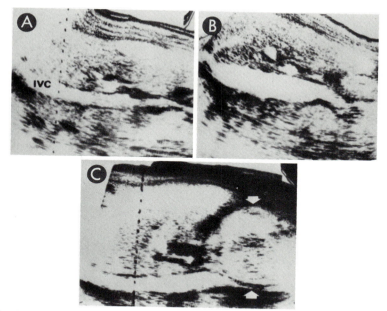

Fig 17.—Ultrasonic venacavography. The inferior vena cava *(IVC)* is shown at rest **(A)** and with the Valsalva maneuver **(B)** in the same normal subject. In **C,** vena caval compression results from a large, round mass *(arrows)* that deforms and narrows the lumen in a patient with metastases from a teratocarcinoma of the testes.

Extension of renal carcinoma into the vena cava has been demonstrated as an intraluminal mass partially filling the vessel.[33] Masses adjacent to the vena cava produce recognizable indentations, and frank compression or obstruction can be seen to explain edema of the lower extremities (Fig 17).[34]

LYMPH NODES

Ultrasound has found wide usage in the staging of malignancy through local tumor identification, size determination and recognition of possible spread. Ultrasound may also prove of utility in evaluating local and distant lymphatic extension of malignancy.

Lymph nodes of normal size are not detectable by ultrasonography. However, when they exceed approximately 2 cm in size, they may be demonstrated as relatively echo-free, lobular masses lying in the distribution of lymphatic chains.[28]

In specific malignancies, such as those arising in the ovaries, testicles, kidneys and high uterine body, the first station lymph node compartment is at the renal pedicle and secondary nodes are found within the mid- and superior aortic lymph node chains. Lower extremity lymphography often inadequately fills superior aortic lymph nodes and leads to difficulty in interpretation. Ultrasound has been valuable in examining the very areas difficult to study by other means. We have encountered enlarged lymph nodes within the superior aortic chain by means of ultrasound; results have been verified by surgery when lymphograms were negative.

Though lymphography remains the most reliable diagnostic tool for demonstration of lymphatic node enlargement, ultrasound offers a complementary examination modality that may discover otherwise inaccessible adenopathy.

KIDNEY

The kidneys are most easily studied with the patient in the prone position. By obliquing the transducer sweep to approximate the longitudinal axis of the psoas muscles, the long axis of both kidneys can be easily depicted. Serial transverse scans, made at 1-cm intervals, complete anatomical imaging. The decubitus position has been useful to expose the kidney for examination by displacing it away from interfering ribs and transverse processes, especially in upper pole disease.

Normally, the kidney is oblong or bean-shaped and is sharply marginated. While the capsule cannot be perceived directly, it forms a clean boundary separating the kidney from perirenal fat. Typically, the internal structure is homogeneously echo-producing peripherally and within this background of low-amplitude echoes, dense, longitudinally oriented echo reflectors are present and represent the collecting system and peripelvic structures (see Fig 19, A).

Obstructive uropathy is manifested by circular echo-free areas representing caliectasis with a central, larger anechoic space, the renal pelvis.[35]

In contradistinction to hydronephrosis, where the echo-free obstructed calixes and pelves are central within the kidney, polycystic kidneys are identified by their contour deformation as

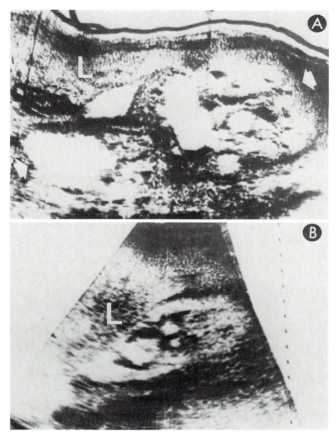

Fig 18. – Polycystic kidney. **A,** an enormous polycystic kidney *(arrows)* extends from under the liver *(L)* to the anterior abdominal wall. Kidney contour is markedly deformed, and renal parenchyma is replaced by multiple, sonolucent, cystic spaces of various sizes. **B,** in moderate hydronephrosis, kidney contour and parenchyma are preserved while dilated collecting structures produce centrally placed sonolucent rings. Both studies are longitudinally oriented.

well as by their enlargement and demonstration of circular cystic spaces distributed throughout the kidney (Fig 18).[36]

Renal masses greater than 2 cm are readily identifiable. Confirmation of the solid or cystic nature of such masses can be achieved with great rapidity and accuracy. A cyst typically is well circumscribed, lacks internal echo reflectors and transmits sound well. Cyst puncture, using either ultrasound or fluoroscopy for localization and guidance, allows aspiration and instillation of a radiopaque contrast agent. Clear, straw-colored fluid, negative cytology and a smooth internal contour virtually exclude the presence of carcinoma.

Renal carcinomas are ultrasonically typified by the presence of a mass usually deforming the renal contour, containing dense internal reflectors and frequently lacking a circumscribed periphery. Occasionally, a solid tumor with a central necrotic core will be sonolucent internally. However, such masses lack totally smooth internal margins and they will, in addition, usually lack good transmission of the sound beam beyond the posterior wall of the lesion (Fig 19).[37-39]

Fig 19.—Renal mass lesions (longitudinal scans). **A,** the normal kidney is bean-shaped, smoothly marginated and contains dense central echoes arising from the collecting system and hilar structures. **B,** solid mass lesions *(arrows)* deform the kidney contour, contain echoes and transmit sound poorly. **C,** renal cysts also deform contour but are sonolucent internally, have sharply demarcated walls and show augmented sound transmission.

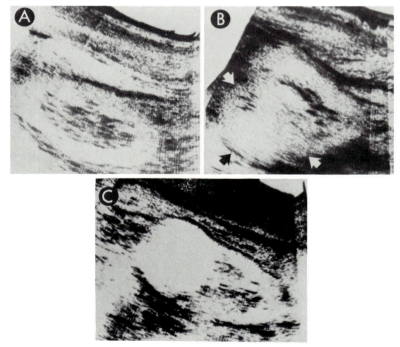

Other solid lesions of the kidney may mimic primary carcinoma. Of these, hamartomas and xanthogranulomatous pyelonephritic masses can be confused with malignancy. Renal abscesses usually contain fewer stromal elements and are therefore less echo-dense than tumors. Hematomas are frequently sub- or extracapsular in position and when studied in the acute state lack internal echo. However, they will absorb some energy and thereby transmit less beyond the mass. Organizing hematomas theoretically may mimic carcinoma. The history of the patient is of extreme use in categorizing these nonmalignant masses. Histories of tuberous sclerosis, recent trauma or pyelonephritis must be considered when interpreting the ultrasound image.

Those patients harboring either solid renal masses or lesions of indeterminate internal character deserve selective renal arteriography as the next sequential evaluative examination following ultrasound.

Biopsy of the kidney, a frequently performed procedure, utilized fluoroscopic control and urographic contrast agent injection for localization of the kidney prior to the advent of ultrasound. With ultrasound, localization of the kidney for biopsy can be performed simply, accurately and without the need for ionizing radiation or a contrast agent.[40] The patient is placed, prone, in the biopsy position with a wedge-shaped bolster under the midabdomen to support the kidney and restrain its mobility. Longitudinal sections of the kidney are obtained and the inferior pole position marked on the patient's skin surface. In addition, a transverse section is taken to identify the central portion of the lower pole. This localization is performed with the patient in full expiration. The depth of the lower pole of the kidney can easily and accurately be determined, enabling precise biopsy. Precise identification of the position of the lower pole of the kidney avoids the complications that have been described with renal biopsy.

Imaging the pediatric patient with kidney disease has been rewarding.[41] Within the immediate neonatal period, polycystic kidney can be identified as the source of an intra-abdominal palpable mass. Wilms' tumors of childhood contain a recognizable pattern, frequently quite similar to primary renal carcinoma, allowing for identification and recognition; ultrasound may yield information relative to the degree of invasion beyond the renal confine as well as the presence of tumor within the contralateral kidney.[42]

Urographic nonvisualization of a kidney in a child requires further study. Retrograde pyelography and cystography can be performed in an attempt to identify a ureteral orifice within the bladder. Ultrasound of the retroperitoneum in these children may demonstrate severe hydronephrosis, agenesis or hypoplasia as a cause of nonvisualization.

ADRENAL GLANDS

The normal adrenal glands are only occasionally viewed with ultrasound. Their size and position makes routine visualization difficult. However, ultrasound is useful under two circumstances when dealing with adrenal masses. First, and most commonly, ultrasound may be the tool by which one can relate a palpable mass to its adrenal origin. Secondly, categorizing the lesion as cystic or solid is helpful in directing further study of the pa-

Fig 20. — Splenic fossa abscess. An abscess *(arrow)* following splenectomy contains some debris and lies adjacent to the upper pole of the kidney. A 2d sonolucent space adjacent to the abscess represents loculated pleural fluid in the posterior sulcus.

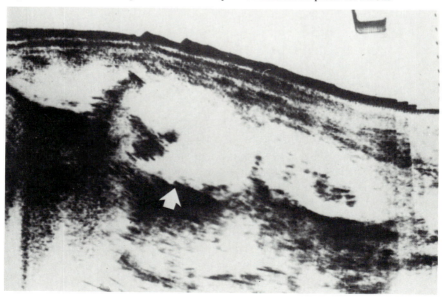

tient.[43] In children the presence of neuroblastoma, when adrenal in location, can be studied without discomfort to the patient.

NONVISCERAL MASSES

Abscesses, primary retroperitoneal tumors and hematomas deform the retroperitoneal space (Fig 20).[44] They may be sonolucent or dense, depending on their nature. Psoas abscesses are typified by asymmetry of the psoas contours, best demonstrated in transverse scans.

Other Applications

THE DISTENDED ABDOMEN

Distention and a taut abdomen often serve as barriers to adequate physical examination. The problem of discriminating among intra-abdominal mass, organomegaly and ascites may be difficult. In addition, it is frequently impossible to ascribe the origin of a suspected abdominal mass to a given viscus.

Ascites presents as a halo of echo-free fluid in which floating bowel can be seen. There is usually great distortion of intra-abdominal contents, presumably as a result of the weight of the fluid and the displacement of structures. When necessary, loculated collections of fluid can be identified and localized for aspiration (Fig 21).[45]

Ultrasound can provide useful diagnostic information regarding the presence, location and size of intra-abdominal abscesses in the pre- or postsurgical period (see Fig 13, C).[46] Though gaseous distention of bowel accompanying abscesses may make their identification difficult, the yield is sufficiently high to justify the use of ultrasound in all suspected cases.

The suspicion of a mass often results in exhaustive clinical and surgical diagnostic procedures. Barium upper and lower gastrointestinal studies, urography, arteriography and laparotomy are frequently performed. The differential diagnosis is long, and the patient work-up is frequently exhaustive, exhausting and expensive. An excellent screening procedure for these patients is abdominal and retroperitoneal ultrasound. If this is carefully performed, many of the diagnostic possibilities can be excluded, and frequently precise diagnosis is possible (Figs 22

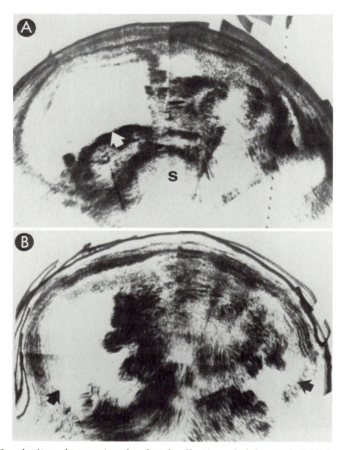

Fig 21. — Ascites. **A,** massive, loculated collection of abdominal fluid *(arrow)* in a patient with diffuse abdominal carcinomatosis. **B,** benign effusions characteristically are bilateral *(arrows)*, and bowel is shown floating freely in the fluid. *s* = spine.

and 23). Confirmation of the pathologic state can then be undertaken logically and rapidly.

Radiation Therapy Planning

With the aid of ultrasound the position of malignant lesions and adjacent normal structures can be mapped upon the patient's surface for optimization of radiation therapy planning.

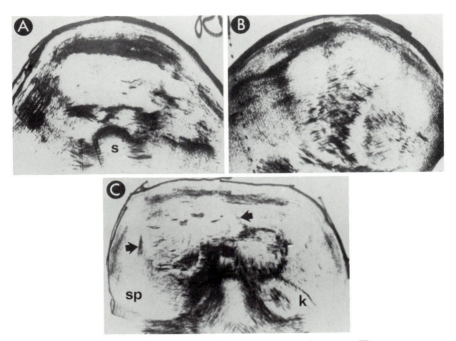

Fig 22. – Ultrasonic characterization of large abdominal masses. Three transverse scans in different patients demonstrate tumor characteristics and anatomical relationships. **A** depicts typical matted lymphomatous nodes in the preaortic chain. Sonolucency without enhanced transmission indicates a solid, homogeneous internal composition. **B,** malignant mesenchymoma is imaged as a multilobulated mass that contains a complex pattern of weak and strong reflectors, indicating the complex nature of the tumor. In **C,** the arrows delineate a large gastric lymphosarcoma in which strong internal echoes represent interfaces produced by enlarged gastric rugae. A mass of nodal metastases is seen anterior to the kidney *(k)*. An enlarged spleen *(sp)* and splenic vein are demonstrated.

The radiotherapist can, therefore, deliver optimal tumor doses while sparing radiosensitive normal structures.[47]

A logical extension of tumor localization is tumor response monitoring. A tumor may be sequentially studied to assess therapeutic response to palliative surgery, chemotherapy or radiation therapy.[48]

PERCUTANEOUS BIOPSY

Fundamental to the treatment of malignancy is rapid and reliable histologic verification of disease. In the past, this usually

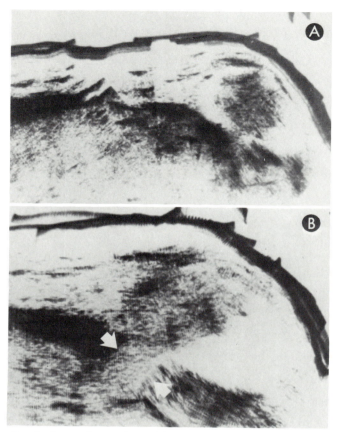

Fig 23. — Inguinal mass in a patient with suspected metastatic carcinoma. **A,** peripherally sonolucent, subcutaneous mass contains indications of mixed tissue composition. **B,** magnified study at a slightly different plane reveals a discontinuity in the abdominal wall through which components of the mass are noted to pass *(arrows)*. At surgery, an inguinal hernia containing bowel and mesentery was found, with focal metastatic deposits in the mesentery from a squamous carcinoma arising in an old appendectomy scar.

required surgical intervention. Recently, the need for such diagnostic surgery has diminished. For example, diagnostic thoracotomy is used only occasionally now that the concept of percutaneous pulmonary biopsy has been accepted. Similarly, percutaneous abdominal biopsy has opened a new vista of diagnosis. A 23-gauge stainless steel needle can be introduced into almost any mass or viscus safely. The aspirate usually yields sufficient cellular material for diagnostic cytopathologic appraisal. Information obtained by ultrasound has been instrumental in localizing suspicious masses for biopsy as well as for observing the path of the needle during the procedure. With this technique, percutaneous pancreatic biopsy has been done safely, and totally without morbidity at European and American institutions.[49, 50] The passage of the fine needle through bowel and liver has not resulted in any significant complications.

Ultrasound and X-Ray Computerized Tomographic Imaging

The emergence of computerized x-ray reconstruction systems for abdominal imaging provides another modality by which cross-sectional images of the abdomen may be obtained.[51] The future role of computerized tomographic (CT) scanning in respect to ultrasound in patient care is yet to be defined and will await the development of the unexploited potential of both. Each technique has advantages and disadvantages but, most importantly, each derives its image on a different physical basis so that the information obtained differs.

Ultrasound detects variations in the mechanical properties of materials so that individual tissues are imaged according to their density and the speed of sound in specific tissues, as well as energy attenuation, which represents a complex of absorption, reflection and scattering. On the other hand, CT scanning recognizes only differences in x-ray absorption, which is dependent on tissue density.

Ultrasound has certain advantages when these two imaging systems are compared. Soft tissue contrast is produced as the result of the unique interaction between sonic energy and the mechanical properties of tissues so that organ architecture and major blood vessels are imaged without contrast injections. Cystic and solid masses can be distinguished relatively easily. The ultrasound examination format permits imaging in longitudinal, transverse and oblique planes. Motion can be faithfully recorded and does not introduce artifacts, which alter the information content of the total image, as in CT scanning. Compact and portable instrumentation is available so that every form of ultrasonic examination can now be performed at the bedside with commercially available devices. Equipment is relatively inexpensive and can be purchased at a small fraction of the cost of CT scanners ($50,000 vs $500,000). Ultrasound images can be inspected and evaluated as they are produced, so that instrument setting, examination planes or minor physiologic interventions such as the Valsalva maneuver can be applied for enhancement of the value of the examination. The ultrasonic signal contains a large, untapped reservoir of information whose eventual utilization should provide us with more precise characterization of tissues in the future. Signal frequency and phase are examples of parameters under investigation and are expected to provide additional tissue-differentiating features for optimal representation of structures and disease processes.

There are some clear advantages in the CT scanning process, however. Bone and gas, which represent barriers through which the ultrasonic beam does not pass in adequate amounts for imaging, represent no significant problem and, in fact, may provide valuable anatomical landmarks. Since CT scans are automated, they can be produced by operators less skilled than those required for ultrasonic imaging. Also, the tonal quality of CT scans corresponds exactly to that of conventional radiologic images, so that surgeons and radiologists feel "at home" and are not required to learn new image interpretation parameters. Radiologic contrast agents are available to provide changes in the imaging parameters of solid organs. Furthermore, CT scanners are capable of presenting the image in a digital readout, which allows quantitation of tissue density characteristics. The recent application of computers to ultrasonic imaging is expected to produce this same capability.

Ultrasound and CT will undoubtedly play complementary roles in abdominal structure imaging. Because of relatively low cost, the avoidance of ionizing radiation and the special imaging capabilities of ultrasonic energy, the ultrasound examination represents the ideal modality for the initial evaluation of patients with abdominal diseases. However, if the ultrasonic examination is complicated by the presence of bowel gas or presents incomplete information, CT scans may be applied in planes designated by the ultrasonic study for further investigation.

Future ultrasonic images may well differ considerably from those of today. Tissue characterization may be significantly enhanced for more precise differentiation of normal and abnormal conditions. Blood flow patterns, imaged by developing Doppler techniques,[52] may be used for evaluation of organ blood supply. Three-dimensional displays may be made by ultrasonic holography[53] or by computer reconstruction from multiple planar images.[54] Scattered, as well as transmitted, ultrasonic energy may also be incorporated to enhance tissue characterization.

The Future

In less than a decade, modern ultrasound has emerged and been developed as a reliable clinical diagnostic modality. It remains without peer in the vast clinical armamentarium in its ability to image abdominal anatomy and pathology safely, rapidly and inexpensively.

The success of this clinical tool is based upon its unique ability to image without ionizing radiation and by different physical principles than those used in other diagnostic methods, thus allowing for realization of information not otherwise easily obtained.

The future of abdominal ultrasound is the predictable extraction of more clinical information than is now available. Three-dimensional, holographic and computerized imaging processes are currently being explored, and their practical clinical applications are forthcoming, thus assuring clinical ultrasound imaging a firm and bright future.

REFERENCES

1. Howry, D. H.: A brief atlas of diagnostic ultrasonic radiologic results, Radiol. Clin. North Am. 3:433, 1965.
2. Holmes, J. H., and Howry, D. H.: Ultrasonic diagnosis of abdominal diseases, Am. J. Dig. Dis. 8:12, 1963.
3. Leopold, G. R., and Asher, W. M.: *Fundamentals of Abdominal and Pelvic Ultrasonography* (Philadelphia: W. B. Saunders Company, 1975).
4. King, D. L. (ed.): *Diagnostic Ultrasound* (St. Louis: C. V. Mosby Company, 1974).
5. Hebert, G., and Gelinas, C.: Hepatic echography, Am. J. Roentgenol. Radium Ther. Nucl. Med. 125:51, 1975.
6. Ross, F. G. M.: Ultrasound in the diagnosis of liver disease, Proc. R. Soc. Med. 67:5, 1974.
7. Pritchard, J. H., Winston, M. A., Berger, H. G., and Blahd, W. H.: Diagnosis of focal hepatic lesions: Combined radioisotope and ultrasound techniques, J.A.M.A. 229:1463, 1974.
8. Rasmussen, S. N., Kardel, T., and Jörgensen, B. J.: Liver volume estimated by ultrasonic scanning before and after portal decompression surgery, Scand. J. Gastroenterol. 10:25, 1975.

JOHN J. CRANLEY

TABLE 1.—SOURCES OF
ARTERIAL EMBOLI IN 405
OPERATIVE PATIENTS

Heart	376 (93%)
Abdominal aortic aneurysm	3
Plastic valve	1
Unknown	25*

*Possibly some of these were of atheromatous origin.

TABLE 2.—CARDIAC STATUS IN
405 PATIENTS TREATED BY
ARTERIAL EMBOLECTOMY

Arteriosclerotic heart disease	253 (62%)
Myocardial infarct	77 (18%)
Rheumatic heart disease	48 (12%)
Atrial fibrillation	356 (90%)

TABLE 3.—INCIDENCE OF RHEUMATIC HEART
DISEASE IN 493 PATIENTS WITH
ARTERIAL EMBOLUS

YEARS	NO. PATIENTS	NO. WITH RHEUMATIC HEART DISEASE
1953–61*	141	38 (27%)
1962–76	352	21 (6%)

*All our data are divided into 2 series, pre- and post-Fogarty embolectomy catheter. The catheter became available in March 1962.

treatment of the primary disease (Table 3). The frequency of emboli due to mitral stenosis has decreased steadily in our experience. Even though the etiology has changed, in 456 embolectomies it was found that emboli continued to lodge in the same sites, 11% in the upper extremities and 89% in the aorta and infra-aortic arteries, most (54%) lodging in the femoral artery. Other vascular surgeons report similar data.

PATHOLOGY

The basic pathology is sudden occlusion of a major artery by the embolus. This sudden impaction results in reduction in distal flow and precipitates a rapidly propagating thrombus. The basic determinant of the outcome is not the embolus but the progressive occlusion of all the important collateral channels as the thrombus propagates distally. Distal thrombosis may not occur in the presence of concurrent liver disease or with early administration of anticoagulant agents, or occasionally for some unknown reason. Survival of the affected limb is possible without treatment, but is not predictable. The first objective is prevention of distal thrombosis. This is best accomplished by giving heparin once the diagnosis is made, regardless of whether or not surgical intervention is planned.

"Arterial spasm." – The smaller caliber of the artery distal to an embolus is the result of normal vasomotor tone in an artery whose intraluminal pressure has been reduced. It is not related to arterial spasm.[5]

DIAGNOSIS

HISTORY. – Sudden onset is the most important fact in the history. A conscious patient can document the moment of onset of symptoms. He may describe sudden pain or numbness. If he is asleep, the onset of symptoms will awaken him. A history of sudden onset helps the clinician distinguish between embolism and acute arterial thrombosis, which has a more insidious onset. The differential diagnosis was of less importance formerly than now, when embolectomy is routinely feasible.

If the embolus is lodged in the femoral artery or proximally, the leg subsequently becomes cold, numb and finally anesthetic. If the site of lodgment is the popliteal artery or an artery of the upper extremity, the patient may notice gradual relief of symptoms some hours after lodgment as collateral circulation begins to supply blood distal to the area of obstruction.

PHYSICAL EXAMINATION. – The examining physician immediately notices the lemon-yellow color of the skin of the extremity. This is diagnostic of total arterial ischemia to the skin. Comparison of the limbs will demonstrate uni- or bilateral occlusion. When bilateral, the skin color is still perceptibly abnormal. The level at which the pulse disappears indicates the site of occlusion. The embolus is present at the bifurcation or below the point of highest palpable pulse. Sudden arterial ischemia with absence of pulses is highly suggestive of arterial embolus. Mottling, coldness and hypesthesia confirm the diagnosis. Attempts to dorsiflex the foot passively help in the detection of rigor mortis of the calf muscles. Minimal rigor is not a contraindication to embolectomy, but if rigor is several hours old and one cannot dorsiflex the foot, the leg is beyond salvage.

Further diagnostic tests are not essential. Arteriography is not justified unless doubt exists. Arteriographic delineation of an embolus is usually clearly distinct from that of obliterative arterial disease with superimposed acute thrombosis. An electrocardiogram can document the presence of atrial fibrillation.

Differential Diagnosis

Acute arterial thrombosis. — The patient with arterial embolus describes the first symptom as sudden pain. In acute thrombosis, the first symptom is numbness. The patient may use the word "sudden" probably not in the sense of "instantaneous" but to describe a symptom extending over a relatively short period, perhaps several hours. On further questioning, he will qualify the symptom as a gradual loss of feeling. Typically, he may have awakened from sleep or arisen from a chair to discover the extremity had become numb. Pain, if present, develops later. In summary, sudden onset of pain is highly indicative of arterial embolism, and gradual numbness indicates acute thrombosis.

Dissecting aortic aneurysm. — Typically, with dissection of the aorta, the patient experiences interscapular pain that radiates down the back. However, the confused or sedated patient may complain only of pain and numbness of his extremity, which symptoms suggest an iliac or femoral artery embolus. We were misled by the first of 3 such patients presenting with absent pulse and acute ischemia of the limb. When we explored for presumed left common iliac embolus, the artery was found to be entirely normal but not pulsating. Arteriotomy showed no clots, only very sluggish blood flow. Autopsy showed that the normal-appearing artery was in reality a total dissection. Occluded by pressure, the true lumen occupied one small segment of the vessel.[5]

Treatment

Heparin. — Heparin is administered as soon as the diagnosis is made to reduce distal thrombosis. It is frequently recommend-

TABLE 4. – OPERATIVE RESULTS RELATED TO SITE OF LODGMENT IN 304 EMBOLECTOMIES WITH CATHETER TECHNIQUE, 1962–76

ARTERY	NO.	% IMPROVED
Axillary	14	100
Brachial	24	96
Aorta	27	97
Iliac	64	94
Femoral	164	93
Popliteal	11	100

ed on the telephone to the referring physician. If the operation can be performed before heparin has lost its effectiveness, the heparin can easily be neutralized by protamine. This is usually not necessary.

EMBOLECTOMY. – The catheter technique is the treatment of choice (Table 4). The time interval between lodgment and removal of the embolus is not the major criterion of operability. If the extremity is viable, it is still possible and desirable to remove the embolus. Embolectomy undertaken 36–72 hours after lodgment has been almost uniformly successful. This paradox rests on the fact that the rate of progression of distal thrombosis varies from individual to individual. In the limb that survives 36–72 hours, distal thrombosis is slow or absent. At times this is due to the fact that the patient is on anticoagulant therapy. Nonoperative treatment of such a patient is not advised since the extremity may become totally ischemic very slowly over a period of a week or two, requiring subsequent amputation. On the other hand, some patients have rigor and other signs of irreversible ischemia within 6–12 hours after lodgment of the embolus. Once rigor is fixed, it is useless to attempt revascularization.

OPERATIVE TECHNIQUE. – Since March 9, 1962,[2] we have not opened the abdomen to remove an aortic or iliac embolus. These have been removed by the inflatable catheter technique through a femoral arteriotomy (Fig 2). Most popliteal emboli have been removed through a similar incision. Some have been extracted through an incision on the medial aspect of the upper third of the leg. Occasionally, more distal exposure may be necessary to clean out the anterior and posterior tibial arteries at the ankle. The catheter technique is simple and safe and can be used in critically ill patients.

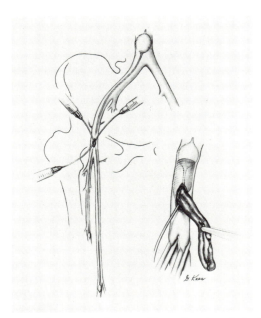

Fig 2.—Catheter embolectomy technique. (From Cranley, J. J.: *Vascular Surgery*, Vol. I, *Peripheral Arterial Diseases* [Hagerstown, Md.: Harper & Row, 1972], chapter 3, p. 102. Used by permission.)

Emboli to upper extremity arteries, formerly treated conservatively, are now treated surgically. Conservative treatment resulted in limb salvage in most instances. Today, however, full restoration of function is the criterion of success.

DISTAL DISCONTINUOUS CLOT. — In the past, brisk back bleeding after embolectomy was erroneously assumed to demonstrate the patency of the distal arterial tree. Surgeons failed to recognize that the artery might be blocked at some distance below the operative site and that backflow was through more proximal collateral channels. The inflatable catheter, inserted distally on completion of embolectomy, proved that distal noncontiguous soft clot was present. At the same time that we were discovering the existence of distal discontinuous clot through the use of the inflatable catheter, the same phenomenon was demonstrated by operative arteriograms following embolectomy by Spencer and Eiseman.[6]

POSTOPERATIVE ANTICOAGULANT THERAPY. — Long-term anti-

coagulant therapy has not been universally endorsed by internists. Many report that patients with chronic atrial fibrillation
present for 20 and more years have not experienced a major
embolus. Our early experience convinced us that once a major
arterial embolus had occurred, the incidence of a 2d embolism
was significantly higher. Therefore, we have recommended that
anticoagulation be continued indefinitely following one major
arterial embolism, unless the patient's cardiac rhythm is restored to normal. Even with prophylaxis, the recurrence rate for
405 patients is just under 6%. This may be an understatement,
because, although 4 instances of fatal embolism to the brain and
8 episodes of mesenteric occlusion have been documented, it is
probable that others have occurred and were not diagnosed.

The fundamental principles of management of a major arterial embolus, then, still include: (1) prevention of distal thrombosis by the immediate use of heparin; (2) early removal of the
embolus; (3) prevention of recurrent emboli by postoperative
anticoagulant therapy for an indefinite time.

LIMB NECROSIS. — This term includes amputated extremities
and those which were irreversibly ischemic at the time of the
patient's death. Prior to the inflatable catheter, the rate in our
series was 20.7% of 152 operated limbs and, with the use of the
catheter, 6% of 304 extremities.

MORTALITY AND SURVIVAL

Survival has been significantly improved since the use of the
inflatable catheter (Table 5). Heart failure continues to be the
chief cause of death (Table 6), although the incidence has
dropped from 15% of 133 patients before the catheter was available to 10% of 302 patients treated since 1962.

TABLE 5.—OPERATIVE RESULTS IN 405 PATIENTS

	WITHOUT CATHETER NO.	%	WITH CATHETER NO.	%
Survived, improved	79	59.5	210	79
Survived, with amputation	8	6.0	6*	2
Death in 30 days	46	34.5	56	20

*Three other patients had amputation prior to death.

TABLE 6. – CAUSES OF DEATH IN
30 DAYS IN 102 PATIENTS OF 405
UNDERGOING ARTERIAL
EMBOLECTOMY, 1953 – 76

CAUSES OF DEATH	NO. PATIENTS
Heart failure	48
Myocardial infarct	8
Cerebrovascular accident	8
Multiple emboli	5
Pulmonary embolus	4
Miscellaneous	29
Total	102 (25%)

ARTERIAL EMBOLI TO THE VISCERA

Recovery from embolectomy is often complicated by further emboli to the visceral circulation. Independent visceral embolization frequently remains occult and is discovered only at autopsy. Premortem diagnosis has occasionally been reported when emboli lodge in the superior mesenteric artery. The first successful extraction was reported in 1951.[7] The incidence of restoration of the mesenteric circulation following embolectomy continues relatively low.

Sudden onset of severe abdominal pain in a fibrillating patient or one who has had a recent embolectomy should be an indication for early surgical exploration. The outcome of mesenteric vascular occlusion is determined first and foremost by its duration. Waiting for signs of peritonitis reduces the chances of successful extraction. The treatment of choice is exploration and embolectomy by the catheter technique, followed by re-exploration of the operative site the following day, if there is any doubt of the normalcy of the bowel.[8] Rarely, a superior mesenteric arteriogram may be helpful. Anticoagulant therapy should begin 6 – 12 hours postoperatively and continue indefinitely.

Renal artery emboli. – When the site of lodgment is the renal artery, the prognosis is most grave. The diagnosis is difficult. If, however, it is made, embolectomy is indicated.

Arteriogenic Emboli

Emboli that originate in the wall or lumen of an artery and lodge at a point of narrowing in the distal arterial tree are included under the term "arteriogenic." Such emboli are either fibrinous or atheromatous in nature. If fibrinous, the material may be the entire plaque or, more frequently, a portion of the plaque.

ATHEROEMBOLI. — It has been suggested that larger atheromatous emboli, resulting from dislodgment of one or several major plaques, should be called atheroemboli.[9] Such emboli are known to attain sufficient size to occlude a major systemic artery and to cause clinically apparent major dysfunction of the affected organ.

CHOLESTEROL EMBOLI. — The smaller emboli, high in crystalline content and the product of erosion of atheromatous plaques, are sometimes referred to as cholesterol emboli.[9] Flory[10] preferred the term "erosion" to "ulceration," since the lesions are not produced by an inflammatory process and have no etiologic or histologic resemblance to ulcers. They are debris carried away from plaques by the bloodstream. Erosion of the intimal surface of atheromatous plaques is commonly seen in arteries with advanced arteriosclerosis.[10]

HISTORICAL REVIEW

The phenomenon of atheromatous embolus was mentioned for the first time in 1862 by Panum in his discussion of Dahleruf and Fenger's report of a fatal ruptured atheroma in the coronary artery of the famous Danish sculptor Thorwaldsen.[11] Soft atheromatous material, considered to have embolized from the proximal ulcerated area, filled the lumen of the artery distal to the lesion. In 1896 Doch[12] described the first case in American literature, also a coronary occlusion; the patient died from multiple cholesterol-rich emboli. In early 20th-century textbooks atheromatous embolization was regarded as a curiosity. It remained for Flory to recognize the pathologic significance of arterial occlusions produced by emboli from eroded aortic atheromatous plaques in the small and medium-sized arteries in the kidneys, spleen, pancreas and thyroid.[10, 13] These arteries measured from 55 to 900μ in diameter. The arterial lumen revealed empty space in the shape of cholesterol crystals (the cholesterol being dissolved out by the usual microscopic preparation) partly surrounded by foreign-body giant cells. The latter finding suggested that emboli containing large cholesterol crystals had lodged in the arterial wall of such vessels and undergone organization. Independently in 1947 Meyer published a classic description of cholesterol emboli and the reactions associated with their lodgment in the arterial walls of vessels ranging in size from 150 to 200μ[14]. The process of embolization and reaction results in obliteration of the lumen.

ARTERIAL ORIGIN OF ATHEROEMBOLI. — Embolization to the femoral artery of a large arterial plaque presumed to come from the aorta was reported in 1952.[15] Embolectomy was successful. The embolus was described as a large irregular calcareous mass, not adherent to the intima, that measured $1 \times 0.7 \times 0.5$ cm. At its proximal end was an adherent fresh clot approximately 1 cm long. The wall of the femoral artery was not sclerotic, and the intima was smooth. The pathologic findings were compatible with those of an embolus consisting of a detached calcific arterial plaque.

EMBOLIZATION TO THE VISCERA. — Thurlbeck and Castleman reported atheroemboli to the kidneys after aortic surgery.[16] In their autopsy studies of patients succumbing after aneurysmectomy or direct arterial surgery for arteriosclerosis of the abdominal aorta with occlusion, 17 (77.3%) of 22 patients had acute embolization of atheromatous material to the kidneys. Four patients had multiple renal emboli and died in uremia. In the control group of nonoperative patients, embolization to the kidneys of atheromatous material from the aorta was found in 13 (31%) of 42 patients with large aneurysms and in 6 (28%) of 38 with severe aortic atherosclerosis, ulceration and mural thrombi.

EMBOLIZATION TO THE EXTREMITIES: THE "BLUE TOE SYNDROME."—Zak and Elias[17] in 1949 described a patient with gangrene involving the toe, who at postmortem examination was found to have atheromatous emboli in the kidneys, spleen and pancreas. The atheromatous embolic origin of the occlusion of the toe could not be proved, as no examination was made of the peripheral vessels. In 1959, two reports appeared documenting atheromatous embolization to the extremities. Sayre and Campbell[18] published an autopsy report of a patient showing severe arteriosclerosis with widespread atheromatous embolization that was most marked in the kidneys and brain. This patient also had arterial insufficiency of the extremities, conjectured to be on the basis of embolization. Hoye et al.[19] reported on a patient with bilateral gangrene of the toe tips; all peripheral pulses were palpable and there was arteriographic proof that the main arteries of both extremities, while narrowed, were not occluded. At operation, the popliteal artery was found to be patent. Nevertheless, bilateral amputation was necessary. Examination of the tissue in the region of the cutaneous ulcers showed evidence of embolic occlusion with typical cholesterol clefts in the occluding thrombi in arteries quite near to the ulcers. A few small arteries found with partially recanalized lumens suggested prior embolization. In 1960, reporting further from this same hospital, Gore and Collins[13] found 6 examples of embolization of atheromatous material peripherally among 34 consecutive autopsies on persons aged 60 years or more. The arterial channels involved by atheroemboli were in arteries less than 1 mm in diameter in the kidneys, brain, pancreas and intestinal tract. There were also 4 patients with an extremity amputated for arterial insufficiency. In each instance it was demonstrated that atheromatous material had contributed to the process and in 2 patients had caused ulceration.[13] Reports confirming such phenomena are becoming numerous.[20-28] Recently, the problem has been brought into complete focus for the surgeon interested in peripheral vascular diseases.[29-31]

DIAGNOSIS

ARTERIOEMBOLI TO THE BRAIN. — These emboli produce a sudden onset of focal ischemia, usually one-sided contralateral weakness or numbness of the face and an extremity, more commonly the upper extremity. Aphasia may be present if the dominant hemisphere is involved, as may also intermittent loss of vision in one eye (amaurosis fugax). Depending on the size of the embolus, the attack may be transient or persistent. If all symptoms and signs have disappeared within 24 hours, the attack is referred to as a transient ischemic attack (TIA). If they persist longer, it is referred to as a "completed stroke."

ARTERIOEMBOLI TO THE LOWER EXTREMITY. — The diagnosis can usually be made by the presence of the "blue toe syndrome," with all peripheral pulses present. It has been suggested that other signs of atheroemboli may include livedo reticularis[28] and arterial ulceration of the skin. Some arterial ulcers of the leg, occasionally called hypertensive ischemic ulcers, may indeed, as in Wagner and Martin's report,[29] be due to emboli rather than to localized thrombosis of the arterioles of the skin.

MUSCLE BIOPSY. — Anderson and Richards[21, 28] stress the importance of muscle biopsy obtained from the gastrocnemius and quadriceps groups in the diagnosis of atheroembolism. Using the technique of tissue sections, a histologic diagnosis can be established in clinically suspect patients. A high frequency of atheroembolism to the musculature of the lower extremity was observed in correlative postmortem studies in patients with erosive aortic atheromatosis. In this study[28] muscle biopsy was positive in all but 1 patient, disclosing atheroemboli in other organs and tissues. Atheroemboli have been implicated as a causative factor in hypertension, renal failure, cerebral encephalomalacia, acute pancreatitis, duodenal ulcer and myocardial infarction, as well as in gangrene of the extremities. It is also suggested[21] that they might be involved in the clinical manifestations of polyarteritis nodosa, as was true of a patient with multiple-system cholesterol embolization associated with a necrotizing angiitis present in various tissues, including skeletal muscle. Anderson recommends muscle biopsy to prove the diagnosis.[21, 28]

ARTERIOEMBOLI TO THE VISCERA. — Small atheroemboli or cholesterol emboli, like those implicated in the cause of multiple-system disease, for example, polyarteritis nodosa,[21, 28] cannot be diagnosed at the present time from clinical symptoms and signs; however, they are a frequent finding in autopsy studies of patients with erosive aortic atheromatosis.

TREATMENT

CEREBRAL EMBOLI. — There is no true treatment of cerebral embolism. Management is mainly supportive. Many surgeons use heparin in an effort to prevent propagation of the thrombus. Others recommend dextran to reduce platelet adhesiveness and to lower blood viscosity. Treatment of arterial emboli to the brain must be prophylactic. Presence of one clearcut transient ischemic attack is, in our opinion, indication for complete study, including arteriography. Routine checking of the carotid arteries for the presence of bruits and the use of noninvasive methods, such as oculoplethysmography and carotid phonoangiography, help in the selection of asymptomatic patients for cerebral angiography, followed by appropriate surgical therapy.

PERIPHERAL ARTERIOEMBOLI. — If the site of lodgment is a major artery, after embolectomy the source of the arteriogenic embolus is sought. If the point of origin is a proximal erosive aorta, endarterectomy is done. If a mural thrombus in the wall of an aneurysmal artery is the source of the embolus, the aneurysm is resected and an arterial graft is inserted. Wagner and Martin[29] reported a right femoral embolectomy followed by endarterectomy 5 days later. Kwaan et al.[30] reported 2 cases of repeated right femoral embolism due to microscopically confirmed atheromatous emboli. The toes had to be amputated. After the patients recovered from right femoral embolectomy, aortoiliac endarterectomy was done. Close scrutiny of the lower aorta and iliac arteries is recommended[31] in an effort to find the source of the embolization. When found, the area is either endarterectomized or excised. In some patients with multiple small emboli, end-to-end anastomosis is recommended rather than bypass grafting.[31]

THE "BLUE TOE SYNDROME". — In our experience, some patients with the "blue toe syndrome" may improve under conservative management or after lumbar sympathectomy, only to return after a lapse of several years with a similar episode. This phenomenon calls for a concerted effort to determine the source of the emboli, whether it be erosive plaque in a proximal vessel, or a mural thrombus in a major arterial aneurysm. Biplane arteriography of the aorta, with complete visualization of the lower extremities, is required. Muscle biopsy, as recommended by Anderson and Richards,[21, 28] may be used if doubt still exists. Once found, the source of the emboli should be eradicated by appropriate surgical procedures.[29-31]

ATHEROMATOUS EMBOLI INDUCED BY HEPARIN THERAPY. — Unexplained multiple arterial embolization has been reported in patients being treated with heparin for a condition that of itself could not possibly be expected to cause arterial emboli.[25, 32-35] On extraction, the emboli proved to be light in color and seemingly composed of fibrinous platelets. They were believed to have originated in an erosive aorta, since there was no apparent cardiac source in any of the patients. The heparin had been administered by the subcutaneous or intramuscular route. Thromboelastographic evaluation[35] seems to implicate this mode of delivery of the drug. We have recently encountered this phenomenon and documented the presence of heparin-induced antiplatelet antibodies in a patient on intravenously administered heparin. Anticoagulant therapy (Dicumarol) has likewise been implicated as a causative factor in cholesterol embolization.[27]

REFERENCES

1. Mosney, and Dumont, J. Embolie fémorale au cours d'un retrécissement mitral pur: Artériotomie; guérison, Bull. Acad. Natl. Med. (Paris) 66:358, 1911.
2. Fogarty, T. J., Cranley, J. J., Krause, R. J., Strasser, E. S., and Hafner, C. D.: A method for extraction of arterial emboli and thrombi, Surg. Gynecol. Obstet. 116: 241, 1963.
3. Cranley, J. J., Krause, R. J., Strasser, E. S., Hafner, C. D., and Fogarty, T. J.: Peripheral arterial embolism: Changing concepts, Surgery 55:57, 71, 1964.
4. Cranley, J. J., Krause, R. J., Strasser, E. S., and Hafner, C. D.: Catheter technique for arterial embolectomy: A seven-year experience, J. Cardiovasc. Surg. 11:44, 1970.
5. Cranley, J. J.: *Vascular Surgery,* Vol. I, *Peripheral Arterial Diseases* (Hagerstown, Md.: Harper & Row, 1972), chapter 3, Peripheral Arterial Embolism.
6. Spencer, F. C., and Eiseman, B.: Delayed arterial embolectomy: A new concept, Surgery 55:64, 1964.
7. Stewart, G. D., Sweetman, W. R., Westphal, K., and Wise, R. A.: Superior mesenteric artery embolectomy, Ann. Surg. 151:274, 1960.
8. Rutledge, R. H.: Superior mesenteric artery embolectomy: Review of the literature and case report, Ann. Surg. 159:529, 1964.
9. Eliot, R. S., Kanjuii, V. I., and Edwards, J. E.: Atheromatous embolism, Circulation 30:611, 1964.
10. Flory, C. M.: Arterial occlusions produced by emboli from eroded aortic atheromatous plaques, Am. J. Pathol. 21:549, 1945.
11. Panum, P. L.: Experimentelle Beitrage zur Lehre von der Embolie, Virchows Arch. [Pathol. Anat.] 25:308, 1862.
12. Doch, G.: Some notes on coronary arteries, M. & S. Reports 75:1, 1896, cited in Hoye, S. J., Teitelbaum, S., Gore, I., and Warren, R.: Atheromatous embolization: A factor in peripheral gangrene, N. Engl. J. Med. 261: 128, 1959.
13. Gore, I., and Collins, D. P.: Spontaneous atheromatous embolization: Review of the literature and a report of 16 additional cases, Am. J. Clin. Pathol. 33:416, 1960.
14. Meyer, W. W.: Cholesterolkrystallembolie kleiner Organarterien and ihre Folgen, Virchows Arch. [Pathol. Anat.] 314:616, 1947.
15. Venet, L., and Friedfeld, L.: Avulsion and embolization of a calcific arterial plaque: Femoral embolectomy, Surgery 32:119, 1952.
16. Thurlbeck, W. M., and Castleman, B.: Atheromatous emboli to the kidneys after aortic surgery, N. Engl. J. Med. 257:442, 1957.

17. Zak, F. G., and Elias, K.: Embolization with material from atheromata, Am. J. Med. Sci. 218:510, 1949.
18. Sayre, G. P., and Campbell, D. C.: Multiple peripheral emboli in atherosclerosis of the aorta, A.M.A. Arch. Intern. Med. 103:799, 1959.
19. Hoye, S. J., Teitelbaum, S., Gore, I., and Warren, R.: Atheromatous embolization: A factor in peripheral gangrene, N. Engl. J. Med. 261:128, 1959.
20. Snyder, H. E., and Shapiro, J. L.: A correlative study of atheromatous embolism in human beings and experimental animals, Surgery 49:195, 1961.
21. Anderson, W. R.: Necrotizing angiitis associated with embolization of cholesterol: Case report, with emphasis on the use of muscle biopsy as a diagnostic aid, Am. J. Clin. Pathol. 43:65, 1965.
22. Edwards, E. A., Tilney, N., and Lindquist, R. R.: Causes of peripheral embolism and their significance, J.A.M.A. 196:133, 1966.
23. Retan, J. W., and Miller, R. E.: Microembolic complications of atherosclerosis: Literature review and report of a patient, Arch. Intern. Med. 118:534, 1966.
24. Crane, Chilton: Atherothrombotic embolism to lower extremities in arteriosclerosis, Arch. Surg. 94:96, 1967.
25. Barker, C. F., Rosato, F. E., and Roberts, B.: Peripheral arterial embolism, Surg. Gynecol. Obstet. 123:22, 1966.
26. Maurizi, C. P., Barker, A. E., and Trueheart, R. E.: Atheromatous emboli: A postmortem study with special reference to the lower extremities, Arch. Pathol. 86:529, 1967.
27. Moldveen-Geroniumus, M., and Merriam, J. C.: Cholesterol embolization: From pathologic curiosity to clinical entity, Circulation 35:946, 1967.
28. Anderson, W. R., and Richards, A. McD.: Evaluation of lower extremity muscle biopsies in the diagnosis of atheroembolism, Arch. Pathol. 86:535, 1968.
29. Wagner, R. B., and Martin, A. S.: Peripheral atheroembolism: Confirmation of a clinical concept, with a case report and review of the literature, Surgery 73:353, 1973.
30. Kwaan, J. H. M., Vander Molen, R., Stemmer, E. A., and Connolly, J. E.: Peripheral embolism resulting from unsuspected atheromatous aortic plaques, Surgery 78:583, 1975.
31. Mehigan, J. T., and Stoney, R. J.: Lower extremity atheromatous embolization, Am. J. Surg. 132:163, 1976.
32. Weismann, R. E., and Tobin, R. W.: Arterial embolism occurring during systemic heparin therapy, A.M.A. Arch. Surg. 76:219, 1958.
33. Roberts, B., Rosato, F. E., and Rosato, E. F.: Heparin — a cause of arterial emboli? Surgery 55:803, 1964.
34. Kaup, H. A., and Roberts, B.: Arterial embolization during subcutaneous heparin therapy: Case report, J. Cardiovasc. Surg. 13:210, 1972.
35. Rosato, F. E., Rosato, E. F., Roberts, B., and Knisely, R. F.: Thromboelastographic evaluation of the method of heparin administration, Am. J. Surg. 113:750, 1967.

Advances in Microsurgery

ROLLIN K. DANIEL and WILLIAM M. SWARTZ

*Department of Plastic Surgery, Royal Victoria Hospital, Montreal, Canada;
Department of Plastic Surgery, Rhode Island Hospital, Providence,
Rhode Island*

> *Microsurgery is a most seductive craft — with a skill, beauty,
> sensitivity and mystique of its own . . . .*[161]

> *Microsurgery is a surgical technique clinically applicable in
> every surgical specialty.*[37]

Microsurgery may be defined as surgery performed under
magnification; the "purist" restricts it to surgery using the operating microscope, while the "generalist" includes loupes and
other ocular aids. Execution of fine work is not limited by hand
coordination, but rather by the ability of the eye to guide the
hand. Therefore, improved visual acuity is mandatory and requires both increased magnification and illumination. Due to
current emphasis on preservation and restoration of function,
surgeons in all specialties must now attempt repair of small critical structures, including the body's sensory organs and luminal
components. As a result, surgeons are turning to microsurgery
as it permits "an extension of Halstedian surgical principles to
delicate tissues where gentle handling and exceedingly accurate
approximation is of paramount importance."[80]

Historical Evolution

In 1921, Nylen[112] utilized a monocular measuring microscope
to operate on 2 patients with chronic otitis and thus became the
first surgeon to employ an operating microscope clinically. Sub-

sequently, binocular magnification, adequate illumination and stable support were added, which resulted in otolaryngology's becoming the first surgical specialty committed to microsurgery.[43] Following mass production of the Zeiss OpMi 1 operating microscope in 1953, ophthalmologists quickly expanded the applications and indications for ocular microsurgery.[67,157]

In the 1960s new horizons were opened by extending microsurgery into the realm of microvascular[80] and microneural[140] surgery. These developments represented a dramatic break from the traditional techniques of otolaryngology, with its emphasis on bony dissection, as well as from ophthalmology with its bloodless, complex suturing. Neurosurgeons were attracted by the microscope's increased magnification and improved illumination. The execution of many procedures shifted from "blind feel" to "direct vision." New procedures for treating cerebral aneurysms and revascularizing the ischemic cerebrum were devised.[128, 164] Plastic surgeons, too, were intrigued by microsurgery, as it promised replantation of amputated parts, distant transfer of composite tissues and increasingly accurate peripheral nerve repairs.[14, 17, 19] Many of the procedures devised by reconstructive microsurgeons are now being done by hand surgeons, who routinely employ 2.5–4.5× loupe magnification for virtually every hand repair except where the higher magnification of an operating microscope is required.[37, 81, 87] Cardiovascular surgeons rely on loupe magnification for inserting aortocoronary bypass grafts.

In the 1970s microsurgical techniques are being implemented on a limited basis in several other specialties. Urologists are finding microsurgery valuable for vasovasotomy, orchidopexy and renal bench surgery.[137] Gynecologic surgeons are attempting anastomosis of fallopian tubes with increasingly satisfactory results. Orthopedic surgeons are being challenged by new bone-grafting techniques, including the free bone transfer procedure plus potential epiphyseal and whole joint transfers.[153, 159] Surprisingly, however, vascular, general and pediatric surgeons have employed the operating microscope on only a limited basis, despite its obviously unlimited application to peripheral vessels, the biliary tract and congenital anomalies.[80]

It is interesting to observe that each surgical specialty has followed a similar evolutionary pattern since adoption of the operating microscope. The first generation of microsurgeons developed basic surgical techniques in the research laboratory, which were applied on an ever-expanding clinical basis by the second generation and accepted as established procedures by the third generation. This progression required over 30 years in otolaryngology, but only 15 years in ophthalmology and less than a decade in plastic surgery and neurosurgery.

When one considers the progressive geometric influence that microsurgery is having on surgery, the following conclusions become apparent. First, microsurgery is now a technique clinically applicable to every surgical specialty and thus must become an integral part of every surgical resident's training. Second, integrated multiple-discipline microsurgical teaching laboratories must be established (Fig 1). Due to the critical nature of most conditions requiring microsurgery and the requisite manual dexterity, conventional intraoperative surgical teaching is not possible. Rather, the neophyte must master microsurgery in the laboratory, using basic experimental models and exercises developed for each specialty. That this training must occur during the residency years is made evident by responses to questionnaires, which indicate that utilization of microsurgical techniques was not dictated by the surgical procedure but rather

Fig 1.—A multidisciplinary microsurgery laboratory. (Courtesy of Harry J. Buncke, Jr., San Francisco, California.)

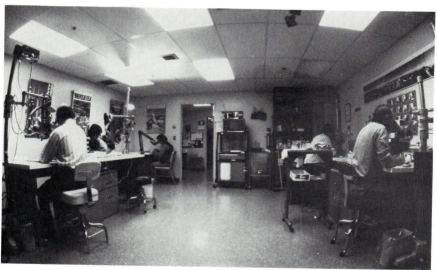

correlated with the surgeon's age and previous microsurgical training.

In this chapter we attempt to summarize the current trends in microsurgery by listing the developments occurring in the established microsurgical specialties (otolaryngology, ophthalmology), by emphasizing the recent advances of the maturing microsurgical specialties (plastic surgery, hand surgery, neurosurgery) and by forecasting the breakthrough in urology.[137]

Equipment

MAGNIFICATION SYSTEMS

Ocular aids, including both loupes and operating microscopes, have recently undergone dramatic changes. The conventional single-lens 2.3× spheroprism system mounted on a metal outrigger (Beebe loupe) has been replaced by achromatic doublet operating telescopes with greater magnification (2.5–6.0×) and a more comfortable working distance (10–21 in.).[89] The latter can be mounted on a "flip-top" bar for easy displacement (Keeler) or set low in the bifocal area permitting maximum view of the wound (Designs for Vision).

As discussed elsewhere, an operating microscope incorporates three ocular systems: an *objective lens,* which establishes the working distance; a *binocular assembly,* which is the primary determinant of base magnification, and a *magnification changer,* which permits selection of different magnification settings.[37] Although otolaryngologists remain satisfied with the Zeiss OpMi 1 model operating microscope, other surgical specialists have found its manual focus, fixed-stage magnification and restriction to use by a single surgeon unacceptable. Therefore, a new generation of "zoom" microscopes has evolved with the following advantages: (1) a mechanized foot-controlled focusing device; (2) a foot-controlled variable magnification system that permits selection of optimal rather than fixed magnification, and (3) a variety of beam splitters that permit the participation of an active surgical assistant rather than a static observer. The frequently inadequate illumination provided by heat-producing 50-w incandescent lamp bulbs has been replaced by the brilliant illumination of fiberoptic light sources.

As each surgical specialty has adopted the operating micro-

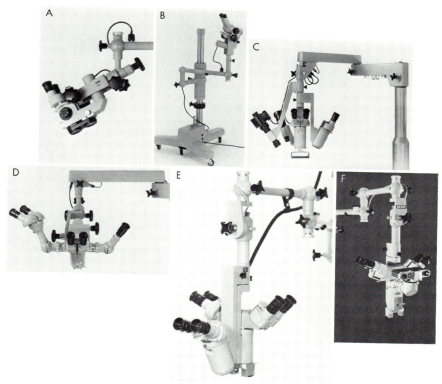

Fig 2.—Operating microscopes. **A,** a standard manual OpMi 1 as used in otolaryngology. **B,** inverse positioning of the OpMi 1 for gynecologic examination. **C,** a zoom OpMi 8 with external illumination for ophthalmic surgery. **D,** a zoom OpMi 6 with observation tubes for neurologic surgery. **E,** an OpMi 8 with 3 binocular heads for plastic and reconstructive microsurgery. **F,** an OpMi 7 with horizontal beam splitter for hand surgery. (Photographs courtesy of Carl Zeiss Ltd., Toronto, Canada.)

scope, additional changes and modifications have been necessary to meet the demands of the operating field, patient position and surgical technique (Fig 2). Ophthalmologists prefer zoom magnification with the assistant sitting at 90 degrees and external illumination from 2 sources to minimize glare from the reflective corneal surface. For neurosurgeons, the restrictive confines of the cerebral depths preclude the use of an active surgical assistant and demand coaxial illumination and maximum positional flexibility, with either manual or zoom magnification acceptable. Plastic surgeons and hand surgeons generally prefer the face-to-face 180-degree position with surgeon and assistant peering through a common horizontal beam splitter plus motorized focusing and magnification. Future microscope developments will increase positional flexibility, especially in the binocular assembly and light sources.

MICROINSTRUMENTS

In contrast to standard surgical instruments, microinstruments are designed for utilization with an operating microscope and are characterized by precision tips, light weight, balanced proportions, graded pinch closure and nonreflective surfaces (Fig 3). Optimal application requires a gentle thumb-index pinch mechanism guided by direct vision rather than by feel.

The tissue-handling characteristics and operative techniques of each surgical specialty demand specific microinstruments. The bony confines of the middle ear forced otolaryngologists to devise a wide variety of curettes, drills and chisels. The tough sclera of the eye and single suture technique required ophthal-

Fig 3.—Microinstruments. **A,** jewelers' forceps. **B,** microscissors. **C,** clamp approximators for occluding blood flow and approximating retracted vessels. **D,** knives for microsurgery (razor blade chip holder, razor blade breaker, diamond knife, *top to bottom*).

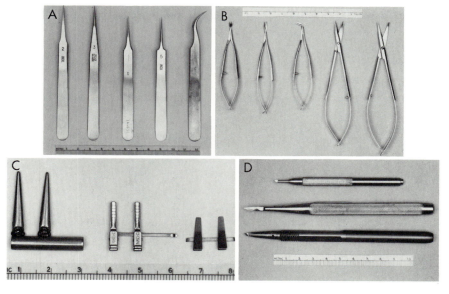

mologists to develop numerous types of spring-handle scissors, razor blade knives and tying forceps. The deep recesses of the brain necessitated long bayonet-shaped instruments for the neurosurgeon. Retraction of several blood vessels and the high risk of thrombosis obliged microvascular surgeons to evolve atraumatic clamp approximators and increasingly finer sutures.[3] At the present time, microinstrument sets suited for each surgical specialty have become commercially available and are described in various microsurgical texts.[37, 128, 157]

MICROSUTURES

A suture is composed of a needle and suture material, with most manufacturers restricting the term "microsutures" to those incorporating 8-0 or smaller suture material (Fig 4). Virtually all microsutures are swaged to monofilament nylon, although ophthalmologists continue to search for an absorbable microsuture material.

The greatest variation among specialties occurs in the cutting tip and shape of the microneedle used. Ophthalmologists favor a "spatulated" needle with its sharp point and trapezoid configu-

Fig 4.—Microsutures. **A,** microneedles; *top,* 70 μ, curved and straight; *bottom,* 130 μ, curved and straight. **B,** sutures tied around a human hair (6-0, 7-0, 8-0, 9-0, 10-0).

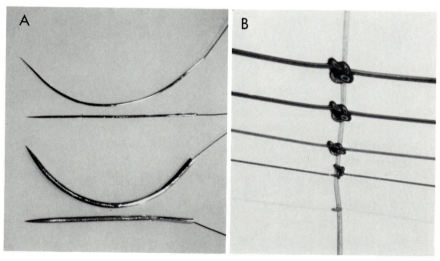

human digital vessels encountered in replantation surgery and to the cutaneous vessels of free tissue transfers. Since many microsurgeons use this model both for achieving proficiency and for research purposes, a detailed discussion of the anastomotic technique will be presented (Fig 6). It can be applied in clinical microsurgery with limited modification.

END-TO-END ANASTOMOSIS OF 1.0-MM ARTERY. — *Preparation of the vessel.* — In the anesthetized rat, a longitudinal incision is made perpendicular to the inguinal ligament on the medial surface of the thigh to expose the femoral artery and vein. Dissection and isolation of the vessels is performed under 6–10× magnification, utilizing microscissors and jewelers' forceps. Once the femoral vessels are exposed, the collateral branches are coagulated with a bipolar coagulator and the femoral artery separated from the femoral vein. Exposure of an adequate length of vessel, at least 1.5 cm, is essential to provide room for the clamp approximator and possible revision of the anastomosis. A contrasting background material is slipped behind the vessel to permit better visual contrast and to isolate it from the surrounding tissue. The operative field is kept constantly moist with warm heparinized saline to prevent vessel desiccation and spasm. Excess fluid is removed by capillary action through a 2 × 2-in. gauze sponge placed in a dependent corner of the wound. The vessel is then bathed in lidocaine or bupivacaine to reverse any neurogenic spasm. A clamp approximator is then applied to prevent bleeding from the cut vessel and allow approximation of retracted vessel ends. The vessel is then cut perpendicularly with sharp scissors; oblique cuts are not necessary except in the case of vessel size discrepancies. Excess adventitia is teased from the vessel end with jewelers' forceps and gently pulled over the lumen. This adventitial "foreskin" is cleanly circumcised; any remaining adventitia will retract, leaving an uncluttered lumen. Radical excision of adventitia is contraindicated and physically impossible. The lumen of the vessel is then irrigated with a stream of warm heparinized saline to remove any blood clots. The vessel lumen is mechanically dilated by gently inserting a polished no. 5 jewelers' forceps, then spreading the forceps apart in a controlled fashion. Detailed preparation and atraumatic manipulation of the vessel is mandatory.

Placing the guide sutures. — The clamp approximator is then adjusted to overcome vessel retraction, which in turn permits utilization of finer suture material. Guide sutures are placed at 16× magnification, and 2 methods are available, each having certain advantages. Cobbett[29] prefers to place 3 guide sutures 120 degrees apart with the appropriate sutures in between (at least 2) to seal the anastomosis. Traction on 2 of the guides allows the front wall to fall away from the back wall, thereby minimizing accidental anterior-posterior wall sutures. The second method consists of placing the guide sutures 180 degrees apart and then halving the distance between these sutures until the anastomosis is completed. As originally proposed by Carrel,[22, 23] the guide sutures permit traction on the vessel and serve as reference points to ensure equal spacing of sutures. Additional interrupted sutures are inserted to coapt the lumen. Each suture must be accurately placed to prevent inversion or buckling of the vessel, which would decrease lumen size and/or expose collagen to circulating platelets. Continuous running sutures are *not* used in vessels smaller than 2 mm. Once the operator is satisfied, the anastomosis is wrapped with a piece of Saran wrap to reduce oozing.[100]

Release of the clamps. — The distal clamp is removed first, followed by the proximal clamp. Blood should immediately cross the anastomosis and dilate it evenly without any areas of indentation. A slowly filling anastomosis indicates partial obstruction due to improperly placed sutures, vessel spasm or adventitia inside the lumen. Minimal ooze can be controlled by gentle pressure, while a jet of blood mandates additional sutures. Bathing the vessel with lidocaine relieves vascular spasm and improves flow, provided there is no mechanical obstruction.[146]

Assessing patency of anastomosis. — The surgeon must be absolutely certain that the anastomosis is fully patent. Pulsations distal to the anastomosis are indicative of vessel patency.[2] The "radical pressure test" is a method for assessing true patency and requires gentle occlusion of the vessel distal to the anastomosis with a no. 2 jewelers' forceps and then, with a second forceps, milking the blood distal to the occluding forceps. The second forceps holds the vessel in occlusion, and the first forceps is then released. Blood should immediately fill the evacuated vessel segment. If filling is sluggish, the anastomosis is partially occluded, while total absence of flow indicates complete occlusion. We have recently observed clinically that systemic fluorescence permits a noninvasive atraumatic technique for as-

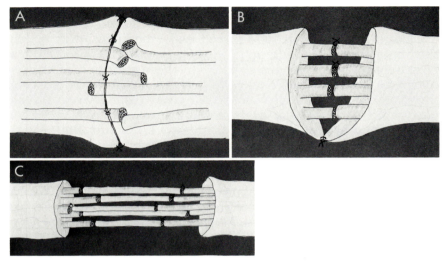

Fig 7.—Microneural techniques. **A,** epineurial repair with overriding, buckling and straddling of the enclosed fascicles. **B,** perineurial repair in which optimal fascicular alignment can be obtained. **C,** fascicular nerve grafting.

cy can be overcome by surgically creating different types of neuroma in experimental groups. Such pretreatment allows surgical experience with scar dissection under magnification, isolation and preservation of fascicles in continuity and careful excision of neuromatous tissue.

MICROINSTRUMENTS. — Peripheral nerve microsurgery does not require the numerous vascular clamps and clamp approximators of microvascular surgery. However, special microinstruments are necessary for proper execution of nerve repairs, and the novice must learn to handle and protect them. Defective microinstruments are mute testimony to rough handling and careless storage. Commercial jewelers' forceps are frequently too traumatic, and the tips must be made finer by using a grinding stone under magnification to achieve the desired tip shape. Vannas type microscissors are preferred for epineuriectomy and interfascicular dissection. For clinical work, fine spring-handled slightly curved iris scissors are an alternative. However, for dissections in secondary clinical nerve repairs the diamond knife, with its nondulling blade, is optimal for dissecting neuromas in continuity, intraneural excision of peripheral nerve tumors, intraneural neurolysis and interfascicular dissection prior to nerve grafting.[155] However, the cost ($400) of the diamond knife makes it a secondary choice to the more available and cheaper razor blade chip for most microsurgeons.

An angled nerve spatula with blunt edges is invaluable as a tool to manipulate, retract and separate fascicles. Additional manipulators include the dissecting microneedles used by neurophysiologists, which are valuable for experimental nerve repairs. These manipulators can be homemade by grinding the tips of readily available "mosquito pins." Cotton tip applicators, black polyethylene background material, wooden spatulas, fine (32-gauge) tubing and blunt needles of various sizes complete the microinstrument armamentarium of the peripheral nerve microsurgeon.

Higher magnification is often necessary for precisely identifying the supportive connective tissue layers within the nerve trunk. Fascicular identification and orientation demands high magnification ($25-40\times$), while intraneural dissection and suture placement dictates a $16-25\times$ magnification. Knot tying is done at $16\times$, while $10\times$ is reserved for initial mobilization of the nerve trunk and insertion of the background material.

The microsutures employed in peripheral nerve surgery are similar to those of microvascular surgery. The $100\text{-}\mu$ needle series is preferred for epineurial repairs, the $70\text{-}\mu$ needle for perineurial repairs and fascicular nerve grafting while the $50\text{-}\mu$ needle is ideal for experimental perineurial repairs and nerve grafting procedures.

Peripheral nerve repair. — Prior to attempting microsurgical nerve repairs, the novice microsurgeon must gain expertise in controlling intraneural bleeding by simple cotton tip pressure and suctioning. One must never apply the suction tip directly onto the nerve; always interpose a cotton tip interface. Mushrooming and lateral bulging must be promptly handled by prevention or correction. Quick stump opposition with subsequent fibrin clot formation eliminates mushrooming, while lateral bulging secondary to faulty suture placement can be corrected by suture removal and revision.

Probably the cheapest and best experimental model for practicing microsurgical nerve repairs is the sciatic nerve of the rat. Since it is a trifascicular nerve, the various procedures, including epineurial and perineurial repairs plus placement of nerve grafts, can be done. A step-by-step guide to experimental micro-surgical nerve repairs is now available for the interested reader.[37]

Once technical expertise has been achieved in the experimental laboratory, clinical peripheral nerve repair becomes possible. Gentle handling of the neural tissue and very accurate approximation of the severed nerve ends under magnification are the keys to optimal nerve repairs. A motionless, bloodless field can be achieved by a combination of general or block anesthesia plus a pneumatic tourniquet. The tourniquet is required for the initial exploration of the lesion, preparation of the nerve ends, interfascicular dissection and fascicular identification. The actual nerve suture can be achieved with or without a tourniquet. However, meticulous hemostasis during the repair and prior to skin closure must be the rule in either case.

If the lesion is a complete severance, marking sutures are placed on an undisturbed segment of the proximal and distal stumps well away from the site of injury. These sutures are of great assistance in orienting the nerve ends prior to repair. If the lesion is in continuity, one should always start the dissection in normal nerve tissue and proceed towards the site of pathology. A longitudinal incision is made proximally and distally in the normal-looking epineurium. Epineuriectomy is then carefully performed towards the neuroma until the epineurium becomes indistinguishable from the entrapping scar. Fascicular groups are isolated at this level and carefully traced into the lesion. The integrity of the perineurial sheath of each bundle is an invaluable guide in carrying out this dissection. If a bundle is involved in the neuroma, the continuity of its surrounding perineurium will be disrupted and replaced by scar tissue. Fascicles that have escaped the injury can be carefully preserved and dissected through the lesion into the distal stump. Every effort should be made to preserve intact bundles so that remaining function can be spared. Entrapping scar secondarily compressing intact fascicles is carefully excised, a procedure referred to as "intraneural neurolysis." At times only an external neurolysis is required, which implies simple isolation of the nerve from the scarred epineurium and surrounding tissue. The decision of which procedure to perform is determined by clinical symptomatology and intraoperative findings.

EPINEURIAL REPAIR. — This is the conventional procedure for surgically anastomosing severed peripheral nerves. A standard epineurial repair involves the following steps: (1) adequate exposure of the lesion under tourniquet control; (2) insertion of marking sutures; (3) preparation and trimming of the cut nerve ends; (4) nerve mobilization proximally and distally to overcome tension, and (5) placement of the first two guide epineurial sutures at 12 o'clock and 4 o'clock positions, with suture tails left long to facilitate nerve rotation for posterior wall anastomosis. The indications for the correct placement of these guide sutures include: longitudinal epineurial vessels, position of mesoneurium and fascicular topography in proximal and distal stumps. The remaining steps are: (6) completion of anterior wall repair and (7) nerve rotation with posterior wall exposure and completion of posterior wall repair.

In execution of this repair, optimal nerve alignment is ensured by small bites of the epineurium of the proximal and distal nerve ends in exactly equidistant location from the first two guide sutures. However, control of the orientation of the intraneural bundles is minimal and is the leading cause of failure.[10, 46, 144] Main advantages of the epineurial repair include: (1) short operative time; (2) minimal magnification; (3) suture placement limited to the epineurial sheath, and (4) technical simplicity. Its disadvantages include: (1) compromised fascicular alignment; (2) the fact that emphasis on simple coaption of nerve ends fosters extensive mobilization of the nerve or insertion of a greater number of larger sutures to overcome tension.

PERINEURIAL REPAIR. — The term "perineurial suture" is used interchangeably with "fascicular" and "funicular" suture. It refers to the surgical manipulation of corresponding fascicular bundles in the proximal and distal stumps to achieve optimal fascicular alignment.

Fascicular suture was first advocated by Langley and Hashimoto in 1917,[94] but with little clinical implementation. Subsequently, Sunderland[143] realized the value of this technique, but the requisite technical aids were not then available. Following introduction of the operating microscope to peripheral nerve surgery, the nerve fascicle became amenable to surgical manipulation and the fascicular suture technique was used clinically for the repair of peripheral nerve injuries.[12, 13, 93, 105, 129, 140]

Although various techniques have been advocated for fascicular suture, the procedure usually involves the following: (1)

resection of the epineurium from the proximal and distal stumps; (2) careful intraoperative sketching of the cross-sectional fascicular pattern, and (3) placement of a single 10-0 suture through the perineurial sheath of corresponding bundles.[10, 51, 79, 101, 140] If there is mild separation ($\leq$ 2 cm) of the cut nerve ends, reinforcing epineurial sutures may be required.

Evidence for the superiority of perineurial suture over the conventional epineurial repair is not without controversy. Clinical studies have reported improved functional restoration by the use of magnification and microsurgical techniques.[46, 56, 57, 103] Objective clinical evidence of the superiority of perineurial neurorrhaphy versus the conventional epineurial repair is missing, and this has prompted many to be reticent in accepting a far more laborious technique.[87] However, experimental data are available comparing the 2 methods of suture.[10, 11, 21, 51, 52, 162, 163] Methods of study have included subjective observations, histologic work, biochemical assay, nerve conduction, muscle tension and electromyography. Five[10, 51, 52, 162, 163] of these 7 studies report superior results subsequent to fascicular repair, while 2[11, 21] recent studies found no difference between the 2 types of repair. A very recent electrophysiologic and ultrastructural report favors perineurial repairs over epineurial repairs.[119]

Despite existing controversy, the evidence accumulated to date points to the following conclusions: (1) there is significantly more myelination present in the distal stump of nerves repaired with perineurial suture; (2) correct fascicular alignment is enhanced, and (3) functional recovery is superior. The ultimate advantage is optimal fascicular alignment, while the disadvantages include the extent of surgical trauma and intraneural introduction of foreign suture material.

NERVE GRAFTING. — Tension at the anastomosis is known to be a detrimental factor for successful regeneration, as it provokes scar formation with strangulation of outgrowing axons.[106, 129] In the late 1960s the primary source of connective tissue proliferation was shown experimentally to be the epineurium.[10, 102] The dilemma for surgeons faced with the repair of large nerve defects has been whether to mobilize extensively and stretch the nerve ends to bridge the gap, thus achieving end-end repair with a single anastomosis, or to eliminate tension by bridging with a nerve graft but forcing the regenerating axons to penetrate two anastomoses, rather than one.[156]

Millesi's experimental and clinical work led to the following observations: (1) connective tissue proliferation was directly related to the amount of tension at the anastomosis; (2) the major source of connective tissue proliferation was the epineurium; (3) scar invasion of the suture line took place only in the presence of tension; (4) postoperative stretching provoked secondary scarring, thus compromising successful recovery.[103-108]

On the basis of these findings, Millesi[104] advocated the placement of autografts for any nerve defect greater than 2 cm by the technique of interfascicular nerve grafting. Briefly, this procedure involves the following: (1) epineuriectomy of proximal and distal stumps; (2) dissection of groups of fascicles under magnification, starting always in normal tissue and working towards the lesion; (3) transection of fascicular groups at various levels; (4) making an intraoperative drawing of the cut surfaces of the proximal and distal stumps, and (5) placement of sural nerve grafts to connect corresponding fascicular groups by a single 10-0 stitch.

Millesi and co-workers'[108] exceptionally good clinical results have been confirmed by other surgeons who have adopted this technique, thus establishing autologous nerve grafting as an effective clinical technique for restoring neural continuity.[47, 130]

In summary, the introduction of microsurgical techniques into the management of peripheral nerve lesions has broadened horizons and provided new hope for patients afflicted with severe motor and sensory deficits. This exciting beginning should serve as a stimulus for further clinical and experimental work on the pathophysiology of the injured nerve until the time that our surgical efforts at repairing peripheral nerve injuries consistently lead to restoration of normal function.

Otolaryngology

During the past 50 years, otomicrosurgery has become the only technique for correcting the myriad problems of the middle ear.[43, 71] Restoration of hearing may be achieved in selected patients by excision of sclerotic stapes and optional replacement with a prosthesis. Repair of the injured tympanic membrane or its reconstruction with temporal muscle fascia is not possible. Suture or decompression of the facial nerve within the temporal bone can be done, but only with the aid of an operating microscope. Resection of tumors within the auditory canal, especially glomus tumors of jugular vein origin, can be done with sparing of important structures. Of great interest has been development of endolymphatic surgery to effect decompression or shunting in cases of Meniere's disease.

Despite this extensive experience with the operating microscope in the middle ear, otolaryngologists have only recently crossed the intervening 15 cm to reach the larynx. Kleinsasser,[88] Jako[84] and Taub et al.[150] pioneered the development of diagnostic and operative endolaryngeal microsurgery. This system requires both the suspension laryngoscope, which frees the surgeon's hands while ensuring stability, and the operating microscope, which provides the essential magnification and illumination. Anesthesia is instilled via a no. 26 French endotracheal tube, or a combination of intravenous anesthesia and laryngeal insufflation is used, which permits free access to the entire region. With endolaryngeal microsurgery, more refined diagnostic and surgical procedures are possible for the differentiation and treatment of laryngeal neoplasms, both benign and malignant. Of special interest is addition of the surgical carbon dioxide laser, which permits pinpoint destruction of tumor tissue without impinging on critical normal structures.[85, 86]

Ophthalmology*

Although ophthalmologists have long utilized magnification for slit-lamp examination, they did not employ the operating microscope until 1946. The pioneering work of Perritt,[125] Barraquer et al.,[7] Harms and MacKensen,[67] Troutman[157] and others, coupled with mass production of the modern operating microscope, ensured widespread ophthalmic application. The Ophthalmic Microsurgery Study Group was formed and served as a forum for stimulating development of new instruments, sutures and surgical procedures (a precedence that each specialty should follow during its early microsurgical years). Of additional interest is the development by Troutman[157] of a series of graded exercises with which the ophthalmologist can perfect microsurgical techniques prior to clinical application. These practice exercises utilize human donor eyes unsuitable for

---

*Pertinent information supplied by Richard C. Troutman, 755 Park Avenue, New York, NY 10021.

transplantation, thereby permitting dramatic simulation of clinical conditions.

Initially, microsurgery allowed refinement of existing operative techniques, including corneal wound closure and connection of pterygia with restoration of a smooth corneal-scleral transition. Exact wound apposition is critical in the cornea to prevent epithelial invasion leading to glaucoma or induced astigmatism. Anterior segment surgery includes extraction of cataracts, corneal transplants and iridectomy. Again the critical problems are exact wound apposition, suture placement and depth of bite, which are critical in preventing leakage of aqueous humor. It must be emphasized that ophthalmic suturing techniques are especially varied and complex in comparison to the standard single interrupted suture. For example, the radially placed double continuous suture is frequently employed in cataract surgery and consists of radial bites placed clockwise followed by equidistant bites placed counterclockwise and parallel to reduce torque on the original radial bite with the knot buried in the suture tract. Microsurgery is now opening up the posterior segment of the eye for vitrectomy as well as developing new techniques for correction of glaucoma and optical surgery of the cornea.

Reconstructive Plastic Surgery

Plastic surgeons were pioneers in developing both microvascular (Buncke)[14] and microneural (Smith,[140] Millesi et al.[107]) techniques. An initial decade of failure and frustration has been rewarded by clinical triumphs in the past 5 years. Buncke's original experimental rabbit ear replantation, monkey toe-to-thumb transfers and free skin flap transfers are now being implemented clinically.[16-19] The initial microsurgical investigations into peripheral nerve repair by Smith[140] and nerve grafts by Millesi et al.[107] are now being performed routinely (see section on hand surgery).

Perhaps the greatest benefit of microsurgery to plastic surgery has occurred with introduction of free tissue transfers as a replacement for multistaged reconstructive techniques. Since the early work of Alexis Carrel,[22, 23] surgeons have dreamed of transferring composite blocks of tissue to distant sites for immediate reconstruction with viability restored by means of vascular

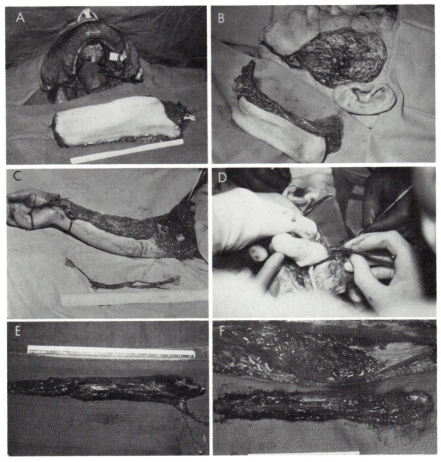

Fig 8. — The spectrum of free tissue transfers. **A,** a free groin flap used to reconstruct floor of mouth, hypopharynx and upper cervical esophagus following resection of a T₄N₂Mo recurrent carcinoma of the tongue. **B,** a composite free flap with pleura to replace oral lining, rib for mandible and chest skin for cheek. **C,** a 20-cm segment of radial sensory nerve isolated with preservation of the vasa nervorum for median nerve grafting. (Courtesy of Ian Taylor, Melbourne, Australia.) **D,** a free toe transfer to the hand. (Courtesy of Harry J. Buncke, Jr., San Francisco, California.) **E,** an isolated segment of the pectoralis major for free muscle transfer. **F,** an 18-cm segment of fibula prior to free transfer for femoral reconstruction.

anastomoses. Initial success was achieved in the early 1960s by Hiebert and Nakayama, who transferred intestinal segments to the neck for esophageal reconstruction.[37] In 1965, Krizek[91] successfully transferred large canine abdominal skin flaps to the neck with end-to-side cuff anastomosis of the cutaneous arteries and veins. Buncke and Schultz' experimental rabbit ear replantations and toe-to-thumb transfer in the rhesus monkey demonstrated that composite tissues could survive following end-to-end anastomosis of a single 1-mm artery and vein.[17, 18] The first clinical toe-to-hand transfer was reported by Cobbett in 1966, and the first free skin flap transfer reported by Daniel and Taylor in 1973.[36] The principles of free tissue transfers have been extended to omentum, bone,[153, 159] muscle, nerve[152] and various combinations (Fig 8).[16]

Execution of a free tissue transfer consists of three basic steps: (1) preparation of recipient vessels, (2) isolation of the donor tissue and (3) the vascular anastomoses. The recipient artery must possess a strong perfusion pressure, while the recipient veins must offer adequate drainage through either the superficial or deep venous system. The donor tissue is selected to permit functional reconstruction of the recipient site defect with isolation on only those blood vessels that will be anastomosed, but must result in acceptable donor site morbidity. Vascular anastomosis of 1 artery and vein is essential, with end-to-end technique preferred. Interest in free tissue transfers has been stimulated anew by success with free skin flap transfers, which will be discussed in depth.

Free Skin Flap Transfers

A free skin flap transfer permits the reconstructive microsurgeon to achieve skin coverage in 6–10 hours rather than the 3–6 months required by conventional techniques. A free flap can be employed wherever a tubed pedicle flap or a complicated direct flap would once have been used, or where local or direct flaps have previously failed. In addition to replacing conventional techniques, free flaps can be modified to incorporate sensation (neurovascular free flaps)[40] or bone (compound osseous-cutaneous flaps),[16] to offer a wide range of new imaginative procedures. Contraindications to free flap transfers include advanced arteriosclerotic vascular disease, diabetes, old age and damaged vessels in the recipient site.

Extensive preoperative evaluation of the donor and recipient site must precede a free flap transfer. The general condition of the patient is thoroughly evaluated, including a history and physical examination to ascertain any contraindications to long-duration anesthesia (6–12 hours). The condition of the recipient vessels may be evaluated by palpation, Doppler probe[5] and arteriography, especially in the traumatized lower extremity.[37]

DONOR SITES.—The requirements of a donor site for free flap transfers include the following: (1) the selected tissue must be able to survive on a single artery and vein; (2) the donor site must suffer minimum morbidity and disfigurement and must not be compromised by previous surgery.

Currently, free flap donor sites are divided into 2 groups on the basis of whether their supplying vessels are direct cutaneous or musculocutaneous arteries. These vessels are distinguished by differences in length, areas of distribution, diameter, anatomic location and physiologic importance.[34] Direct cutaneous arteries course parallel to the skin surface and permit elevation of large flaps (30 × 20 cm) on a single artery of diameter suitable for anastomosis (0.8–1.5 mm).

Flaps supplied by direct cutaneous arteries can be subdivided into regional and arterial flaps. Regional flaps incorporate at least 2 arteriovenous systems, with the dominant one selected intraoperatively, and include the iliofemoral (groin), deltopectoral and axillary flaps. Arterial flaps are designed along the course of a single direct cutaneous artery and include the scalp (superficial temporal artery), retroauricular area (postauricular artery) and foot (dorsalis pedis artery). Musculocutaneous arteries represent the terminal candelabra skin branches of segmental vessels supplying the muscle mass. Therefore, isolation of these flaps for distant transfer requires incorporation of a significant muscle mass to ensure preservation of the numerous small musculocutaneous arteries. Although musculocutaneous flaps can be isolated in virtually any area of the body, principal donor sites are the intercostal, gracilis and gluteal regions.[37, 120]

ILIOFEMORAL FLAP.—The most widely used free flap is the iliofemoral (groin) flap, which straddles the inguinal ligament and is supplied by 2 arteriovenous systems: the superficial circumflex iliac (SCIA) and superficial inferior epigastric (SIEA).[36]

The anatomic interrelationship between these 2 systems, including their variability, dominance and origin, has been carefully defined in 100 cadaver dissections.[151] The SCIA and the SIEA have variable points of origin, with one or the other being the dominant regional artery. The SCIA is always present, while the SIEA is frequently diminished or absent. Venous drainage is via the superficial inferior epigastric vein (SIEV), which empties into the saphenous bulb, and by paired venae comitantes that course with their respective cutaneous arteries to form a 1-mm vein that enters the undersurface of the femoral vein. These detailed anatomic studies were essential before clinical procedures on patients could be attempted and have permitted design of safer operative techniques.[117]

Flap design. — The central axis of the flap parallels the expected course of the SCIA, extending from a point 5 cm below the inguinal ligament along the femoral artery to the anterior superior iliac spine. Isolation of the flap proceeds from lateral to medial, incorporating the sartorius muscle fascia at its lateral edge. Dissection continues medially until the origins of both the SCIA and SIEA have been identified, then the SIEV is traced to its entrance into the saphenous bulb. In the event that suitable vessels cannot be identified (a rare occurrence), the lateral-to-medial dissection allows utilization of the iliofemoral flap as a conventional groin flap.

In transferring the flap, a single artery is sufficient to nourish flaps as large as 30×20 cm. As many veins as possible should be anastomosed to provide adequate drainage and minimize flap congestion. The principal advantages of the iliofemoral flap include its multiple arterial and venous systems, its large size, primary donor site closure and relative hairlessness. Disadvantages include its thickness, poor color match and short vascular stalk. In addition, the area has frequently been involved in previous surgical procedures such as inguinal herniorrhaphies and vein stripping. This flap has been utilized to resurface traumatic soft tissue losses of the upper and lower extremity,[36, 76] to release burn contractures of the neck,[61] to reconstruct soft tissue losses of the face[62] and to restore the oral cavity during ablative cancer operations.[37, 59, 123] In major microsurgical centers, success rates approaching 80–90% are being achieved, with most failures restricted to the initial attempts.[8, 37, 63, 76, 115 135]

THE DELTOPECTORAL FLAP. — Since 1965 the mainstay of head

and neck reconstructive surgery has been the medially based deltopectoral flap, as originally described by Bakamjian.[6] With microsurgical technique, this flap can be converted to a free deltopectoral flap with primary elevation and insertion in a distant site.[62] The major blood supply to the deltopectoral flap comes from the perforating branches of the internal mammary artery, with the second anterior thoracic perforator being the largest (0.8–1.2 mm). Venous drainage is by paired venae comitantes (1.2–2.0 mm), which course with the cutaneous arteries.[38] The axis of the free deltopectoral flap is placed over the 3d rib, and the flap is raised from lateral to medial beneath the deep fascia of the pectoralis major, with intraoperative selection of either the 2d or 3d perforator. Although a single artery has sufficient perfusion pressure to supply a flap of this size, the venous drainage is often marginal and the flap often becomes congested in the postoperative phase. The largest deltopectoral flap in Harii's series was 19 × 19 cm, which covered half the face.[62]

Advantages of the free deltopectoral flap are its acceptable color match for facial skin and its relative thinness. As a free flap, it is not subjected to the kinks and twists of its pedicle counterpart or limited in its site of application. Disadvantages include a short vascular stalk and a donor site disfigurement, which may be unacceptable in female patients.

SCALP FLAPS.—Free scalp flaps are used to reconstruct the hairline in patients with cicatricial alopecia, and are supplied by the temporal vessels.[64] The superficial temporal artery is easily palpated in front of the tragus and averages 1.0–1.8 mm in size, with venous drainage through the superficial temporal vein (0.8–1.5 mm). A narrow flap is preferred in this area to permit primary closure of the donor site.

A retrocuricular free flap based on the posterior auricular branch of the superficial temporal artery has been used by Fujino et al.[50] to reconstruct soft tissue loss on the nose. The authors stress the good color match of this flap, its thinness and its inconspicuous donor site.

FOOT FLAP.—Island flaps based on the dorsalis pedis artery were developed by McCraw and Furlow[98] to cover soft tissue defects over the malleoli and exposed Achilles tendon. Daniel et al.[40] converted it to a neurovascular free flap to provide sensation in an anesthetic hand by anastomosing the superficial peroneal nerve to the appropriate digital nerve, thereby ensuring correct cortical localization. The flap is centered over the dorsalis pedis artery, which lies directly on the tarsal bones, providing numerous (4–5) small branches to the skin in its distal portion. The flap must be carefully dissected to prevent inadvertent separation from its requisite artery. Venous drainage is through the greater saphenous vein.

Advantages of the dorsal foot flap include its constant anatomy with a terminal 2-mm artery plus superficial and deep draining veins. It is innervated by an expendable sensory nerve, which can be used to provide sensation within the recipient site. Also, the flap is quite thin, with minimal subcutaneous tissue and available size up to 10 × 10 cm.

The major disadvantages are the difficult dissection and a significant donor site morbidity, whose long-term sequelae remain to be determined. For hand injuries requiring small areas of critical sensation, we prefer the first web space, with progression onto the dorsum if additional skin coverage is required.[37]

INTERCOSTAL FLAPS. — The intercostal free flap, supplied by the intercostal artery, vein and nerve, provides a readily available building block of compound tissue to fulfill a variety of reconstructive requirements. The rib may be included in the flap and used to restore bone continuity where overlying skin is lost, or, by anastomosing the intercostal nerve to a suitable recipient sensory nerve, sensation can be provided as well as skin coverage.

Blood supply to the intercostal flap is via the posterior intercostal artery, which arises from the thoracic aorta, courses over the vertebral bodies and enters the costal groove along the inferior border of the rib. Perforating musculocutaneous arteries supply the intercostal muscles, periosteum and skin. The major blood supply to the rib itself is via the medullary artery, a branch of the intercostal that arises 2 cm proximal to the costal groove. Sensory supply is via major named cutaneous branches (dorsal, lateral, anterior) of the intercostal nerve as well as minor branches. The size of this free flap appears virtually limitless. Daniel et al.[39] have raised a 25 × 12 cm intercostal neurovascular island flap 5 interspaces wide with intact sensation. As neurovascular island flaps supplied by a single intercostal bundle, these flaps have been utilized to provide sensation, padding and skin coverage in paraplegic patients with pressure sores.[39] Buncke and Furnas[16] have utilized this compound flap, including the rib, to reconstruct traumatic defects in the lower extremity, providing both an immediate free vascularized bone graft and skin coverage in 1 operation rather than a multistaged 6–12-month procedure. Advantages of the intercostal free flap include its reconstructive multipotential; the large amount of tissue available, and the inconspicuous donor site defect following primary closure.

THE GRACILIS FLAP. — The flap is isolated with the gracilis muscle, whose nutrient artery is a branch of either the profundus femoris or the medial circumflex femoral vessels, which enter the gracilis muscle in its upper third. Arterial diameter is 1.2–1.8 mm, and the accompanying venae comitantes are 1.5–2.0 mm. The motor nerve to the gracilis muscle accompanies the sensory nerve and originates from the obturator nerve. The gracilis flap can nourish compound musculocutaneous flaps up to 33 × 10 cm.[65] If the motor nerve to the muscle is not anastomosed, it will undergo significant atrophy over 2–3 months, but will remain thicker than other free flaps. Currently, the free gracilis flap is preferred to the free intercostal flap because of the former's consistent venous drainage.[37]

FREE MUSCLE TRANSFERS

The transfer of intact, functional muscle tissue by microneurovascular techniques permits restoration of muscle function by replacing traumatized or paralyzed muscle groups. Experimental work in dogs by Tamai et al.,[149] Kubo et al.[92] and Daniel and Terzis[37] has convincingly demonstrated that transferred muscle will recover normal function as defined by electromyography at 3 weeks and be normal histologically at 3 months, provided the dominant neurovascular bundle is repaired. Muscles selected for transfer should have a single neurovascular supply whenever possible, and the transfer should produce minimal donor site deformity. Suitable muscles for distant transfer include the lateral portion of the pectoralis major, the extensor digitorum brevis and the gracilis muscle.

Clinical application was achieved by Harii et al.[66] who used the gracilis muscle to reanimate the corner of the mouth in a patient with facial paralysis, and by Ch'en,[26] who used the lateral pectoralis major to reconstruct the forearm following Volkmann's ischemia. Ikuta et al.[75, 78] have also reported use of the pectoralis major muscle transferred on a branch of the thoracicoacromial artery, its accompanying veins and dominant nerve to obtain flexion of the thumb and 4 fingers in a patient with severe Volkmann's ischemic contracture. Subsequently, they used the gracilis muscle to reconstruct the digital flexors in a similar patient and used the anterior interosseous nerve as the recipient motor nerve. These authors stress the importance of selecting as a recipient a pure motor nerve rather than a mixed nerve, and placing the nerve suture as close to the muscle as possible. Additional technical considerations include placing the muscle under sufficient tension to give adequate excursion without causing muscle ischemia.

FREE BONE TRANSFERS

Reconstructive and orthopedic surgeons have long been faced with the necessity of restoring bony continuity under conditions of poor tissue coverage due to trauma or irradiation. Conventional reconstructive techniques require skin and soft tissue coverage by local or distant flaps followed by bone grafting. Survival of the bone graft is entirely dependent upon the vascularity of the recipient tissue bed and is unpredictable in many cases.[14] Numerous investigators have confirmed that much of the bone graft dies and becomes a skeletal framework for new bone formation via creeping substitution.[99] Recent experimental studies by Östrup[121, 122] led to development of the free, living bone graft transferred by microvascular anastomoses. Östrup's extensive research has resulted in definition of the following principles for successful free bone transfers: (1) Survival of the bone graft depends upon successful arterial and venous anastomoses. (2) Linear bone formation in the graft is comparable to that in the rest of the skeleton. (3) The quality of the recipient bed does not influence survival, including radiated tissue beds. (4) Union between graft and bed is similar to that in fracture healing, with both bones contributing to callus formation. (5) Free bone transfers are not replaced by creeping substitution.[121]

Clinical application of these principles was first achieved by Taylor et al.,[153] who transferred a 22-cm fibular segment on its nutrient peroneal vessels to the opposite leg for reconstruction of a tibial defect. Using a similar technique, Weiland and Daniel have replaced the distal radius following resection of a giant cell tumor and proximal femur following resection of a chondrosarcoma. Bony union is followed by bone hypertrophy in lower extremity transfers.[159] Buncke and Furnas utilized a free rib transfer to reconstruct a tibial defect in a child, and a compound osseous-cutaneous flap to reconstruct a compound skin tibial defect.[16]

At present, the free rib graft is designed to include the nutrient artery, which is essential for rib survival. This dissection necessitates isolating the vascular pedicle proximal to the costovertebral angle. Care must be taken not to sacrifice the major artery to the lumbar spinal cord—the artery of Adamkiewicz—which arises from the dorsal branch of T7 to L4. Disadvantages include a difficult dissection requiring a formal thoracotomy with its attendant risks. Applications of free rib transfer include compound flaps for reconstructing mandibular defects with options for oral lining and/or skin coverage even in irradiated tissue beds.[37]

Hand Surgery

REPLANTATION SURGERY

Since 1965 replantation of severed digits has become a clinical reality due to refinements of microsurgical techniques, instrumentation and sutures.[90] Although early experimental work in the field began with replantation of canine limbs in 1906 by Carrel and Guthrie,[23] clinical replantation surgery had to await the development of controlled anesthesia, blood transfusion and antibiotics. In 1960 Lapchinski[95] of the USSR and Snyder et al.[141] of the United States successfully replanted canine extremities and renewed surgical interest in this field. These investigations paved the way for the first clinical replantation of the upper extremity by Malt et al.[97] in 1962 and by Ch'en Chung-Wei et al.[26] in 1963. These triumphs were soon followed by replantation of amputations at the wrist and midpalm, but attempts at the digital level failed. Buncke and Schultz[19] provided the essential techniques experimentally by replanting the thumb and index finger of a rhesus monkey with anastomosis of a single artery (0.7 mm) and vein (0.7 mm). Clinical confirmation came in 1965 when Tamai[90] replanted a completely amputated thumb. Currently, success rates of 80–93% for digital replantation are being reported from major microsurgical hand centers.[4, 114, 147] Thus, the efforts of the past decade have permitted the hand surgeon to shift his criteria of success from survival to function of the replanted hand unit with greater emphasis on primary repair of all structures (Fig 9).

Fig 9.—Hand surgery. **A,** severe hand injury with incomplete and complete amputations of all 4 fingers. **B,** hand 3 weeks following replantation despite 24 hours of ischemia in the ring finger. **C,** neuroma of the ulnar nerve following a primary epineurial repair (note resection of epineurium proximal and distal to the lesion). **D,** revision of the nerve anastomosis with a fascicular repair under high magnification. **E,** an extensive lesion of the brachial plexus. **F,** reconstruction of the brachial plexus with multiple sural nerve grafts. (Brachial plexus graft performed by Andrew Weiland, Johns Hopkins University, Baltimore, Md.)

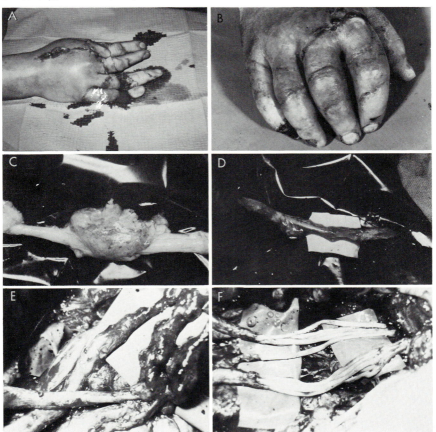

INDICATIONS FOR REPLANTATION.—The decision to replant a severed digit or extremity must take into consideration the general health and condition of the patient, the technical feasibility of successfully replanting the part, the relative importance of the lost part and the wishes of the patient. First, and most important, is a thorough evaluation of the traumatized patient, as associated head and chest injuries are often present. Provided adequate cooling is instituted immediately, the severed part may be replanted as long as 12–24 hours following amputation.[145] Advanced diabetes and arteriosclerotic vascular disease are absolute contraindications to replantation, while relative contraindications include significant peptic ulcer, recent myocardial infarction and pulmonary problems.

Technical considerations include the mechanism of injury and the level of amputation. Cleancut or mild crush amputations can usually be replanted with a minimal amount of bone shortening and debridement. More severe crush injuries must be carefully evaluated under the operating microscope to assess fully the damage to important structures. Severe crush and avulsion amputations require extensive shortening and debridement before healthy tissue is found. Often nerves and vessels are stripped from the proximal stump, making replantation impractical.

The number of digits and the level of amputation determine the priorities for replantation. Multiple digital amputations proximal to the distal interphalangeal joint and all individual thumb amputations should be replanted whenever possible. Single digit amputations should *not* be replanted except for extenuating circumstances such as in children, a ring finger in a woman or occupational requirements. All amputations proximal to the metacarpal phalangeal joints should be replanted whenever possible. Finally, the patient must be informed of the long and difficult operation ahead, the chances of survival of the replanted part and the need for additional procedures to achieve a *limited* return of function.

PREOPERATIVE PREPARATION.—Care of the amputated part must begin immediately to minimize warm ischemia time. The part should first be copiously rinsed with normal saline, dried and wrapped in sterile gauze and then sealed in a plastic bag. The watertight bag is covered with ice. On arrival at the replantation center, the patient is resuscitated. Subsequently, the amputation stump is inspected, and then the severed part is evaluated in the operating room under magnification. If replantation is delayed, the part may be stored up to 24 – 36 hours at 4 degrees Celsius and replantation carried out when the patient is stable. The patient is given antitetanus coverage and systemic antibiotics, and cross-matched for 2 or more units of whole blood.

OPERATIVE TECHNIQUE. — General anesthesia or regional blocks with long-acting agents such as bupivacaine (Marcaine) combined with intravenous sedation may be used. Thorough debridement and identification of the neurovascular structures in the amputated part prior to induction of anesthesia substantially shortens anesthesia time.

Since finger amputations are a far more frequent occurrence than major limb amputations, the technique for digital replantation will be discussed in depth. Modifications in operative technique are only necessary in more proximal lesions above the muscle mass of the mid forearm. The basic sequence is as follows: (1) identification and debridement of all structures; (2) bone fixation; (3) extensor tendon repair; (4) dorsal vein anastomoses; (5) flexor tendon repair; (6) digital artery anastomosis; (7) digital nerve repairs, and (8) skin closure.

Digital arteries are easily located by first identifying the larger digital nerves at the lateral edges of the flexor tendon. At times, it is difficult to identify collapsed veins. These may be found by milking the blood proximally until it is seen to ooze from the cut vessel ends just beneath the superficial fascia. Irrigating the digital artery with cold, heparinized Ringer's lactate will mark the veins by runoff of clear fluid. Alternatively, veins may be identified after revascularization of the digit.

Perfusion of the amputated part with heparinized Ringer's lactate remains a controversial issue among hand surgeons. Shimizu et al.,[136] in a study of crush amputations of rabbit ears, concluded that crush amputations should be perfused prior to replantation to wash out thrombi within the vascular bed. However, Harashina and Buncke[58] showed that perfusion of the amputated rat limb reduced the replantation survival rate by 20% as compared with that of nonperfused limbs. Currently, the severed part is perfused in severe crush or avulsion injuries, double-level injuries and when dorsal veins have not been identified. If perfusion is done, a soft Silastic catheter is gently introduced into the vessel lumen and cold, heparinized Ringer's lactate allowed to perfuse the part under gravity pressure.

The bone ends are shortened to permit neurovascular anastomoses *without tension*. Usually 5–8 mm of shortening is sufficient in digital amputations and 3–8 cm for limb replantation. Fixation by K-wire, interosseous wiring or small plates with screws has been advocated.[77] If the amputation is through a joint, arthrodesis in a position of function is recommended. Following bone fixation, the entire extensor mechanism including the lateral bands is meticulously repaired.

The venous anastomoses are then performed, with a ratio of 2 veins for each arterial anastomosis, thereby ensuring adequate venous drainage. If proximal dorsal veins are too severely damaged, volar veins are repaired or veins rotated from adjacent fingers. The veins are sutured under 25× magnification with 8–10 sutures of 10-0 nylon. Proximal clamps are left in place to prevent back bleeding and stasis of blood at the anastomosis site. The dorsal skin is loosely approximated to allow access to the venous anastomosis. If there is substantial skin loss, a split-thickness skin graft may be placed directly over the venous repairs.

The arterial anastomoses are then done. The proximal digital artery is debrided until pulsatile flow is observed. Failure to ensure strong pulsatile proximal flow is the most common cause of failure in digital replants. Both digital arteries are inspected and the least damaged vessel repaired. The vessel ends are carefully debrided of traumatized tissues and anastomosed with 8–10 sutures of 10-0 nylon. Perfusion of the digit may be restored prior to digital nerve repair, depending on the surgeon's preference. The vascular clamps are released, veins first and then arteries, and the finger is observed for rapid capillary filling and hyperemia. If vascular spasm occurs, it may be overcome by bathing the artery with Xylocaine or Marcaine. Anticoagulation is routinely used in replantation surgery and begun before release of the arterial clamps. It is continued for 2 weeks, as thrombosis may occur at any time from a few hours to 12 days postoperatively.

Both digital nerves are repaired by means of a peripheral fascicular technique under magnification. If nerve avulsion has occurred, then secondary nerve grafting is necessary. The quality of functional recovery is related to sensory restoration, and every effort is made to achieve accurate *primary* nerve repairs. Primary repair of the flexor profundus tendon is also done. In severe crush injuries or avulsions, a Silastic rod may be inserted as a secondary procedure for subsequent tendon grafts. The vascular anastomoses are then checked for patency. If thrombosis has occurred, the anastomosis is resected, followed by revision or insertion of a vein graft taken from the dorsum of the foot. The skin is then loosely approximated with 6-0 nylon.

POSTOPERATIVE CARE. — The replanted part is kept exposed for continued observation and supported in a volar plaster slab. The patient is given systemic heparin by continual intravenous drip maintaining the partial thromboplastin time at 2 times normal for 10 days to 2 weeks. Aspirin, 10 grains twice a day, is given by mouth or suppository and continued for 3 weeks. In severe crush injury, sympathetic blocks are instituted to relieve spasm in the proximal vessels.

Early postoperative complications include arterial or venous occlusion. Arterial insufficiency is heralded by a change in color, a drop in temperature of the digit, a mottled appearance and decreased turgor in the digital pulp. Venous occlusion is signaled by increasing cyanosis, edema and turgor of the digital pulp. Objective methods of monitoring postoperative circulation have included the plethysmograph,[158] the Doppler probe and the thermocouple.[9] Baudet[9] considers venous occlusion to have occurred when the temperature of the digit falls 5 degrees below that of the rest of the hand, whereas a quick falloff in temperature correlates with arterial occlusion. However, none of these objective methods is totally reliable. Therefore, clinical judgment acquired by constant vigilance is the best method of assessing subtle circulatory changes in the replanted digit. If the signs of circulatory embarrassment mentioned earlier are detected, immediate re-exploration of both the arterial and venous anastomoses is indicated.

Postoperative management includes early active and passive exercise of the digit as soon as clinical bony union has occurred, usually by 4–6 weeks. Physical and occupational therapy is important to maintain supple joints and prepare the patient for any secondary tendon or nerve grafts needed. Tenolysis of the extensor and flexor tendons as well as capsulotomy are often

nerve, internal carotid artery, posterior communicating artery, posterior cerebral artery, basilar artery, cerebral peduncle and pons may all be surrounded by tumor overgrowth and adhesions, it is mandatory that these structures be carefully isolated and preserved.[164] It is now possible to spare important hypothalamic vessels and other microstructures that would otherwise have been irreparably damaged. Tumors, including chordomas, chondromas, epidermoids, dermoids and meningiomas, that may lie along the clivus can now be approached via the transclival route with the aid of the microscope.[109, 142]

Perhaps the greatest achievement in the microsurgical removal of intracranial tumors is the resection of acoustic neurinomas. House[72] introduced microtechniques for surgery of the cerebellopontine angle and demonstrated that small intracanalicular tumors could be removed without damage to the facial nerve.[69] Although there are now 5 accepted approaches to this region (subtemporal-transsphenoidal, transtentorial, translabyrinthine, combined translabyrinthine and suboccipital, suboccipital), the surgeon must utilize microsurgical techniques to visualize and preserve such delicate structures as the lower cranial nerves, facial nerve and anteroinferior cerebellar artery, as well as to remove tumor from the brain stem.

SPINAL CORD TUMORS

The most significant gains in microsurgery of spinal cord tumors have been in radical removal of intramedullary tumors. Despite the exploits of a few surgeons, including Von Eiselsberg and Horrax, who were able to remove intramedullary tumors, it was not until Greenwood[53-55] introduced the bipolar coagulating forceps in 1940 and described the necessary surgical techniques that removal of intramedullary neoplasms was deemed feasible. Now, with the high magnification and illumination afforded by the operating microscope, resection of intramedullary tumors is possible for many lesions, including diffuse hemangiomas, ependymomas and some discrete astrocytomas.

VASCULAR DISEASE

However, it is in the area of vascular diseases of the central nervous system that microsurgical techniques are now enabling the neurosurgeon to make his greatest gains. Included under this heading are arteriovenous malformations (AVM), aneurysms and cerebral revascularization for occlusive cerebrovascular disease. These three entities show a dramatic progression, not only in surgical technique but in understanding of the anatomy and physiology of basic pathophysiologic processes.

The AVM, spinal or intracerebral, causes symptoms by rupturing to form a hematoma with mass effect by a "steal" phenomenon. Recent advances in regional cerebral blood flow (rCBF) have corroborated the "steal" theory in intracerebral lesions.[41] From a neurosurgical standpoint, the advent of microsurgical techniques permits not only isolation of the feeding and draining components of these lesions but also their total removal, despite their location surrounding the brain stem or within the substance of the spinal cord.

The next great advance in vascular neurosurgery is the obliteration of intracranial aneurysms. In the past 10 years, surgeons have approached aneurysms at the anterior circle of Willis and on the basilar artery with greater appreciation of the delicate structures that must be and can be protected with the use of an operating microscope. Interest in this surgery has forced neurosurgeons to return to the dissecting laboratory to learn more about the anatomy of these structures on a finer scale than previously necessary. An example of this new enthusiasm in microneurosurgical anatomy is the extensive work of Rhoton and his colleagues, who have precisely determined the microarchitecture of the anterior cerebral-anterior communicating artery complex.[124] Understanding of the anatomy of this complicated region and its surgery was pioneered by Yasargil.[164, 165] Drake[45] introduced the microsurgical approach to aneurysms of the basilar artery. In each of these regions the surgeon must operate between and around small perforating vessels, cranial nerves and major vessels, isolate the offending arm and then obliterate the aneurysm while sparing the surrounding microanatomic structures.

Perhaps the most exciting aspect of microneurosurgery is that of cerebral revascularization. It is in this area that the neurosurgeon has applied his technical imagination, his anatomic inquisitiveness and his appreciation of neurovascular physiology to the treatment of a specific disease entity—occlusive cerebrovascular disease.[25, 44, 132] At the present time, 450,000 new strokes occur yearly, 80% of which are due to occlusive cerebro-vascular disease.[24] It is estimated that 2,000,000 persons in America are presently disabled and unemployable as a result of stroke. The majority of such persons are aged under 65 and are thus in the preretirement or productive years.[24]

The current approach to correct this circulatory insufficiency entails microvascular anastomosis of the superficial temporal branch of the external carotid artery in an end-to-side fashion to a cortical branch of the middle cerebral artery. Patient selection must be stringent and should include individuals with occlusive or stenotic lesions of the major extracranial vessels or of their intracranial branches whose lesions are inaccessible to regular vascular procedures, i.e., completely occluded internal carotid artery(ies), cavernous carotid stenosis, middle cerebral artery stenosis and vertebral-basilar lesions.[24] In each case the patient must display signs of hypoperfusion and poor collateral formation. This is indicated by the presence of transient cerebral ischemia (TIA), reversible ischemic neurologic deficit and physiologic evidence of hypoperfusion by diminished regional cerebral blood flow (rCBF).[24, 126, 132] At this writing the author has evaluated 2 patients for cerebral collateral augmentation who presented with TIA and unilateral occlusion of the internal carotid arteries. Both had diminished but marginal rCBF. Neither patient elected to have surgery. On re-examination 2 months later, neither patient was having TIAs and both had normalized their rCBF.[126] Other patients who underwent a bypass procedure had incapacitating TIA and marked to moderate reduction in their rCBF.[42] Perhaps we will be able to define a level of reduction in rCBF that is absolutely critical to proper maintenance of cerebral perfusion and thus identify the patient population that cannot create its own collateral blood supply and will require a bypass operation.

Urology*

Urology will probably become the next surgical specialty to reap the clinical rewards of microsurgical techniques. As noted by Silber, the operating microscope enables the urologist to de-

---

*Pertinent information supplied by Sherman J. Silber, Ballas Parkway Medical Center, 522 N. New Ballas Road, Suite 280, St. Louis, MO 63141.

sign experimental models for investigating the riddles of transplantation plus clinical procedures for solving complex urologic conditions.[137]

EXPERIMENTAL MODELS

Following development of a rat renal transplant model by Fisher and Lee,[48] widespread investigation of the rejection phenomenon became possible. In their model, the donor kidney is isolated on the cuffed renal artery, renal vein and ureter, with the recipient vessels being the aorta and vena cava. After transplantation the kidney is revascularized by an end-to-side anastomosis, inserting the cuff of the renal vessels into excised ellipses in the larger vessels. The operating microscope, microinstruments and 7-0 silk were initially used. Subsequently, numerous technical modifications have been added, which have improved both survival rates and physiologic duplication. Additional research into renal growth, renal hypertrophy and acute renal failure have been reported.

The urologist interested in reaping the rewards of clinical microsurgery must master microsurgical repair of the vas deferens, as well as microvascular techniques. The best experimental model for the urologist to use while learning microvascular surgery is rat renal transplantation. Experimental emphasis on 1-mm vessels facilitates clinical repair of larger vessels; also, it may prove a stimulus for increasing urologic research. Vas deferens repairs can be practised initially on excised surgical specimens, but the absence of repeated obscuration by seminal fluid and blood precludes exact clinical similarity. Anastomosis of the rat vas deferens is an excellent experimental model and the one recommended by Silber.

CLINICAL PROCEDURES

As has occurred in other specialties, the urologist trained in microsurgery will be able to refine conventional techniques as well as developing new surgical procedures for correcting problems previously considered unsolvable.

VASOVASOTOMY. — The vas deferens consists of a thin mucosalined tube with an internal diameter of 0.5 mm surrounded by a thick muscularis layer. The tube provides an unobstructed

2. Acland, R. D.: Signs of patency in small vessel anastomosis, Surgery 72: 744, 1972.
3. Acland, R. D.: New instruments for microvascular surgery, Br. J. Surg. 59:181, 1972.
4. American Replantation Mission to China: Replantation surgery in China, Plast. Reconstr. Surg. 52:476, 1973.
5. Aoyagi, F., et al.: Detection of small vessels for microsurgery by a Doppler flow meter, Plast. Reconstr. Surg. 55:372, 1975.
6. Bakamjian, V. Y.: A two stage method for pharyngoesophageal reconstruction with a primary pectoral skin flap, Plast. Reconstr. Surg. 36:178, 1965.
7. Barraquer, J. I., Barraquer, J., and Lihmann, H.: A new operating microscope for ocular surgery, Am. J. Ophthalmol. 63:90, 1967.
8. Baudet, J., et al.: Ten free groin flaps, Plast. Reconstr. Surg. 57:577, 1976.
9. Baudet, J.: Panel discussion on replantation surgery, American Society of Plastic and Reconstructive Surgery, Boston, October 1976.
10. Bora, F. W., Jr.: Peripheral nerve repair in cats: The fascicular stitch, J. Bone Joint Surg. [Am.] 49:659, 1967.
11. Bora, F. W., Pleasure, D. E., and Didizian, N. A.: A study of nerve regeneration and neuroma formation after nerve suture by various techniques, J. Hand Surg. 1:138, 1976.
12. Brunelli, G.: Attnali orientamenti per la riparazione dei nervi della mano, Riv. Chir. della Mano 7:40, 1969.
13. Buncke, H. J.: Digital nerve repairs, Surg. Clin. North Am. 52:1267, 1972.
14. Buncke, H. J.: The Suture Repair of 1.0 Mm. Vessels, in Donaghy, R.M.P., and Yasargil, M. G. (eds.): *Microvascular Surgery* (Stuttgart: Georg Thieme, 1967).
15. Buncke, H. J., and Blackfield, H. M.: The vasoplegic effects of chlorpromazine, Plast. Reconstr. Surg. 31:353, 1963.
16. Buncke, H. J., and Furnas, D.: Free Compound Bone-Skin Transfer, in Daniel, R. K., and Terzis, J. K. (eds.): *Reconstructive Microsurgery* (Boston: Little, Brown & Company, 1977).
17. Buncke, H. J., and Schultz, W. P.: Immediate Nicoladoni procedure in the rhesus monkey, or hallux-to-hand transplantation utilizing microminiature vascular anastomoses, Br. J. Plast. Surg. 19:332, 1966.
18. Buncke, H. J., and Schultz, W. P.: Total ear reimplantation in the rabbit utilizing microminiature vascular anastomoses, Br. J. Plast. Surg. 19:15, 1966.
19. Buncke, J. D., Buncke, C. M., and Schultz, W. B.: Experimental digital amputation and reimplantation, Plast. Reconstr. Surg. 36:62, 1965.
20. Bunnel, S., and Boyes, J. H.: Nerve grafts, Am. J. Surg. 44:64, 1939.
21. Cabaud, H. E., Rodkey, W. G., McCarroll, H. R., Mutz, S. B., and Niebauer, J. J.: Epineurial and perineurial fascicular nerve repairs: A critical comparison, J. Hand Surg. 1:131, 1976.
22. Carrel, A.: The results of the transplantation of blood vessels: Organs and limbs, J.A.M.A. 51:1662, 1908.
23. Carrel, A., and Guthrie, C. C.: Complete amputation of the thigh with replantation, Am. J. Med. Sci. 131:297, 1906.

24. Chater, N., and Peters, N.: Neurosurgical microvascular bypass for stroke, West. J. Med. 124:1, 1976.
25. Chater, N. L., Spetzler, R. F., and Touvemaclur, K.: Microvascular bypass surgery. Part 1: Anatomic studies, J. Neurosurg. 44:712, 1976.
26. Ch'en, C. W., Ch'en, Y. C., and Pao, Y. S.: Salvage of the forearm following complete traumatic amputation: Report of a case, Chin. Med. J. 82: 632, 1963.
27. Clodius, L.: Microlymphatic Techniques, in Daniel, R. K., and Terzis, J. K. (eds.): Reconstructive Microsurgery (Boston: Little, Brown & Company, 1977).
28. Clodius, L., and Wirth, R.: A new model for chronic lymphedema of the extremities, Chir. Plastica 2:115, 1974.
29. Cobbett, J. R.: Small vessel anastomosis, Br. J. Plast. Surg. 22:16, 1967.
30. Cohen, B. E., May, J. W., Daly, J. S., and Young, H. H.: Successful clinical replantation of an amputated penis by microneurovascular repair, Plast. Reconstr. Surg. 59:276, 1977.
31. Cordeiro, A. K.: Linfoedemo primario anastomose linfo-venosa. Presented at 16th Brazilian Congress for Angiology, November 1969.
32. Cormann, J. L., Anderson, J. T., Taubman, J., Stables, D. P., Halgrimson, C. G., Popontzer, M., and Starzl, T. E.: Ex vivo perfusion, arteriography, and autotransplantation procedures for kidney salvage, Surg. Gynecol. Obstet. 137:659, 1973.
33. Danese, C., Bower, R., and Howard, J.: Experimental anastomoses of lymphatics, Arch. Surg. 84:6, 1962.
34. Daniel, R. K.: The Anatomical and Hemodynamic Characteristics of the Cutaneous Circulation and their Influence on Skin Flap Design, in Grabb, W. C., and Meyers, B. (eds.): Skin Flaps (Boston: Little, Brown & Company, 1975).
35. Daniel, R. K., and Entin, M. A.: Microsurgery bibliography, Clin. in Plast. Surg. 3:159, 1976.
36. Daniel, R. K., and Taylor, G. I.: Distant transfer of an island flap by microvascular anastomoses, Plast. Reconstr. Surg. 52:111, 1973.
37. Daniel, R. K., and Terzis, J. K.: Reconstructive Microsurgery (Boston: Little, Brown & Company, 1977).
38. Daniel, R. K., Cunningham, D. M., and Taylor, G. I.: The deltopectoral flap: An anatomic and hemodynamic approach, Plast. Reconstr. Surg. 55: 275, 1975.
39. Daniel, R. K., Terzis, J. K., and Cunningham, D. M.: Sensory skin flaps for coverage of pressure sores in paraplegic patients, Plast. Reconstr. Surg. 58:317, 1976.
40. Daniel, R. K., Terzis, J. K., and Midgley, R.: Restoration of sensation to an anesthetic hand by a free neurovascular flap from the foot, Plast. Reconstr. Surg. 57:275, 1976.
41. Deshmukh, V. D., and Mayer, J. S.: Personal communication.
42. Deshmukh, V. D., Mayer, J. S., Naritomi, J. L., Peters, N. D., et al.: Diagnostic and prognostic value of noninvasive regional cerebral blood flow (rCBF) in stroke. Presented at the 2d Joint Meeting on Stroke and Cerebral Circulation, Miami, Fla., February 1977.
43. Dohlman, G. F.: Carl Olof Nylen and the birth of the otomicroscope and microsurgery, Arch. Otolaryngol. 90:161, 1969.

44. Donaghy, R. M. P., and Yasargil, M. G.: Extra-intracranial blood flow diversion. Presented to the American Association of Neurological Surgeons, Chicago, Ill., April 1968.
45. Drake, C. G.: Surgical treatment of ruptured aneurysms of the basilar artery, J. Neurosurg. 23:457, 1965.
46. Edshage, S.: Peripheral nerve suture: A technique for improved intraneural topography, Acta Chir. Scand. [Suppl.] 331:1, 1964.
47. Finseth, F., Constable, J., and Cannon, B.: Interfascicular nerve grafting, Plast. Reconstr. Surg. 56:492, 1975.
48. Fisher, B., and Lee, S.: Microvascular surgical techniques in research surgery, Surgery 58:904, 1965.
49. Fry, W. J., Ernst, C. B., Stanley, J. C., and Brink, B.: Renovascular hypertension in the pediatric patient, Arch. Surg. 107:692, 1973.
50. Fujino, T., et al.: Free skin flap from the retroauricular region to the nose, Plast. Reconstr. Surg. 57:338, 1976.
51. Goto, Y.: Experimental study of nerve autografting of funicular suture, Arch. Jap. Chir. 36:478, 1967.
52. Grabb, W. C., et al.: Comparison of methods of peripheral nerve suturing in monkeys, Plast. Reconstr. Surg. 46:31, 1970.
53. Greenwood, J.: Total removal of intramedullary tumors, J. Neurosurg. 11:616, 1954.
54. Greenwood, J.: Surgical removal of intramedullary tumors, J. Neurosurg. 26:275, 1967.
55. Greenwood, J.: Spinal Cord Tumors, in Youmans, Julien R. (ed.): Neurological Surgery, Vol. 3 (Philadelphia: W. B. Saunders Co., 1973), pp. 1514–34.
56. Hakstian, R. W.: Funicular orientation by direct stimulation: An aid to peripheral nerve repair, J. Bone Joint Surg. [Am.] 50:1178, 1968.
57. Hakstian, R. W.: Perineurial neurorrhaphy, Orthop. Clin. North Am. 4:956, 1973.
58. Harashina, T., and Buncke, H.: Study of washout solutions for microvascular replantation and transplantation, Plast. Reconstr. Surg. 56:542, 1975.
59. Harashina, T., et al.: Reconstruction of the oral cavity with a free flap, Plast. Reconstr. Surg. 58:412, 1976.
60. Hardy, J. S., and Wigser, M.: Transsphenoidal surgery of the pituitary fossa tumors with televised radiofluoroscopic control, J. Neurosurg. 23:612, 1965.
61. Harii, K., and Ohmori, K.: Free skin flap transfer, Clin. in Plast. Surg. 3:111, 1976.
62. Harii, K., Ohmori, K., and Ohmori, S.: Free deltopectoral skin flaps, Br. J. Plast. Surg. 53:231, 1974.
63. Harii, K., Ohmori, K., and Ohmori, S.: Successful clinical transfer of ten free flaps by microvascular anastomoses, Plast. Reconstr. Surg. 53:259, 1974.
64. Harii, K., Ohmori, K., and Ohmori, S.: Hair transplantation with free scalp flaps, Plast. Reconstr. Surg. 53:410, 1974.
65. Harii, K., Ohmori, K., and Sekyuchi, J.: The free musculocutaneous flap, Plast. Reconstr. Surg. 57:294, 1976.

66. Harii, K., Ohmori, K., and Torii, S.: Free gracilis muscle transplantation with microneurovascular anastomoses for the treatment of facial paralysis, Plast. Reconstr. Surg. 57:133, 1976.
67. Harms, H., and Mackensen, G.: *Ocular Surgery under the Microscope* (Chicago: Year Book Medical Publishers, Inc., 1966).
68. Hayhurst, J. W., and O'Brien, B. McC.: An experimental study of microvascular technique, patency rates, and related factors, Br. J. Plast. Surg. 28:128, 1975.
69. Hitselberger, W. E., and House, W. F.: Surgical approaches to acoustic tumors, Arch. Otolaryngol. 84:286, 1966.
70. Holmes, W., and Young, J. Z.: Nerve regeneration after immediate and delayed suture, J. Anat. 77:63, 1942.
71. Holmgren, G.: Some experiences in surgery of otosclerosis, Acta Otolaryngol. (Stockh) 5:460, 1923.
72. House, W. F.: Surgical exposure of the internal auditory canal and its contents through the middle cranial fossa, Laryngoscope 71:1363, 1961.
73. Howard, J. M., Danese, C., and Laine, Q. B.: Experimental lymphatic anastomoses, J. Cardiovasc. Surg. 5:694, 1964.
74. Hulka, J. F., and Davis, J. E.: Vasectomy and reversible vasoocclusion, Fertil. Steril. 23:683, 1972.
75. Ikuta, Y.: Free Muscle Transfer, in Daniel, R. K., and Terzis, J. K. (eds.): *Reconstructive Microsurgery* (Boston: Little, Brown & Company, 1977).
76. Ikuta, Y., et al.: Free flap transfers by end-to-side arterial anastomoses, Br. J. Plast. Surg. 28:1, 1975.
77. Ikuta, Y., and Tsuge, K.: Microbolts and microscrews for fixation of small bones of the hand, Hand 6:261, 1974.
78. Ikuta, Y., Kubo, T., and Tsuge, K.: Free muscle transplantation by microsurgical technique to treat severe Volkmann's contracture, Plast. Reconstr. Surg. 58:407, 1976.
79. Ishikawa, F.: Experimental study on nerve suture, especially about the funicular suture of the peripheral nerves, Med. J. Hiroshima Univ. 14:359, 1966.
80. Jacobson, J. H.: Microsurgery, *Current Problems in Surgery* (Chicago: Year Book Medical Publishers, Inc., February 1971).
81. Jacobson, J. H.: Microsurgical technique in repair of the traumatized extremity, Clin. Orthop. 29:132, 1963.
82. Jacobson, J. H., and Suarez, E. L.: Microsurgery in the anastomosis of small vessels, Surg. Forum 11:243, 1960.
83. Jacobson, S.: Studies of the blood circulation in lymphedematous limbs, Scand. J. Plast. Reconstr. Surg. [Suppl. 3], 1967.
84. Jako, G. J.: Laryngoscope for microscopic observation, surgery and photography, Arch. Otolaryngol. 91:2, 1970.
85. Jako, G. J.: Laser surgery of the vocal cords, Laryngoscope 82:2204, 1972.
86. Jako, G. J., and Polanyi, T. G.: Carbon Dioxide Laser Surgery in Otolaryngology, in Kaplan, I. (ed.): *Laser Surgery* (Jerusalem: Jerusalem Academic Press, 1976).
87. Kleinert, E. H., and Griffin, J. M.: Technique of nerve anastomosis, Orthop. Clin. North Am. 4:907, 1973.
88. Kleinsasser, O.: A larynx-microscope for early diagnosis and differential-

diagnosis of carcinoma of the larynx and oral cavity, J. Laryngol. Rhinol. Otol. 40:276, 1961.

89. Koetting, R. A.: A survey of telescopic lenses for dentistry and surgery, Optom. Weekly 3:619, 1971.

90. Komatsu, S., and Tamai, S.: Successful replantation of a completely cut-off thumb, Plast. Reconstr. Surg. 42:374, 1968.

91. Krizek, T. J., et al.: Experimental transplantation of composite grafts by microsurgical vascular anastomoses, Plast. Reconstr. Surg. 36:538, 1965.

92. Kubo, T., Ikuta, Y., and Tsuge, K.: Free muscle transplantation in dogs by microneurovascular anastomoses, Plast. Reconstr. Surg. 57:495, 1976.

93. Kurze, T.: Microtechniques in neurological surgery, Clin. Neurosurg. 11: 128, 1964.

94. Langley, J. N., and Hashimoto, M.: On the suture of separate nerve bundles in a nerve trunk and on internal nerve plexuses, J. Physiol. 51:318, 1917.

95. Lapchinski, A. G.: Recent results of experimental transplantation of preserved limbs and kidneys and possible use of this technique in clinical practice, Ann. N.Y. Acad. Sci. 64:539, 1960.

96. Littler, J. W.: Neurovascular pedicle transfer of tissue in reconstructive surgery of the hand, J. Bone Joint Surg. [Am.] 38:917, 1956.

97. Malt, R. A., and McKhann, C.: Replantation of severed arms, J.A.M.A. 189:716, 1964.

98. McCraw, J. B., and Furlow, L. T.: The dorsalis pedis arterialized flap, Plast. Reconstr. Surg. 55:177, 1975.

99. McDowell, F.: The free living bone graft (editorial), Plast. Reconstr. Surg. 55:612, 1975.

100. McLean, D. H., and Buncke, H. J.: The use of the Saran wrap cuff in microsurgical arterial repairs, Plast. Reconstr. Surg. 51:624, 1973.

101. Michon, J., et Massé, P.: Le moment optimum de la suture nerveuse dans les plaies du membre supérieur, Rev. Chir. Orthop. 50:205, 1964.

102. Millesi, H.: Zum Problem der Überbrückung von Defekten peripherer Nerven, Wien. Med. Wochenschr. 118:182, 1968.

103. Millesi, H.: Microsurgery of peripheral nerves, Hand 5:157, 1973.

104. Millesi, H.: Treatment of Nerve Lesions by Fascicular Free Nerve Grafts, in Michon, J., and Moberg, E. (eds.): *Traumatic Nerve Lesions* (Edinburgh: Churchill Livingstone, 1975).

105. Millesi, H., Ganglberger, J., and Berger, A.: Erfahrungen mit der Mikrochirurgie peripherer Nerven, Chir. Plast. Reconstr. 3:47, 1967.

106. Millesi, H., Meissl, G., and Berger, A.: Entwicklungstendenzen in der Operativen Wiederherstellung durchtrennter peripherer Nerven, Medicinska Naklada Zagreb 161, 1970.

107. Millesi, H., Meissl, G., and Berger, A.: The interfascicular nerve grafting of the median and ulnar nerves, J. Bone Joint Surg. [Am.] 54:727, 1972.

108. Millesi, H., Meissl, G., and Berger, A.: Further experience with interfascicular grafting of the median, ulnar and radial nerves, J. Bone Joint Surg. [Am.] 58:209, 1976.

109. Mullan, S. R., Naunton, J., Hekmat-Panah, G., and Vailati, T.: The use of the anterior approach to ventrally placed tumors in the foramen magnum and vertebral column, J. Neurosurg. 24:536, 1966.

110. Nielubowicz, J., and Olszewski, W.: Surgical lymphaticovenous shunts in patients with secondary lymphoedema, Br. J. Surg. 55:440, 1968.
111. Nielubowicz, J., and Olszewski, W.: Experimental lymphovenous anastomosis, Br. J. Surg. 55:449, 1968.
112. Nylen, C. O.: The microscope in aural surgery: Its first use and later development, Acta Otolaryngol. 116:226, 1954.
113. O'Brien, B. M.: Replantation of digits. Presented at American Society of Plastic and Reconstructive Surgeons meeting, Boston, October 1976.
114. O'Brien, B. M., et al.: Clinical replantation of digits, Plast. Reconstr. Surg. 52:490, 1973.
115. O'Brien, B. M., et al.: Free flap transfers with microvascular anastomoses, Br. J. Plast. Surg. 27:220, 1974.
116. O'Brien, B. M.: Replantation and reconstructive microvascular surgery, Ann. Roy. Coll. Surg. 58:171, 1976.
117. Ohmori, K., and Harii, K.: Free groin flaps: Their vascular basis, Br. J. Plast. Surg. 28:238, 1975.
118. Orcutt, T. W., Foster, J. H., Richie, R. E., Wilson, J. P., and Howell, D. W.: Bilateral ex vivo renal artery reconstruction with autotransplantation, J.A.M.A. 228:493, 1974.
119. Orgel, M. G., and Terzis, J. K.: Epineurial vs. perineurial repair: An ultrastructural and electrophysiological study of nerve regeneration, Plast. Reconstr. Surg. 1977. (In press.)
120. Ortichochea, M.: The musculocutaneous flap method: An immediate and heroic substitute for the method of delay, Br. J. Plast. Surg. 25:106, 1972.
121. Östrup, L.: The Free Living Bone Graft (Linkopink: Medical Press, 1976).
122. Östrup, L., and Fredrickson, J.: Distant transfer of a free, living bone graft by microvascular anastomoses: An experimental study, Plast. Reconstr. Surg. 54:274, 1974.
123. Panje, W., et al.: Reconstruction of the oral cavity with a free flap, Plast. Reconstr. Surg. 58:415, 1976.
124. Perlmutter, D., and Rhoton, A. L.: Microsurgical anatomy of the anterior cerebral-anterior communicating-recurrent artery complex, J. Neurosurg. 45:259, 1976.
125. Perritt, R. A.: Recent advances in corneal surgery, Am. Acad. Ophthalmol. Otolaryngol. course no. 288, 1950.
126. Peters, N., and Deshmukh, V.: Unpublished data.
127. Phadke, G. M., and Phadke, A. G.: Experience in the reanastomosis of the vas deferens, J. Urol. 97:888, 1967.
128. Rand, R. W.: Microneurosurg (St. Louis: C. V. Mosby Company, 1969).
129. Samii, M., and Wallenborn, R.: Tierexperimentelle Untersuchungen über den Einfluss der Spannung auf den Regenerationserfas nach Nervennaht, Acta Neurochir. 27:87, 1972.
130. Samii, M.: Modern Aspects of Peripheral and Cranial Nerve Surgery, in Krayenbuhl, H. (ed.): Advances and Technical Standards in Neurosurgery (New York: Springer-Verlag, 1975), Vol. 2.
131. Schmidt, S.: Anastomosis of the vas deferens: An experimental study, J. Urol. 81:203, 1959.
132. Schniedek, P., Grutzl, O., et al.: Selection of patients for extra-cranial

intra-cranial arterial bypass surgery based on rCBF measurements, J. Neurosurg. 44:303, 1976.

133. Seddon, S. H.: *Surgical Disorders of the Peripheral Nerves* (Edinburgh: Churchill Livingstone, 1975).

134. Sedlacek, J.: Lymphovenous shunt as supplementary treatment of elephantiasis of lower limbs, Acta Chir. Plast. 11:157, 1969.

135. Serrafin, D., *et al.*: Fourteen free groin flap transfers, Plast. Reconstr. Surg. 57:707, 1976.

136. Shimizu, T., *et al.*: Fundamental study on the irrigation of the part in digit replantation. Presented at the meeting of the Japanese Orthopaedic Society, April 1975.

137. Silber, S. J.: Microsurgery in clinical urology, Urology 6:150, 1975.

138. Silber, S. J.: Perfect anatomic reconstruction of vas deferens with a new microscopic surgical technique, Fertil. Steril. 1977. (In press.)

139. Sixth People's Hospital, Shanghai: Replantation of severed organs: Clinical experience in 217 cases involving 373 fingers, Chin. Med. J. 1:184, 1975.

140. Smith, J. W.: Microsurgery of peripheral nerves, Plast. Reconstr. Surg. 33:317, 1964.

141. Snyder, C. C., Knowles, R. P., Mayer, P., and Hobbs, J.: Extremity replantation, Plast. Reconstr. Surg. 26:251, 1960.

142. Stevenson, G. C., Staney, J. J., Perkins, R. K., and Adams, J. E.: A trans-cervical trans-clinical approach to the ventral surface of the brain stem for removal of a clivus chordoma, J. Neurosurg. 24:544, 1966.

143. Sunderland, S.: *Nerves and Nerve Injuries* (Edinburgh and London: E. & S. Livingstone, Ltd., 1968).

144. Sunderland, S.: The intraneural topography of the radial, median and ulnar nerves, Brain 68:243, 1945.

145. Swartz, W. M., et al.: The effects of prolonged ischemia in the replanted rat leg: A biochemical and morphologic study of microvascular techniques, Surg. Forum. In press.

146. Swartz, W., Brink, R., and Buncke, H.: Prevention of thrombosis in arterial and venous microanastomoses by using topical agent, Plast. Reconstr. Surg. 58:478, 1976.

147. Tamai, S.: Multiple Digit Replantation, in Daniel, R. K., and Terzis, J. K. (eds.): *Reconstructive Microsurgery* (Boston: Little, Brown & Company., 1977).

148. Tamai, S.: Personal communication.

149. Tamai, S., *et al.*: Free muscle transplants in dogs with microsurgical neurovascular anastomoses, Plast. Reconstr. Surg. 46:219, 1970.

150. Taub, H. G., Scazco, A. N., and Shipman, W. F.: Microscopic suspension laryngoscopy, Ann. Otol. Rhinol. Laryngol. 69:1134, 1960.

151. Taylor, G. I., and Daniel, R. K.: The anatomy of several free flap donor sites, Plast. Reconstr. Surg. 56:243, 1975.

152. Taylor, G. I., and Ham., F. J.: The free vascularized nerve graft, Plast. Reconstr. Surg. 57:413, 1976.

153. Taylor, G. I., Miller, G., and Ham, F.: The free vascularized bone graft, Plast. Reconstr. Surg. 55:533, 1975.

154. Terzis, J.: Sensory mapping, Clin. in Plast. Surg. 3:59, 1976.

155. Terzis, J., Faibisoff, B. A., & Williams, H. B.: A diamond knife for micro-surgical repair of peripheral nerves, Plast. Reconstr. Surg. 54:102, 1974.
156. Terzis, J., Faibisoff, B. A., and Williams, H. B.: The nerve gap: Suture under tension vs. graft, Plast. Reconstr. Surg. 56:166, 1975.
157. Troutman, R. C.: *Microsurgery of the Anterior Segment of the Eye.* Vol. 1, *Introduction and Basic Techniques* (St. Louis: C. V. Mosby Company, 1974).
158. Webster, M., and Patterson, J.: The photoelectric plethysmograph as a monitor of microvascular anastomoses, Br. J. Plast. Surg. 29:182, 1976.
159. Weiland, A. J., Daniel, R. K., and Riley, L. H., Jr.: Application of the free vascularized bone graft in the treatment of malignant or aggressive bone tumors, Bull. Johns Hopkins Hosp. 140:85, 1977.
160. Williams, H. B., and Terzis, J.: Single fascicular recordings: An intra-operative diagnostic tool for the management of peripheral nerve lesions, Plast. Reconstr. Surg. 57:562, 1976.
161. Wilmot, T. J.: Otological balance, Proc. Roy. Soc. Med. 67:331, 1974.
162. Wise, A. J., Topulzu, C., Dairo, P., and Kaye, I. S.: A comparative analysis of macro- and microsurgical neurorrhaphy techniques, Am. J. Surg. 117:566, 1969.
163. Yamamoto, K.: A comparative analysis of the process of nerve regeneration following funicular and epineurial suture for peripheral nerve repair, Arch. Jap. Chir. 43:276, 1974.
164. Yasargil, M. G.: *Microsurgery: As Applied to Neurosurgery* (Stuttgart: Georg Thieme Verlag, 1969).
165. Yasargil, M. G., Fox, J. L., and Ray, M. W.: The Operative Approach to Aneurysms of the Anterior Communicating Artery, in *Advances in Neurosurgery,* Vol. 2, 1975, p. 114.

Injuries to the Metacarpal Bones and Joints

RICHARD J. SMITH and CLAYTON A. PEIMER

Hand Surgery Service, Department of Orthopaedic Surgery, Massachusetts General Hospital, Harvard Medical School, Boston, Massachusetts

The metacarpals are the keystones of the longitudinal and transverse arches of the hands.[21] They position and stabilize the fingers and thumb, while permitting variations of grip and versatility of motion. This versatility is lost if there is a malunited metacarpal fracture, a stiff or unstable metacarpophalangeal (MP) or carpometacarpal joint or metacarpal loss and shortening. The treatment of injuries to the metacarpals and their adjacent joints is crucial to restore function to the injured hand.

Anatomy

METACARPALS AND CARPOMETACARPAL JOINTS

The 2d and 3d metacarpals form a rigid pillar in the center of the hand, while the 1st, 4th and 5th metacarpals are mobile at their bases and allow the palm to be cupped and the thumb and little fingers to be brought into opposition.

The *2d metacarpal* is usually the longest. Its large, forked base holds the trapezoid firmly between its ulnar and radial styloid process. There is virtually no motion at the metacarpal-trapezoid joint. The radial styloid process articulates with the trapezium, and the ulnar styloid articulates with the base of the 3d metacarpal and capitate. Stout ligaments envelop these articulations and further support and immobilize the 2d metacarpal. The extensor carpi radialis longus inserts at the dorsum of the metacarpal base and the flexor carpi radialis at its volar side. The shaft is cylindric and has a gentle volar curve in the region of the neck. The head is large and somewhat irregular with a smooth, convex articular surface that is greater in the volar-dorsal direction than from side to side. On sagittal section, the head is asymmetric and is smaller dorsally than volarly. On coronal section the dorsal half of the metacarpal head is narrower than the volar half. The volar portion of the metacarpal head is, therefore, both wider and more rounded than its dorsal aspect.

The *3d metacarpal* is a little smaller than the 2d. Its concave proximal surface articulates with the capitate. A radial styloid process extends dorsally to articulate with the 2d metacarpal and trapezoid; on the ulnar side, 2 facets are present for the 4th metacarpal articulation. These complex bony articulations and strong intermetacarpal ligament stabilize this joint and allow little motion. The shaft, neck and head are similar to those at the 2d metacarpal. The adductor muscle takes origin from a longitudinal volar crest on the shaft and the extensor carpi radialis brevis inserts at its base.

The *4th metacarpal* base is divided into a radial and ulnar portion by a prominent ridge. The radial facet articulates with the capitate and the 3d metacarpal. The ulnar facet articulates with the radial half of the hamate and the 5th metacarpal. An arc of 15–20 degrees of flexion-extension is permitted by these articulations. The 4th metacarpal head and shaft are very similar to those of the 3d metacarpal.

The *5th metacarpal* articulates at its base with the ulnar half of the hamate and, by a small facet, with the 4th metacarpal. The proximal articular surface of the 5th metacarpal is saddle-shaped with a convexity in the volar-dorsal direction and a concavity in the radial-ulnar direction. At this joint 25–40 degrees of flexion and extension are permitted. A small ulnar styloid process gives origin to the abductor digiti quinti muscle. A volar ridge marks the attachment of the opponens digiti quinti muscle. The 5th metacarpal head is similar to those of the adjacent fingers.

The *1st metacarpal* is the shortest and the broadest of the five. It has a prominent volar ridge to which attaches the opponens pollicis muscle. The 1st metacarpal base is saddle-shaped, convex in the transverse direction and concave dorsovolarly. It articulates with the distal end of the trapezium, which is convex dorsovolarly and concave from side to side. The radius of curvature of the distal end of the trapezium is greater than that of the 1st metacarpal base. Thus, the metacarpal base may rotate, relatively free of constraint, in the shallow distal trapezial articular surface. A snug, congruent saddle joint would permit motion in only 2 planes, flexion-extension and abduction-adduction. Although circumduction may be produced by combining these motions, rotation would not be possible. Thus, the loose but sturdy ligaments and the relatively incongruous articulation of the metacarpal-trapezial joint permits pronation of the thumb.[34] Because of the lack of skeletal stability, only the strong capsule at the base of the 1st metacarpal stabilizes the joint. It includes thick anterior and posterior oblique ligaments that extend from the ulnar styloid of the 1st metacarpal base to the base of the 2d metacarpal and the trapezoid. These ligaments are so strongly attached to the bone that a sudden injury is much more likely to cause an avulsion fracture than a ligament tear. With loss of these basal ligaments, the thumb metacarpal is unstable.[17]

The head of the 1st metacarpal is less spherical than those of the other metacarpals and may be quite flat and quadrilateral, limiting MP joint flexion. The transverse diameter of the volar half of the 1st metacarpal head is broader than that of the dorsum, as with the finger metacarpals.

Metacarpophalangeal Joints

The spherical head of each of the metacarpals articulates with a concave shallow base of the proximal phalanx. Unlike the interphalangeal joints, which permit only flexion and extension, the MP joint of each of the fingers and of the thumb permits both flexion-extension and abduction-adduction. Minimal rotation is also permitted.

The stability of the MP joint is dependent almost entirely upon the soft tissues that surround and support it. The dorsal capsule of the MP joint is thin and often almost translucent. It is reinforced by the extensor digitorum communis, the proper digital extensors of the index and little fingers, and, in the thumb, by the extensor pollicis brevis. The dorsal capsule offers little support, and principally serves to contain the joint synovium.[36]

The collateral ligaments to the radial and ulnar side of each of the joints may be up to 3 mm in thickness and 8 mm wide. Proximally, they are attached to a depression at either side of the metacarpal head and course distally and volarly to attach to the base of the proximal phalanx volar to the axis of motion. Because the metacarpal head is larger volarly than dorsally, both in its sagittal and coronal planes, the collateral ligaments become progressively tighter as the MP joints flex. In extension, these ligaments are relatively lax and permit abduction, adduction and slight rotation of the fingers and thumb. When the fist is clenched, the ligaments are tight, permitting only a few degrees of lateral deviation at the MP joints.

In addition to preventing excessive lateral deviation, the collateral ligaments also support the proximal phalanges dorsally and prevent their volar subluxation. With the collateral ligaments intact, contraction of the flexor tendons and of the intrinsic muscles results in flexion of the MP joints, and the collateral ligaments act like hinges about which the phalanx rotates. If these ligaments are lost, the extrinsic and intrinsic flexors will translocate the proximal phalanx volarly rather than flexing it.

The accessory collateral ligaments lie adjacent and just volar to the collateral ligaments. They run from the metacarpal head volarly and distally to the lateral rims of the volar plate. These ligaments help with lateral stabilization of the MP joint, particularly when the joint is in extension. They also support the volar plate and the adjacent flexor tendons and pulley at the midline of the MP joint.

The volar capsule is thickened distally into a fibrocartilaginous plate, which is firmly attached to the volar rim at the base of the proximal phalanx. Laterally, the plate is supported by the accessory collateral ligaments. The cartilaginous plate lies beneath the metacarpal head, and more proximally thins into a membranous layer attached loosely to the neck of the metacarpal. The membranous portion of the volar capsule folds beneath the metacarpal head with MP joint flexion. In the thumb, the little finger and occasionally the index finger the volar plate is reinforced by small sesamoid bones.

The volar plates of the 4 fingers are interconnected by transverse fibers known as the deep transverse metacarpal ligament. The entire capsular structure is reinforced by the tendons of the intrinsic and extrinsic muscles that surround these joints.[51]

Metacarpal Fractures

EXTRA-ARTICULAR FRACTURES OF THE METACARPALS OF THE FINGERS

FRACTURES OF THE METACARPAL NECK. — Closed fractures of the neck of the metacarpal are among the most common fractures of the hand. They are usually the result of a blow, and have been called "boxer's fractures." The 4th and 5th metacarpals are most frequently involved. Typically, patients will complain of pain at the dorsum of the hand, particularly while making a fist. The rounded prominence of the knuckle is lost, and in its place a protuberance is seen about 1 cm proximal to the fracture site. Volar angulation of metacarpal neck fractures is due to 2 factors: (1) The impact usually occurs at the dorsum of the metacarpal head with a resultant vector force on the metacarpal head that is directed in both a volar and proximal direction causing impaction of the volar cortex; (2) the interosseous and intrinsic muscles lie volar to the axis of MP motion and hold the metacarpal head flexed. With metacarpal head acutely flexed, the MP joint tends to hyperextend.

If the fracture is not adequately reduced and is allowed to heal in its position of deformity, pain may develop in the palm when the protruding metacarpal head is pressed against a tightly grasped object. There may be limitation of motion of the MP joint, particularly if the proximal phalanx has been allowed to remain hyperextended. Many patients will be concerned about the loss of the normal knuckle contour and the bony protuberance at the fracture site. If there is a rotational component to the fracture, overlapping of the fingers can also be quite disabling.

Due to the mobility of the 4th and 5th metacarpals at the carpometacarpal joints, a fracture that has healed with a mild flexion deformity will cause little functional disability.[30] With grasp, the 4th or 5th metacarpal head will be pushed dorsally to the limits of carpometacarpal joint motion. Angulation of more than 10–15 degrees of the 2d or 3d metacarpals, however, may be quite uncomfortable; with grasp, the patient may complain that he feels as though there is a marble in his palm.

Many methods of treatment of this fracture have been described, including traction, manipulation and surgery.[49] We believe a displaced closed metacarpal neck fracture should be

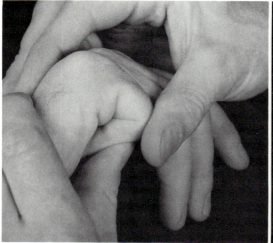

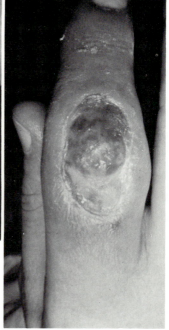

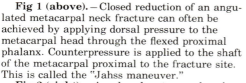

Fig 1 (above). — Closed reduction of an angulated metacarpal neck fracture can often be achieved by applying dorsal pressure to the metacarpal head through the flexed proximal phalanx. Counterpressure is applied to the shaft of the metacarpal proximal to the fracture site. This is called the "Jahss maneuver."

Fig 2 (right). — A reduced metacarpal neck fracture should never be immobilized with a proximal interphalangeal joint acutely flexed or in any type of pressure cast. This patient developed a deep ulcer involving skin, subcutaneous tissue and the extensor apparatus of the proximal interphalangeal joint as the result of a pressure cast.

treated by closed means if at all possible.[32] After infiltration of the fracture hematoma with 2–3 ml of local anesthetic, the MP and proximal interphalangeal joint are acutely flexed. The surgeon's fingers are placed proximal to the fracture site dorsally and his thumbs apply upward and dorsal pressure at the head of the flexed proximal phalanx. Most frequently, the base of the proximal phalanx will act as a buttress, reducing the metacarpal head into its normal position by this "Jahss maneuver" (Fig 1).[32]

Occasionally, it is first necessary to disengage the fracture fragments by applying longitudinal traction to the extended finger. The angulatory deformity is then reduced as described above. Rotatory alignment is tested by allowing all fingers to flex simultaneously and noting whether there is any divergence or overlap of the fingertips. If so, the finger is flexed at the MP joint and rotated back into its neutral position.

It is essential not to immobilize the reduced fracture with the interphalangeal joints flexed or by applying continuous pressure to the proximal phalanx or the dorsum of the metacarpal. Pressure upon the metacarpal shaft and flexed proximal phalanx should only be used for the *reduction* of the fracture and *not* for retaining the reduction once achieved. Prolonged immobilization with the proximal interphalangeal joint flexed or with a pressure cast can be catastrophic and may lead to permanent flexion contraction of the proximal interphalangeal joint, ulceration and loss of dorsal apparatus of the finger or ulceration over the dorsum of the metacarpal (Fig 2). Once reduction has been achieved, the injured and the adjacent fingers are immobilized in a volar gutter-type plaster splint with 20 degrees of flexion at the interphalangeal joints, 50 degrees of flexion of the MP joints and with the wrist in 30 degrees of dorsiflexion. The position is checked with x-rays after the plaster is applied and again after 1 week. Immobilization is maintained for 3 weeks and then protected active motion is encouraged, even if there is no radiographic evidence of bony union. The prolonged use of "Chinese fingertraps" or the use of banjo splints to maintain reduction should be avoided as they risk circulatory damage and extension contracture of the MP and interphalangeal joints.

If fracture reduction cannot be achieved or maintained by the methods described, the surgeon must first determine whether the deformity is acceptable. In a child with an open epiphysis, one may accept up to 30 degrees of volar angulation of 2d and 3d metacarpals and up to 50 degrees of volar angulation of 4th or 5th metacarpals. Remodeling will occur. In adults, there is no disability with up to 15 degrees of volar angulation of the 2d and 3d metacarpals and up to 30 degrees of the 4th and 5th metacarpals.[29, 30] Rotatory deformity cannot be accepted in either children or adults.

If the deformity is not acceptable, then open reduction and internal fixation are preferred over skeletal traction, pressure casts or other so-called conservative measures. Through an appropriate dorsal incision (transverse incisions usually leave better scars), the fracture site is exposed and reduced, and smooth crossed Kirschner wires are inserted. It is best to avoid passing these wires through the MP joints. The hand is splinted for 3 weeks and then active motion begun. The wires may be removed in 4 – 6 weeks.

With boxer's fractures, one must be particularly alert to the presence of a penetrating wound that has entered the joint. Although the patient's primary concern may be the fracture, the opponent's tooth may have entered his MP joint. As the bacteria contained in a human bite are often quite virulent, these injuries require debridement of the wound, irrigation of the joint with antibiotic solution, high levels of antibiotics for 4 or 5 days and secondary closure. Human bite wounds should not be closed primarily.[18]

FRACTURES OF THE METACARPAL SHAFT. — Metacarpal shaft fractures frequently result from direct trauma. With a *transverse fracture* of the metacarpal shaft, the distal portion of the metacarpal is usually flexed, as with the metacarpal neck fractures. Due to the length of the distal fragment, however, the head of the metacarpal will protrude farther into the palm, with 30 degrees of angulation at the midshaft of the metacarpal than it will with 30 degrees of angulation at the metacarpal neck. The acceptable degree of angulation with midshaft fracture is, therefore, less than with neck fractures. In a child, less remodeling will occur with shaft fractures than with fractures closer to the epiphysis. Transverse fractures of the middle third of the metacarpal shaft are less stable than those of the metacarpal neck and are slower to heal, as there is virtually no cancellous bone in this region. We, therefore, advise open reduction and cross-wire internal fixation of metacarpal shaft fractures if there is rotation, or if there is angulation of more than 20 degrees in the 4th or 5th metacarpals or 10 degrees in the 2d or 3d metacarpals (Fig 3). After reduction, the injured finger is immobilized to the adjacent finger (ring with little; index with middle), as has been described for metacarpal neck fractures. In treating fractures of the metacarpal shaft, it is most important to determine the accuracy of rotatory alignment. As little as 10 or 15 degrees of malrotation may cause annoying overlap of the fingers in flexion, which can be disabling. After reduction has been achieved, the fingers must always be tested in flexion to detect any rotational malalignment. Remodeling does not correct rotatory deformity.

Oblique and spiral fractures. — Oblique and spiral fractures of the metacarpal shaft frequently involve more than 1 metacarpal

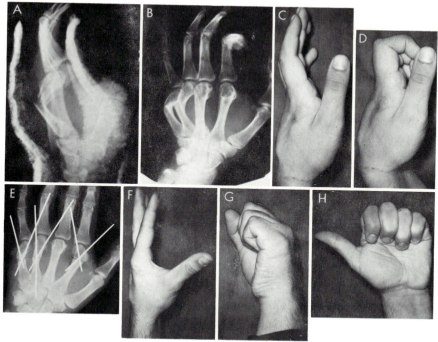

Fig 3. — A, incorrect treatment was rendered to this patient with severely angulated fractures of the shafts of the 4th and 5th metacarpals, dislocation of the base of the 3d metacarpal and a rotated fracture of the 2d metacarpal neck. Fourth and fifth metacarpal shaft fractures require open reduction and internal fixation. Dislocation of the base of the 3d metacarpal could probably have been reduced by volar pressure at the site of the dislocation. The "Jahss maneuver" should have been attempted to reduce the rotated fracture of the 2d metacarpal neck. In addition to the failure of reduction of the bony injuries, the plaster splints have been applied improperly as they immobilize the metacarpophalangeal joints in hyperextension. **B,** the fractures and dislocations healed in malposition. **C,** hyperextension of the metacarpophalangeal joints results in incomplete extension of the proximal interphalangeal joints and a mild "claw-hand" deformity. The dislocation of the base of the 3d metacarpal is seen. **D,** due to prolonged immobilization with the metacarpophalangeal joints in hyperextension, the collateral ligaments have become tight and the patient is unable to make a fist. **E,** reconstructive surgery consisted of metacarpal osteotomy and capsulectomy with resection of the collateral ligaments of the metacarpophalangeal joints. This operating room x-ray shows the osteotomy sites held with multiple crossed Kirschner wires. **F, G,** and **H,** postoperatively, good extension is maintained and flexion is improved. Prolonged disability and multiple surgical procedures could have been avoided by appropriate primary treatment to the fractures.

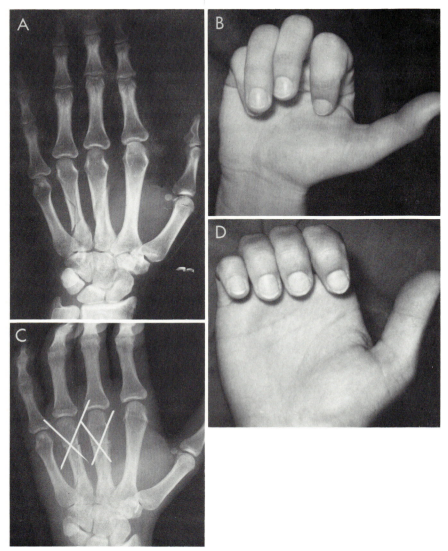

Fig 4. — **A,** spiral fractures of the shafts of the 3d and 4th metacarpals in this young woman appear in relatively good alignment. Mild rotational deformities cannot be properly diagnosed by x-ray examination alone. This fracture had been treated by a volar plaster splint with no attempt at reduction. **B,** the fractures healed with twenty degrees of pronation. Overlapping of the middle and ring fingers was the result of the rotational deformity. She was unable to resume her occupation as a typist and found the deformity disabling. The malrotation could have been detected by examining the fingers in flexion at the time of the original injury. Reduction of the fractures and internal fixation would have avoided this complication. **C,** the deformities were treated by dero-

and are usually the result of twisting or impaction injuries. They are usually not markedly angulated. The principal problems with these fractures are those of rotational malalignment or shortening (Fig 4). We have found it difficult to maintain reduction by closed means following rotatory deformities. Similarly, the shortening that occurs from contraction of the interosseous muscles is difficult to correct and maintain in plaster casts. These injuries usually require open reduction and fixation with crossed Kirschner wires. The use of a compression plate and small screws may also be considered.[15, 28] Normal length should be achieved at the operating table, and traction casts are not necessary postoperatively.

INTRA-ARTICULAR FRACTURES OF THE METACARPALS OF THE FINGERS

FRACTURES OF THE METACARPAL HEAD. — Often these fractures are open and associated with extensive wounds about the dorsum of the hand and the extensor tendons. Whenever possible, restoration of anatomical alignment should be attempted. Usually this is best achieved by the use of multiple Kirschner wires. Even small fragments of cartilage with subchondral bone may be fitted together like a jigsaw puzzle to reconstitute the contour of the metacarpal head. Articular defects caused by crushing or the loss of fragments of bone and cartilage should be allowed to remain open. These defects will fill with fibrocartilage, and the joint may function well despite its poor radiographic appearance. Unlike weight-bearing joints, an incongruous MP joint may be consistent with useful, painless motion. If the extensor tendons have been lacerated, they should be repaired primarily where possible. Although there may be a temptation to immobilize the joint in complete extension when an extensor tendon has been repaired, the hand should be immobilized with 60 degrees of dorsiflexion at the wrist and 45 degrees of flexion at the MP joints. Active MP joint motion should be encouraged after 3 weeks.

---

tational osteotomy with crossed Kirschner wire fixation. **D,** when the osteotomies had healed, normal rotation and alignment of the fingers was restored. Note that under normal circumstances, the index finger is frequently supinated up to ten degrees when in flexion.

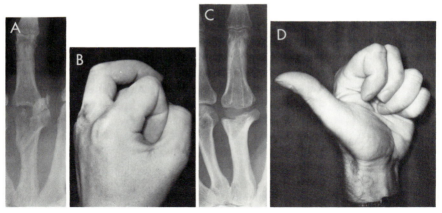

Fig 5.—**A,** this comminuted fracture of the 3d metacarpal head should be treated by open reduction and internal fixation, if possible. This fracture had been allowed to remain untreated. **B,** the fracture healed in poor position resulting in a stiff meta-carpophalangeal joint of the middle finger. **C,** the comminuted fracture fragments were removed and a silicone metacarpophalangeal joint arthroplasty was performed. **D,** excellent (but incomplete) flexion was restored following silicone arthroplasty.

Gross joint destruction with a comminuted fracture of the metacarpal head, as may occur after a machine accident, should be treated by copious lavage, removal of detritus and soft tissue closure. Occasionally, secondary skin closure may be indicated. Passive joint mobility should be maintained by range-of-motion exercises. After all inflammation has subsided, usually within 2 or 3 months, arthroplasty may restore a stable, painless and movable joint (Fig 5). Fifty or 55 degrees of active motion provided by arthroplasty would appear preferable to arthrodesis.[56] Arthroplasty is rarely indicated at the time of injury since wound contamination increases the risk of postoperative infection. In addition, postoperative settling of an implant or prosthesis is less likely to occur if arthroplasty is performed after the multiple microfractures that inevitably occur at the time of injury have healed. With the use of silicone arthroplasty the patient can begin protective active range-of-motion exercises 2 days postoperatively. A lively extension splint, consisting of a soft leather sling suspended from a dorsal outrigger by a rubber band, is used for 3 weeks postoperatively.

FRACTURES OF THE BASE OF THE METACARPAL.—If there is no angulatory deformity, isolated intra-articular fractures of the base of the 2d and 3d metacarpals cause little disability, as these joints are relatively immobile. Occasionally, an avulsion fracture at the base of the 2d or 3d metacarpal may occur secondary to a fall on the dorsum of the hand, resulting in pain and a tender prominence about the insertion of the extensor carpi radialis longus and brevis. If pain persists, the avulsion fragments may be removed secondarily. Intra-articular fractures of the base of the 2d and 3d metacarpal require only supportive treatment with the use of a wrist cock-up splint for 2 weeks. All fingers may be allowed to remain free.

Intra-articular fractures of the base of the 4th metacarpal require accurate reduction since the mobility of this metacarpal on the hamate is sufficient to cause continued pain and disability if a normal articular surface is not restored. If necessary, open reduction and Kirschner wire fixation of the fracture fragment are performed.[27]

Fig 6. – **A,** this roentgenogram shows a "reverse Bennett's" fracture subluxation of the base of the 5th metacarpal. This injury was the result of a fall on the outstretched hand. The intermetacarpal ligament remains attached to a small fragment of bone from the radial side of the 5th metacarpal base. The metacarpal is subluxated proximally and ulnarly by the pull of the extensor carpi ulnaris tendon. **B,** these fracture dislocations are unstable. They usually require internal fixation with 1 or 2 Kirschner wires (as seen here) immobilizing the 5th metacarpal base to the hamate.

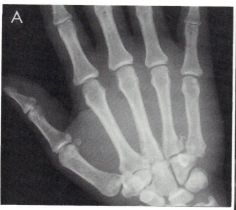
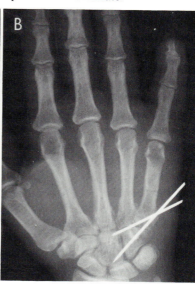

A firm palmar and dorsal ligament fix the radial facet of the base of the 5th metacarpal base to that of the 4th metacarpal. A dorsiflexion injury to the 5th metacarpal will often fracture this radial facet. The remainder of the base of the 5th metacarpal will be unstable and will frequently subluxate ulnarly and dorsally (Fig 6). The pathomechanics of the deformity are similar to those of Bennett's fracture of the base of the 1st metacarpal. Closed reduction of this "reverse Bennett's fracture-dislocation" of the 5th metacarpal may be attempted by traction upon the little finger and digital pressure at the dorsal and ulnar aspect of the metacarpal base. If the metacarpal clicks into place, a plaster splint is applied immobilizing the carpo metacarpal joints of the ring and little fingers in mid flexion with the wrist in 45 degrees of dorsiflexion. Additional x-rays should be taken 1 or 2 days later since the pull of the extensor carpi ulnaris and the abductor digiti quinti may cause redislocation. If the joint is unstable but reduction is readily achieved, a smooth Kirschner wire may be inserted percutaneously through the 5th metacarpal base and proximally into the hamate. If closed reduction cannot be achieved, open reduction is required. The 5th metacarpal base is reduced into the ulnar facet of the hamate and held with a Kirschner wire through the metacarpal and hamate. A second wire is then passed through the metacarpal base into its radial facet fracture fragment.

With internal fixation of the 4th or 5th metacarpal-hamate joint, the metacarpal bases should be flexed to 30–40 degrees. Even if the metacarpal-hamate joints become ankylosed in flexion, excellent function of the hand can be anticipated. However, if the 4th or 5th metacarpal-hamate joints become ankylosed in extension as the result of joint injury or internal fixation, the palm will be flattened and the grip weakened. Painful malunion at the bases of the 4th and 5th metacarpals may be treated by arthrodesis of the metacarpal-hamate joint in the position of about 30 degrees of flexion.

COMPOUND FRACTURES OF THE METACARPALS OF THE FINGERS WITH BONE LOSS

Bullet wounds, shotgun blasts, explosions or heavy machinery accidents all may cause severe injuries to the hand with loss of a portion of one or more metacarpals. With such injuries, the primary goal is to cleanse and debride the wounds. If there has been gross contamination, devitalization of tissues or extensive thermal injuries, skin closure should be delayed.[11, 19, 31, 45]

After thorough lavage and debridement, attention should be directed at maintaining metacarpal length and preventing joint contractures. The use of transverse Kirschner wires has been found valuable in preventing metacarpal collapse. If the appropriate metacarpal length is not maintained, the normal force of the interosseous muscles, flexor and extensor tendons and, ultimately, scar contraction will cause collapse of the fingers and an unsightly and stiff hand. If either the 2d or 3d metacarpal shaft has been lost, a transverse wire is passed between the 2d and 3d metacarpal heads, using the intact metacarpal to splint the one that has been partially destroyed. Similarly, the 4th metacarpal may be used to splint the 5th, and vice versa (Fig 7). With loss of the shaft of both the 2d and 3d or the 4th and 5th metacarpals, transverse wires are passed through the heads and through the bases of the injured metacarpals. These wires are connected to an external device, such as the Roger Anderson or Charnley apparatus, which is then adjusted to restore the proper length. If there has been destruction of all 4 metacarpal shafts, 2 sets of lengthening devices should be used since the insertion of 1 wire through all 4 metacarpals is difficult and would flatten the hand. Relatively stout Kirschner wires or thin Steinman pins will be required to prevent bowing of the apparatus. Longitudinal Kirschner wires are then inserted through each metacarpal neck and into its base to maintain correct alignment. A third set of wires is passed obliquely through each MP joint holding the proximal phalanx in 70 degrees of flexion. By this technique, proper rotatory alignment is achieved, and extension contraction of the MP joint is prevented. In more severe injuries, where the entire metacarpal shaft and head had been lost, the distal transverse wires are placed through the proximal phalanges of the fingers to maintain length. If the patient is seen after shortening has occurred, the same technique is employed, and the metacarpal head-to-base length is gradually restored with the external fixation device (Fig 8).

After any severe injury to the hand, to prevent adduction contraction of the thumb secondary to edema and scarring of the adductor pollicis, the 1st metacarpal is held in maximum pal-

grafts are used. An iliac or fibular bone graft may be used to fill the defect in the 4th or 5th metacarpal shaft. One should be certain that the 4th and 5th carpometacarpal joints are flexed 30–40 degrees when the grafts are inserted.

With loss of all 4 metacarpals, one should not attempt to provide 4 separate bone struts, but rather insert 1 large iliac bone graft, appropriately shaped, to provide stability and to preserve length to all fingers. The graft is fixed to the bases of the proximal phalanges with 45 degrees of flexion. If the metacarpal shaft and head have been lost, no attempt is made to provide MP joint motion. Attempts to achieve MP motion by arthroplasty would appear fruitless.

Only after skin coverage has been achieved and secondary bone grafting has restored stability to the hand is any attempt made to reconstitute the muscle tendon function. With the loss of extensors to the middle or ring fingers, the extensor indicis proprius or extensor digiti quinti proprius may be transferred to the bases of the proximal phalanges. If all 4 extensors have been lost, the flexor digitorum superficialis may be removed from middle and ring fingers, passed through the interosseous membrane proximal to the pronator quadratus muscle and transferred to the dorsal bases of the proximal phalanges.[6] As a final stage in reconstruction of these hands, appropriate tendon transfers are often needed to regain interphalangeal joint extension, which has been lost with destruction of the intrinsic muscles.[8, 47]

FRACTURES OF THE METACARPAL OF THE THUMB

FRACTURES OF THE DISTAL 1ST METACARPAL. — Fractures of the head, neck or shaft of the 1st metacarpal occur less frequently than those of the finger metacarpals. In most instances these fractures are due to a direct blow or angular force. Fracture of the diaphysis or distal metaphysis may usually be treated by closed reduction and immobilization in a thumb spica for 4 weeks. If the fracture is stable and shortening, angulation of more than 20 degrees, significant rotational deformity or displacement of more than 20% of the distal articular surface occurs, the fracture should be treated by open reduction and internal fixation.

FRACTURES OF THE METAPHYSIS OF THE 1ST METACARPAL. — Extra-articular fractures of the first metacarpal may be either transverse or vertical-oblique. Surgery is rarely indicated. Reduction can usually be achieved by closed manipulation with immobilization in a short-arm thumb spica. Accurate anatomical alignment is not necessary for good function. The transverse fracture of the 1st metacarpal shaft is usually stable and up to 20–30 degrees of angulation does not limit thumb motion. The thumb is immobilized for 4 weeks, after which time gentle protected motion is begun.

The most common epiphyseal fractures of the 1st metacarpal are those of type II (Salter and Harris classification). If displaced, they require precise restoration and realignment. If closed reduction is not successful, open reduction and fixation with unthreaded wires may be necessary. Plaster immobilization is used for 4 weeks. If a child is involved, the parents should be aware of the possible disturbances of the growth plate that may occur as a result of some epiphyseal injuries.

FRACTURES OF THE BASE OF THE 1ST METACARPAL. — Because of the position and unusual anatomical features of the 1st metacarpal, the patterns of fractures of its base are different from patterns in fractures of the fingers. Most fractures of the 1st metacarpal base result from a combination of axial and abduction forces sustained in a fall or as the result of a blow. The 1st metacarpal is abducted at rest and with axial force it is pushed proximally. The entire shaft acts as a lever, with the fulcrum at the metacarpal-trapezial joint. Strong carpometacarpal ligaments usually remain intact and produce an intra-articular fracture with separation of the metacarpal from a small medial volar fragment.

Fractures about the base of the 1st metacarpal include intra-articular fracture dislocations (Bennett's and Rolando's fractures) and extra-articular basilar fractures, with either a primarily vertical or transverse component.[25, 40]

Bennett's fracture. — Described in 1882,[4] Bennett's fracture is a vertical avulsion fracture of the ulnar base of the 1st metacarpal, which remains attached to the stout anterior oblique ligaments. The size and shape of the avulsion fragment may vary. Two forces act upon the unsupported 1st metacarpal shaft: (1) the adductor pollicis, attached to the distal portion of the metacarpal, angulates the metacarpal shaft ulnarly, and (2) the abductor pollicis longus displaces the metacarpal base proximally and dorsoradially.

Many methods of treatment of Bennett's fracture-dislocation

have been recommended. These have included immobilization in opposition, application of a cast with padding and pressure at the 1st metacarpal base and skin or skeletal traction,[5, 10, 13, 44, 58] closed reduction with percutaneous pinning[57] and open reduction with pin or screw fixation.[2, 15, 22, 28, 43]

We treat Bennett's fracture by first attempting closed reduction with longitudinal traction upon the extended thumb while countertraction is applied about the wrist by an assistant. Pressure is applied to the radial base of the 1st metacarpal in an ulnar direction. The thumb is placed in opposition, and if the reduction is unstable, a single unthreaded Kirschner wire is passed from the 1st into the 2d metacarpal. The reduction is checked with x-rays and repeat x-rays are taken after 1 and after 7 days to check whether the reduction has been maintained.

If the postreduction roentgenograms fail to reveal anatomical restoration of the articular surface, open reduction is performed. We prefer a J-shape[57] incision overlying the base of the thenar eminence and extending distally over the dorsum of the 1st metacarpal. Special care must be taken to avoid injury to the branches of the superficial radial nerve and princeps pollicis artery. Under direct visualization, a Kirschner wire is passed distally through the fracture of the metacarpal shaft. The fracture is reduced and the wire drilled proximally through the ulnar fragment.

A second wire is then passed through the 1st metacarpal into the base of the 2d metacarpal with the thumb in opposition. X-rays are taken to check the alignment, and wires are cut just beneath the skin. After wound closure, a padded plaster thumb spica cast is applied from the base of the nail to below the elbow. The arm is elevated overnight and additional x-rays are taken prior to discharge and again at 1 week. Immobilization is maintained for 6 weeks, at which time the pins are removed. Gentle active motion is then begun.

Rolando's fracture. — The Rolando fracture, described in 1910, is a comminuted variant of the Bennett's fracture.[50] The most common configuration of the fracture is that of a T or Y with a large ulnar and radial fragment, both of which are separated from the shaft of the metacarpal. There may be extensive comminution of the fragments at the base of the metacarpal without dislocation. In these patients, open reduction is not indicated. The thumb should be placed in opposition in a molded thumb spica plaster cast and immobilization continued for 4 – 6 weeks.

With a grossly comminuted basilar fracture and dislocation of the metacarpal shaft where restoration of the anatomical configuration of the articular fragment is impossible, the dislocation should be reduced by traction and the 1st metacarpal stabilized with a Kirschner wire into the 2d metacarpal base.

If the fracture has resulted in 2 large fragments from the ulnar and radial condyles of the proximal end of the first metacarpal, open reduction and internal fixation are necessary. Under direct visualization, the metacarpal shaft is reduced and pinned onto the ulnar fracture fragment with an unthreaded Kirschner wire. The radial fragment is then reduced and a second wire introduced through it into the metacarpal shaft. A third wire may be passed into the base of the 2d metacarpal to stabilize the 1st metacarpal-trapezial joint in opposition. Immobilization is continued for 6 weeks.

Injuries to the Carpometacarpal and Metacarpophalangeal Joints of the Fingers

DISLOCATIONS OF THE CARPOMETACARPAL JOINTS

Severe, sudden dorsiflexion injuries with force applied to the palm may cause the bases of the metacarpals to be dislocated dorsally. This injury may occur in children with skateboard accidents or in workers by sudden, severe force such as may occur with the explosion of a rubber tire being applied to a wheel rim. The metacarpal shaft is usually angulated volarly, the entire ray displaced proximally, and there is prominence of the metacarpal base beneath the radial wrist extensors, which usually causes considerable pain with attempts at wrist or finger motion. Dislocation of the 2d and 3d metacarpal bases are usually difficult to reduce unless the limb is totally anesthetized. Traction is applied to the dislocated ray by an assistant. The wrist is dorsiflexed and the base of the dislocated metacarpal guided by firm pressure of the surgeon's thumb into its relocated position. Unless these injuries are treated promptly, closed reduction is often impossible to achieve. Open reduction may require clearing the distal articular surface of the trapezoid or capitate with a small Bennett retractor or skid while applying pressure to the dorsum of the base of the dislocated metacarpal.

Dorsal dislocations at the base of the 4th and 5th metacarpals are more frequent than those of the 2d and 3d and usually result from sudden, forceful pressure upon the palm of the hand. If treated early, the dislocations may be reduced by traction upon the ring and little fingers and volar pressure upon the dorsum of the dislocated metacarpal bases. Frequently, the patient and surgeon will be rewarded by a satisfying, audible and palpable click with almost instantaneous relief of pain. Nothing further need be done other than immobilization of the wrist and fingers for a period of 3 weeks. If the patient is seen late, or if closed reduction is not possible, open reduction and internal fixation as described for dislocations of the 2d and 3d metacarpal bases are necessary. Volar dislocations of the base of the 5th metacarpal are rare and may require open reduction.[16, 41]

Dislocations of the Metacarpophalangeal Joints

Sudden hyperextension injuries of the MP joints of the fingers may cause dorsal dislocation of the proximal phalanx, occasionally with rupture of the volar plate. Most frequently, these dislocations may be easily reduced by longitudinal traction upon the dislocated finger. Many reduce spontaneously.

Dorsal dislocation of the proximal phalanx of the index finger may be irreducible by closed means (Fig 9).[33] In these patients, the 2d metacarpal head can be palpated subcutaneously in the distal palm. The index finger is displaced dorsally at the MP joint and is usually ulnarly deviated and mildly supinated. Any attempt at MP joint flexion is painful.

With irreducible MP dislocations of the index finger, the second metacarpal head is trapped in the palm.[3, 26, 33] The flexor tendons lie to its ulnar side, the lumbrical to its radial side, the superficial transverse metacarpal ligament lies volar to the metacarpal neck and the torn volar plate and natatory ligament (skin ligament of the web) lie between the metacarpal head and the base of the dislocated proximal phalanx that is dorsal to it. Occasionally, when the patient is appropriately anesthetized, these dislocations may be reduced without surgery by gentle traction, then flexion of the proximal phalanx. Most frequently, however, open reduction is necessary.

A volar incision is made overlying the metacarpal head. Great care must be taken to avoid injuring the radial digital nerve, which may be pressed against the skin by the 2d metacarpal

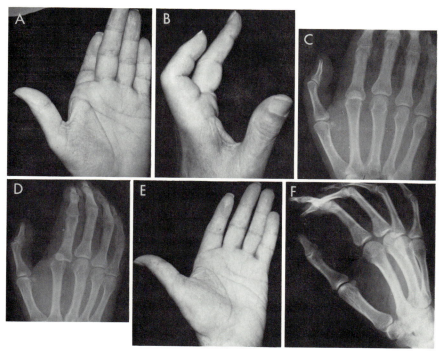

Fig 9. – **A** and **B**, these photographs reveal the typical position of the irreducible, or "complex," fracture-dislocation of the base of the index finger. The metacarpophalangeal joint is mildly hyperextended and the interphalangeal joint flexed. The finger is rotated into supination. The 2d metacarpal head is prominent in the palm and can be seen subcutaneously at the juncture of the midpalmar and thenar flexion crease to the radial side of the palm. **C** and **D**, roentgenograms of the complex dislocation of the metacarpophalangeal joint of the index finger shows superimposition of the base of the proximal phalanx upon the 2d metacarpal head. **E** and **F**, after reduction, normal alignment of the fingers is seen and roentgenograms reveal a normal joint space.

head. Lumbrical and flexor tendons are retracted from about the metacarpal head, and the volar plate and natatory ligament are freed from between the metacarpal head and the proximal phalanx. Longitudinal traction and flexion of the index finger with pressure to the volar side of the 2d metacarpal will usually achieve reduction. The reduced joint is held in 45 degrees of flexion for 3 weeks with a dorsal plaster splint. Active flexion is encouraged in 24–48 hours. If these injuries are treated late, the ulnar collateral ligament may also require transection, as it may have gradually become contracted while the joint was displaced.

LOCKED METACARPOPHALANGEAL JOINTS

Occasionally, after a twisting injury to the index and little finger, the MP joint locks in a flexed position. Extension past 40 degrees, either actively or passively, is not possible, and any attempts at passive extension are accompanied by pain. With injury to the index finger, there is frequently mild supination. With injury to the little finger, there may be mild pronation. Interphalangeal joint flexion and extension is complete.

The locking of the MP joint is usually due to incarceration of the volar plate or its sesamoid about a prominent condyle of the metacarpal head. X-rays are not diagnostic. The condition must not be confused with a locked trigger finger.[1, 9, 20]

Surgery is required to release a locked MP joint. The volar plate is incised at its attachment to the accessory collateral ligament on both its radial and ulnar side, and a transverse incision is made proximally through the membranous portion of the volar capsule. The distal portion of the plate remains attached to the base of the proximal phalanx. Once the plate is freed, full extension is usually restored. The MP joint is splinted in extension for 2 weeks and then active exercises are begun.

CONTRACTURES OF THE METACARPOPHALANGEAL JOINTS

Any injury to the hand that causes edema or ischemia or limits active or passive motion of the fingers may result in stiffness at the MP joints.[59] When the proximal phalanges are in extension or hyperextension, the collateral ligaments are relaxed. When the proximal phalanges are flexed, the collateral ligaments are stretched. If the MP joints of the fingers are permitted to rest in extension or hyperextension after injury, the collateral ligaments will shorten. The metacarpal head is asymmetrical and results in a cam effect with flexion of the proximal phalanx which stretches the collateral ligament. As the volar half of the metacarpal head is wider than its dorsal half, the collateral ligaments must, with flexion, diverge from the midline of the finger. A short, tight collateral ligament, thickened with posttraumatic edema, will have little elasticity and will prevent flexion of the proximal phalanx. With the proximal phalanx extended, the fibrocartilaginous and membranous portions of the volar plate become adherent to the volar half of the metacarpal head, contributing to the fixed extension deformity.

In most cases, after severe injuries about the hand, MP joint extension contracture may be prevented by holding the MP joints of the fingers in 70 degrees of flexion.[48] This is not a "position of function." Rather, it is the position at which mobility is most likely to be preserved and contracture avoided, since the collateral ligaments are stretched to their maximum length. With less severe injuries, MP flexion can be achieved by holding the wrist in mild dorsiflexion and applying a dorsal splint over the MP joints.

In more severe injuries, in those with extensive edema or hematoma or in cases where positioning of the hand may be difficult during the application of a remote pedicle flap, MP joint flexion should be maintained with the use of transarticular smooth Kirschner wires. The wires may be removed in 3 – 4 weeks, at which time active and passive exercises may be instituted. If the patient is first seen after mild extension contracture has developed, a lively flexion splint should be considered. These splints consist of a volar plaster or orthoplast gutter that extends from the midforearm to the midpalm. An outrigger is attached to rubber band flexion slings placed about the dorsum of the proximal phalanges intermittently throughout the day. The patient can adjust the tension on the rubber bands to achieve a maximal flexion force without causing vascular embarrassment or skin injury. Active and passive range-of-motion exercises should be begun as soon as possible.

Often, extension contractures of the MP joints may be prevented by correct attention to the position or length of a plaster cast. Excessive wrist palmar-flexion will increase the tenodesis effect of the extensor tendons, causing them to pull the MP joints into hyperextension. If MP joint flexion is prevented by a plaster cast that extends past the midpalm, extension contracture is almost inevitable. With the MP joints hyperextended, the interphalangeal joints flex, and a stiff clawhand deformity may develop. Disability may be lessened if the 4th and 5th metacarpal are permitted to flex and the thumb to abduct. In summary, when applying a plaster cast after bone or soft-tissue injury, one should, if possible:

Avoid: excessive wrist flexion
extending the plaster past the
    midpalmar flexion crease
flattening the palm
thumb adduction

Try to: end volar plaster at middle palmar flexion crease
mold plaster in palm to flex 4th and 5th metacarpals
keep thumb abducted
trim plaster proximal to trapezio-
    metacarpal joint at thumb

Capsulectomy is often required for established extension contractures of the MP joints that do not respond to conservative care. The collateral ligaments are principally responsible for the extensor contracture in these joints. The dorsal capsule is usually thin and rarely plays a significant role in causing or maintaining MP extension contracture. Dividing the dorsal capsule risks postoperative dislocation of the extensor tendons and may complicate recovery after collateral ligament resection. The "capsulectomy" required for MP extension contractures consists principally of division of the collateral ligaments.

Through a dorsal transverse incision, the ulnar side of the joint is first exposed. The sagittal band that runs from the extensor tendon to the volar plate is identified and retracted proximally. The collateral ligament is divided at the lateral base of the proximal phalanx. Care is taken not to transect the accessory collateral ligament that runs from the metacarpal head to the volar plate. The radial collateral ligament is then transected, and the proximal phalanx manipulated into flexion. If flexion cannot be achieved, a probe is passed between the volar side of the metacarpal head and the volar plate. A recess must be formed to allow free gliding of the base of the proximal phalanx on the metacarpal head. The surgeon must be certain that the MP joint flexes without deviating to either side and without the joint hinging open at the dorsum. If the base of the proximal phalanx does not freely glide on the metacarpal head, the joint must be freed further. Postoperatively, we hold the MP joint in 70 degrees of flexion with a longitudinal or oblique Kirschner wire through the articular surfaces for 3 weeks. After removal of the Kirschner wires, an active flexion splint is used.

INTRINSIC MUSCLE CONTRACTURE OF THE
METACARPOPHALANGEAL JOINT

Ischemic contracture of the interosseous muscles of the hand may follow severe edema.[23, 48, 51] As with Volkmann's ischemic contracture of the forearm, venous drainage from the closed interosseous spaces of the hand may be impeded by edema following severe trauma. Increased pressure causes limited capillary flow. Gradually, the ischemic muscles lose their tone and become fibrotic and scarred. As scar contracts, the interosseous muscles may pull the MP joint into acute flexion and the interphalangeal joints into extension. Impending ischemic contracture may be diagnosed by the intrinsic tightness test: with intrinsic muscle contracture, there will be greater limitation of passive proximal interphalangeal point (PIP) flexion when the MP joint is extended than when it is flexed.

Ischemic contractures of the interosseous muscles may often be prevented by early release of the dorsal fascia overlying the interosseous muscles. Edematous interosseous muscles will often balloon out from between the metacarpals once the dorsal interosseous fascia have been divided.

Once intrinsic contracture has developed, correction of the MP joint flexion contracture requires intrinsic muscle release. If the intrinsic muscles are not paralyzed, they may be relaxed by a subperiosteal muscle slide. The origin of each of the dorsal and volar interossei are freed from their attachments to the proximal half of each metacarpal shaft and allowed to displace distally. The fingers are placed in a "clawed" position for about 2 weeks postoperatively. Frequently, however, with an established intrinsic muscle contracture that has flexed the MP joints, the interossei are fibrotic and nonfunctional. Release requires transection of the interosseous tendons in the region of the metacarpal neck, as well as division of the membranous volar plate and accessory collateral ligament of each finger. Full correction may also require exploration of the dorsum of the joint as well, as the dorsal capsule may become adherent to the metacarpal head.

Injuries to the Carpometacarpal and Metacarpophalangeal Joints of the Thumb

DISLOCATIONS OF THE CARPOMETACARPAL JOINT

Because of the strength of the anterior and posterior oblique ligaments to the ulnar side of the base of the first metacarpal, extension and abduction stress to the thumb will more frequently result in a Bennett's fracture than in a ligament tear without bony injury.[17] Yet, dislocation of the first metacarpal base without fracture does occur infrequently.

The abductor pollicis longus displaces the metacarpal base dorsally and proximally. The adductor pollicis flexes and adducts the metacarpal shaft, and the base projects even further dorsally. Although closed reduction may be readily achieved with an audible snap, the deforming forces and the loss of ligamentous support will usually result in persistent instability. If the reduction can be achieved and maintained by closed means, immobilization should be continued for 6 weeks. If reduction is readily obtained but the base of the metacarpal redislocates or subluxates, percutaneous Kirschner wires should be passed through the base of the 1st metacarpal into the trapezium or 2d metacarpal base. Plaster immobilization should be used for 6 weeks. Even with prolonged immobilization in the reduced position, the thumb may remain unstable. Unfortunately, the initial diagnosis may be overlooked due to a spontaneous reduction of the initial dislocation and normal x-rays. Eaton has described ligament reconstruction in which the distal end of the flexor carpi radialis is divided longitudinally and its radial half is passed through the base of the first metacarpal, beneath the distal end of the abductor pollicis longus and then woven volar to the trapezium and ulnar to the metacarpal base.[17] This is a useful procedure in cases of chronic instability without evidence of arthritis.

In late cases where pain is caused by traumatic arthritis, resection arthroplasty with palmaris longus interposition and shortening of the abductor pollicis longus tendon or silicone arthroplasty may restore painless motion.

Dislocation of the Metacarpophalangeal Joint

Volar dislocation of the MP joint of the thumb is infrequent and may satisfactorily be treated by closed reduction.

Dorsal dislocation of the proximal phalanx of the thumb results from a hyperextension force. The volar plate tears at the moment of dislocation and may become interposed between the base of the proximal phalanx and metacarpal head. This is called a "complex," or irreducible, dislocation. A small sesamoid bone is located within the volar plate of the thumb (usually on the ulnar side) and can be used to identify the location of the volar plate on diagnostic radiographs.

Simple dislocations may be reduced easily by closed manipulation. Care must be taken not to convert the simple dislocation into a complex one. This will occur if the volar plate is interposed within the joint during reduction.[39] The interphalangeal joint is held flexed during the reduction to release tension on the flexor pollicis longus tendon. Longitudinal traction is applied to the proximal phalanx until the base is disengaged and full length restored. Then the base of the phalanx is pushed volarly over the metacarpal head while traction is maintained, reducing the dislocation. Only at this point is the MP joint allowed to flex. Maintaining hyperextension of the MP joint during reduction will usually prevent interposition of the volar plate between the base of the proximal phalanx and the metacarpal head while reduction is being attempted. Following reduction, the thumb is held in 30 degrees of flexion of the MP joint for 3 weeks in a plaster spica cast.

With "complex" dislocations, there is often a skin "dimple" over the volar surface of the joint, as with complex MP dislocations of the fingers. It is not uncommon for the proximal phalanx to lie at the dorsum of the metacarpal head in marked hyperextension in the simple dislocation. In the complex type, the proximal phalanx may lie parallel and dorsal to the metacarpal shaft, with its base at the level of the distal metacarpal metaphysis. With a complex dislocation, an attempt at closed reduction is warranted. If unsuccessful, an open reduction is indicated. Through a volar incision the volar plate is freed from behind the metacarpal head. If the tendons of the flexor pollicis brevis have also trapped the first metacarpal head anteriorly, they need only to be retracted laterally when the volar plate is freed to achieve reduction. Postoperative x-rays should be taken to confirm congruence and absence of an associated volar lip fracture of the proximal phalanx. The thumb is immobilized in 30 degrees of MP flexion for 4 weeks.

COLLATERAL LIGAMENT INJURY (GAMEKEEPER'S THUMB)

In 1955 Campbell described 20 gamekeepers who had instability of the ulnar side of the MP joint of the thumb as the result of repeated stress to the thumb base caused by killing rabbits.[12] "Acute gamekeeper's thumb" is a term that now refers to acute posttraumatic ulnar collateral ligament instability that may result from rupture or avulsion of the ulnar collateral ligament or a fracture of its attachment at the ulnar base of the proximal phalanx. The bony fragment may represent as much as one third of the articular surface of the proximal phalanx.

The acute ulnar collateral ligament injury is most frequently caused by sudden radial deviation-extension of the thumb. Frequently, the thumb is injured by a ski-pole strap during a fall. Two goals of treatment are (1) restoration of joint stability and (2) joint congruity when fracture has occurred.

Following the trauma, the patient will complain of pain localized to the MP joint. There may be diffuse local swelling. A true anteroposterior and lateral x-ray of the joint should be obtained to determine if a nondisplaced fracture is present.[55] If so, the injury may be treated by plaster immobilization in a thumb spica for 4 weeks. A large, displaced or rotated bony fragment should be replaced surgically. If radial pressure upon the injured joint results in more than 45 degrees of lateral deviation as compared to the opposite side, then surgical repair of the collateral ligament is indicated.[35, 46, 52, 53] Surgery is also indicated if the proximal phalanx is subluxated volarly. If there is only mild instability, the injury may be treated successfully by 4 weeks of plaster immobilization in slight flexion and protected activity with a radial gutter splint for an additional 2-3 weeks.[14]

If surgery is necessary, the joint is exposed through a longitudinal dorsoulnar incision with care taken to protect the branches of the superficial radial nerve. The adductor expansion is divided. The collateral ligament is usually ruptured from its distal attachment. Depending upon the surgical findings, the ligament may be sutured, reattached to the base of the proximal phalanx with a pullout suture or the attached articular fragment repositioned and fixed with a Kirschner wire. The adductor expansion is then repaired. Plaster immobilization for 4 weeks is followed by the use of a protective splint for an additional 4–6 weeks.

If these injuries are not treated within 3–4 weeks, the collateral ligament will gradually scar and retract preventing its surgical reattachment to the base of the proximal phalanx.[42] In these cases, collateral ligament reconstruction by means of a tendon graft is usually required.[52] The new ligament should be attached dorsal to the axis of flexion on the metacarpal and volar to this axis on the proximal phalanx to provide dorsal support. Patients who present with x-ray evidence of arthritis will be most successfully managed by arthrodesis in 10 degrees of flexion and 10 degrees of pronation.

The so-called reverse gamekeeper's thumb refers to an injury to the radial collateral ligament similar to that on the ulnar side of the joint. This injury is one-third as frequent as ulnar collateral ligament injuries. The presence of a large articular fragment, marked displacement of an avulsion fragment, marked instability or volar subluxation again are indications for operative repair.

Conclusions

Most frequently it is the junior house officer in the emergency ward or the busy general practitioner who is called upon to treat metacarpal fractures and injuries to the carpal and metacarpal joints. Since many simple metacarpal fractures will heal regardless of treatment, it is often assumed that the treatment of these injuries is of little consequence. The more experienced surgeon has learned, however, that an entire hand may be crippled by the casual handling of a metacarpal fracture or adjacent joint injury. The errors of overtreatment of the metacarpal fracture by taping a finger over a bandage roll and acutely flexing the interphalangeal joints are even more tragic than the inadequate attention that the Bennett's fracture or malpositioned metacarpal fracture may receive. Thorough familiarity with the anatomical details of the metacar-

43. Pfeiffer, K. M.: Advances in osteosynthesis of hand fractures, Handchirurgie 8:17, 1976 (Engl. abstr.).
44. Pollen, A. G.: The conservative treatment of Bennett's fracture – subluxation of the thumb metacarpal, J. Bone Joint Surg. (Br.) 50:91, 1968.
45. Rank, B. K., and Wakefield, A. R.: *Surgery of Repairs as Applied to Hand Injuries* (Baltimore: The Williams & Wilkins Company, 1960).
46. Resnick, D., and Danzig, L. A.: Arthrographic evaluation of injuries of the first metacarpophalangeal joint: gamekeeper's thumb, Am. J. Roentgenol. Radium Ther. Nucl. Med. 126:1046, 1976.
47. Riordan, D. C.: Surgery of the Paralytic Hand, in *A.A.O.S. Instructional Course Lectures* (St. Louis: The C. V. Mosby Company, 1959), vol. 16, p. 79.
48. Riordan, D. C., and Harris, C., Jr.: Intrinsic contracture in the hand and its surgical treatment, J. Bone & Joint Surg. (Am.) 36:10, 1954.
49. Rockwood, C. A., and Green, D. P. (eds.): *Fractures* (Philadelphia: J. B. Lippincott Company, 1975).
50. Rolando, S.: Fracture de la base du premier metacarpien: et principalement sur une variete non encore decrite, Presse Méd., 33:303, 1910.
51. Smith, R. J.: Intrinsic Muscles of the Fingers: Function, Dysfunction, and Surgical Reconstruction, in *A.A.O.S. Instructional Course Lectures* (St. Louis: C. V. Mosby Co., 1975), vol. 24, p. 200.
52. Smith, R. J.: Post traumatic instability of the metacarpophalangeal joint of the thumb, J. Bone & Joint Surg. (Am.) 59:14, 1977.
53. Stener, B.: Displacement of the ruptured ulnar collateral ligament of the metacarpophalangeal joint of the thumb, J. Bone & Joint Surg. (Br.) 44: 869, 1962.
54. Stranc, M. E., and Sanders, R.: Abdominal Wall Skin Flaps, Grabb, W. C., and Myers, M. B. (eds.) in *Skin Flaps* (Boston: Little Brown & Company, 1975).
55. Sutro, C. J.: Pollex valgus (A bunion-like deformity of the thumb corrected by surgical intervention), Bull. Hosp. Joint Dis. 18:135, 1957.
56. Swanson, A. B.: *Flexible Implant Resection Arthroplasty in the Hand and Extremities* (St. Louis: The C. V. Mosby Company, 1973).
57. Wagner, C. J.: A method of treatment of Bennett's fracture dislocation, Am. J. Surg. 80:230, 1950.
58. Watson-Jones, R.: *Fractures and Joint Injuries* (4th ed.; Edinburgh: E. & S. Livingstone, Ltd., 1956).
59. Weeks, P. M., and Wray, R. C.: *Managment of Acute Hand Injuries. A Biological Approach* (St. Louis, The C. V. Mosby Company, 1973).

Adjuvant Oncotherapy: The Treatment of Systemic Micrometastases*

JOHN M. BENNETT

University of Rochester Cancer Center and the Department of Medicine, University of Rochester School of Medicine & Dentistry, Rochester, New York

An adjuvant program may be defined as one that is designed to aid in delaying relapse in a population of cancer patients who have significant risk of occult micrometastases following definitive cancer surgery. The anticipated outcome of improving this "disease-free survival interval" is an increase in the percentage of long-term cures of the particular neoplasm that is so treated. Adjuvant oncotherapy may be either a single modality (i.e., radio-, chemo- or immunotherapy) or a combination of two or more of these treatments.

Effective chemotherapy destroys large numbers of malignant cells, but cytotoxicity follows first-order kinetics, with only a fixed percentage of tumor cells being killed with each treatment. There is some indication that minimally effective agents in advanced diseases may be more beneficial when the tumor cell burden is lower.[1] The proved ability of regional irradiation to control overt nodal relapses provides a means of combining local control with suspected systemic micrometastases.

To date the most successful demonstration of this combined or separate approach has been in the pediatric neoplasms, includ-

*Supported, in part, by USPHS Grants #CA 11083 and CA 11198, from the National Cancer Institute, National Institutes of Health, Bethesda, Md.

ing Wilms' tumor, Ewing's sarcoma and embryonal rhabdomyo-
sarcoma.[2] Another example is the prophylactic use of radioche-
motherapy in preventing CNS relapse in childhood acute lym-
phocytic leukemia.[3] The following sections serve as illustra-
tions of the various forms of adjuvant programs that are currently under active study.

Colon Cancer

Because of the natural tendency for colon cancer to spread
perpendicularly through the bowel, Dukes's classification, as
modified by Oster and Coller, has been of proved value in predicting survival. It has become the mainstay of justifying adjuvant programs. When tumor is confined to the mucosa (A), 5-
year survival ranges from 74–100%. With penetration into but
not through the muscularis (B1), the 5-year survival falls to
60–65%. Extension into the serosa or pericolic fat with negative
nodes (B2) reduces survival further, to 40–60%, and when regional lymph nodes are involved, the figures fall to the 20–40%
range (Dukes's C).[4] In contrast to breast cancer, where regional
lymph node involvement is a marker for systemic spread, as
high as 50% of patients with colorectal cancer may have regional failure alone.[5]

Accurate staging, including assessment of liver involvement
by careful inspection, palpation and direct biopsy of the liver
(5–15% involvement by microscopic assessment) is an important prerequisite for chemoradiation adjuvant programs.

CARCINOEMBRYONIC ANTIGEN AS TUMOR MARKER. —The identification of the colorectal tumor antigen, carcinoembryonic antigen (CEA), permits the possible predictability of tumor biology
that can be of value in observing patients on adjuvant programs.
Of 23 patients who had recurrences, 20 had elevated CEA levels
at the recognition of metastasis and 14 had elevations several
months prior to detection.[6] It is reasonable to follow patients
with serial CEA levels every 6 months. When an elevation is
noted, then liver function studies and a chest x-ray would be in
order. If a patient has been on adjuvant chemotherapy, at least
two consecutive elevations of CEA, 3 months apart, should be
demonstrated before consideration of removal from the particular program. If an elevated CEA is found in a patient who has
not been in an adjuvant program but is at high risk for relapse

(Dukes's B2 or C), then serious consideration should be given for institution of chemotherapy after appropriate laboratory studies and isotope scans are carried out.

ALPHAFETOPROTEIN AS TUMOR MARKER. — Alphafetoprotein (AFP) has been determined in the serum of patients with primary liver carcinoma; teratocarcinomas, and gastric, pancreatic, colon and prostatic tumors.[7] The potential for follow-up with CEA exists.

RADIATION THERAPY AS ADJUNCT IN RECTAL CANCER. — The role of preoperative radiation in the management of rectal carcinoma is well established. Significant regression of primary tumors with approximately 5,000 rads delivered over 5–6 weeks has been demonstrated by Fletcher and co-workers.[8] When the regional nodes are included in the radiation field, the expected incidence of Dukes's B and C specimens is reduced by at least 50%.[9] This translates into a better 5-year survival figure (41% vs 28%) in at least one study published by the V. A. Surgical Adjuvant Group (VASAG).[10]

RADIATION THERAPY AND CHEMOTHERAPY AS ADJUNCT FOR RECTAL CANCER. — In patients with operable rectal cancer one can accurately carry out pathologic staging and eliminate patients for whom no benefit can be expected from adjuvant therapy. A current Eastern Cooperative Oncology Group (ECOG) designed a study (EST4276) to test whether a combination of 5-fluorouracil (5-FU) and methyl-CCNU (semustine) is as effective as bowel radiation for regional control and also for improving survival in patients with Dukes's B and C lesions. A third group of patients will receive both modalities.

ADJUVANT THERAPY FOR NONRESECTABLE RECTAL CANCER. — In patients with nonresectable large-bowel cancer the median survival is approximately 7 months, with 50% of the patients dying of local rather than distant metastases.[11]

Radiation therapy is an effective means of palliation for the subset of patients with rectal or rectosigmoid carcinoma, with relief of symptoms in at least 50% of cases and even occasional (5%) long-term survival.[12]

5-Fluorouracil, a chemotherapeutic antimetabolite, has been the standard agent for the management of advanced bowel cancer for more than 20 years. Yet the percentage of patients who respond has been consistently low (usually 15–20%), and the survival prolongation of the responders is less than 6 months.

Nevertheless, in a program designed to improve local control rates in patients with nonresectable tumors and to treat occult distant micrometastases, Moertel[13] compared radiation therapy (4,000 rads in 4 weeks) with radiation therapy plus just 3 injections of 5-FU. The 5-FU group had control of disease lasting twice as long as the radiation-alone group (10 months vs 5 months). Similar differences were observed in the survival of the two groups (16 months median for the 5-FU group vs 10.5 months for the radiation-alone group).

Recent programs utilizing the nitrosourea drug methyl-CCNU in combination with 5-FU have increased the response rate to 30–40% in patients with both advanced gastric carcinoma and advanced colorectal cancer.[14]

This combination is undergoing present evaluation in adjuvant programs for residual, recurrent or inoperable carcinomas of the rectum or rectosigmoid that are confined to the pelvis. The ECOG is exploring two forms of radiation therapy (standard vs split-course radiation therapy) with initial 5-FU and then the combination of 5-FU and methyl-CCNU for a maximum of 18 months (EST 3276).

CHEMOTHERAPY AS ADJUVANT FOR BOWEL CANCER. — The use of 5-FU as a systemic adjunct in attempts to eradicate microfoci of tumor cells has been studied by the VASAG with 5-year results that suggest some benefit for patients who underwent palliative resections but not for patients who underwent curative resections. The results were not statistically significant.[15] Several other studies have shown either negative or marginal effectiveness at periods of observation ranging from 18 months to 5 years. Hopefully, with potentially better chemotherapeutic regimens, such as 5-FU and methyl-CCNU, large numbers of carcinoma cells can be destroyed in micrometastases and, therefore, delay recurrence and prolong survival.

ADJUVANT THERAPY WITH NONSPECIFIC IMMUNOSTIMULANTS. — The potential for the use of immunotherapy in resected bowel cancer is obvious, just as it is in breast cancer. There is considerable evidence that immunotherapy is effective only when the tumor cell burden is low (10^5 cells or less).[16] Most current trials involve BCG (bacillus Calmette-Guerin), *Corynebacterium parvum* and MER (methanol-extracted residue of BCG). The rationale assumes that there exists a basic antitumor immunity that can be stimulated by these agents.

In addition, these agents can be combined with a tumor cell vaccine or a tumor antigen preparation to try to provoke specific antitumor immunity.

Most current immunotherapy trials for bowel cancer are in a very early stage with short follow-up periods. In the few studies published to date the use of historical rather than prospective controls makes it difficult to provide a meaningful interpretation. However, in one study conducted at M. D. Anderson Hospital[17] a significantly improved disease-free survival ($p<$ .05) has been demonstrated.

Osteogenic Sarcoma

One of the most dramatic examples of combined modality approach to malignancy has been the surgical chemotherapeutic management of osteogenic sarcoma. Prior to 1970 less than 25% of patients were cured by amputation. Formerly, at the Sidney Farber Cancer Center 80–90% of patients relapsed within 3–12 months after control of the primary tumor, almost invariably with pulmonary metastases. With the employment of aggressive chemotherapy, consisting of methotrexate, $3-7.5$ gm/M^2, with citrovorum rescue (MTX-CF), a significant alteration in the disease-free interval has been achieved. Eleven of 12 patients have been free of disease from 6–23 months with a median of 13-plus months.[18]

In another study Cortes and co-workers, utilizing doxorubicin (Adriamycin), an anthracycline antitumor antibiotic, reported that 60% of patients were expected to be disease-free 18 months after surgical resection.[19]

A major question remains to be answered. Does the adjuvant therapy merely delay the development of overt metastases with subsequent death, or are these micrometastases actually eradicated? An additional 3–5 years of follow-up will be necessary to answer this unequivocally, but the fact that many patients are alive and free of disease more than 1 year after discovery must be viewed as highly encouraging.

Lung Cancer

Since the majority of lung cancers are unresectable due to involvement of mediastinal and scalene nodes, the role of adjuvant programs continues to be very restrictive. In the past several years, however, considerable interest has developed in the use of combined modalities in small cell carcinoma of the lung (30–40% of all cases). No matter what the initial clinical pathologic stage of this cell type, the survival figures at 1 year are below 10%. The surgical mortality rate exceeds the surgical survival rate.[20] With apparent localized disease, close to 50% of patients will have bone marrow involvement.[21]

Since small cell carcinoma is highly sensitive to both radiation and chemotherapy, programs of regional radiation to encompass gross disease and chemotherapy to treat presumptive occult micrometastases have been developed. Two cooperative groups, the Radiation Therapy Oncology Group (RTOG) and the ECOG are currently exploring this combined approach versus the more standard treatment of radiation followed by chemotherapy at relapse (cyclophosphamide and a nitrosourea agent, lomustine [CCNU]. Prophylactic brain irradiation has been recommended by some because of the known high incidence of cranial metastasis (about 20%).

Brain Tumors

In contrast to other carcinomas, brain tumors have stimulated little interest among chemotherapists until very recently. The combination of inability to define a tumor response coupled with a lack of active agents has delayed progress in the treatment of such very aggressive tumors, particularly glioblastoma multiforme (astrocytomas, grade IV). The mainstay of therapy has been surgical resection followed by supervoltage radiation.

In the past 5 years, however, interest in the use of 2 nitrosourea agents, carmustine (BCNU) and CCNU, has become evident, since these agents readily enter normal brain tissue. In one study the use of BCNU as an adjunct improved survival from 37 weeks with radiation alone to a median of 40 weeks, not a striking difference, but suggestive of activity.[22] This slight increase in median survival is accompanied by a significant prolongation of useful life for approximately 20% of the BCNU-treated patients. In a disease that is as aggressive as glioblastoma multiforme a shift in the survival curve of only 1 month must be viewed as encouraging.

Nonseminomatous Testicular Cancers

Although a rare tumor, the social and economic impact of this cancer on a young and middle-aged male population demands an aggressive approach to staging and combined modality therapy. Following diagnosis, whole lung tomograms and bipedal lymphangiograms are usually performed. Most American urologists perform extensive retroperitoneal lymphadenectomy, and Staubitz and co-workers have demonstrated that this procedure is satisfactory to sterilize the area, obviating the need for radiation therapy.[23]

The dramatic regressions of pulmonary metastasis achieved with bleomycin and vinblastine by Samuels and associates with a significant number of complete remissions[24] and the previously demonstrated effectiveness of actinomycin D[25] in teratocarcinomas provide a unique opportunity to destroy foci of micrometastases that exist in from 20–40% of patients with stage B disease. Skinner has demonstrated an improvement in the 5-year survival figures for all stages with a combined adjuvant program of chemotherapy and regional radiation.[26] For stage A patients with a 5-year survival of 85–90% with surgery alone, the role of adjuvant therapy is not as well defined.

Breast Cancer

Cancer of the breast is the commonest malignant disease in women, with approximately 90,000 cases diagnosed annually in the United States. More than 50% have died of it up to now, regardless of therapy, with a higher rate in the first 3 years. The cause of this failure is occult metastasis present at the time of initial treatment, clearly demonstrated by Schabel and co-workers.[27] Even in the most favorable group of patients with no cancer in the axillary nodes, less than 70% will survive 10 years and the death rate for the subgroup, age 40–60, is 2–3 times greater than that of the general population.[28]

Early adjuvant trials were based on the assumption that tumor cells were released into the circulation at the time of surgery. Treatment consisted only of several days, usually with only a single agent, and results generally have been inconclusive. Based on the 53% response rate of advanced breast cancer with a 3-drug combination of cyclophosphamide, methotrexate and 5-fluorouracil (CMF) achieved by the ECOG, Bonadonna initiated the Milan trial of adjuvant treatment of breast cancer in 1973.[29]

Utilizing a life-table analysis at 24 months, 42% of the group of women who received radical mastectomy alone and had 4 or more positive nodes were disease-free in contrast to 95% of the CMF group. The percent of local recurrences in the CMF group is similar to that in the radiotherapy series.[29] The role of radiation therapy in preventing local recurrences in patients with positive axillary nodes is under reexamination. Concern has been raised that a "depression of natural defence mechanisms" by radiation may produce a higher than expected mortality in this group.[30] Hopefully, coordinated, carefully designed clinical studies will answer this concern, for this is the most efficient and quickest way to improve the quality of care for patients with breast cancer.

Summary

This review has not been encyclopedic but rather has highlighted those specific diseases where adjuvant programs have been introduced in the past 5 years. It is obvious that more and more patients with stage I and II disease are being referred by primary care physicians and surgeons for consideration of adjuvant oncotherapy programs.

The burden of the responsibility for the care and decision making is slowly shifting toward a multidisciplinary approach by a team of specialists. The goals must include optimal therapy with acceptable toxicity; the hopeful translation of improvement in disease-free survival into cures, and an awareness, by the establishment of a national data registry, of the potential long-term complications of these programs, including second malignancies.

REFERENCES

1. Fisher, B., et al.: L-PAM in the management of primary breast cancer, N. Engl. J. Med. 292:117, 1975.
2. Rosen, G., et al.: Disease free survival in children with Ewing's sarcoma treated with radiation therapy and adjuvant four day sequential chemotherapy, Cancer 33:384, 1974.

3. Price, R. A., and Johnson, W. W.: The central nervous system in childhood leukemia, Cancer 31:520, 1973.
4. Copeland, E. M., Miller, L. D., and Jones, R. S.: Prognostic factors in carcinomas of the colon and rectum, Am. J. Surg. 116:875, 1968.
5. Burt, C. A.: Carcinoma of the ovaries secondary to cancer of the colon and rectum, Dis. Colon Rectum 3:352, 1960.
6. Herrera, M., Chu, T. M., and Holyoke, E. D.: Carcinoembryonic antigen (CEA) as a prognostic and monitoring test in clinically complete resection of colorectal carcinoma, Am. Surg. 183:5, 1976.
7. Waldmann, T. A., and McIntire, K. R.: The use of a radioimmunoassay for alphafetoprotein in the diagnosis of malignancy, Cancer 34:1610, 1974.
8. Fletcher, W. S., Allen, C. V., and Dunphy, J. E.: Preoperative irradiation for carcinoma of the colon and rectum, Am. J. Surg. 109:76, 1965.
9. Kligerman, M. M.: Preoperative irradiation of rectosigmoid carcinoma including its regional lymph nodes, Am. J. Roentgenol. Radium Ther. Nucl. Med. 114:498, 1972.
10. Roswit, B., et al.: Preoperative irradiation for carcinoma of the rectum and rectosigmoid colon, Cancer 35:1597, 1975.
11. Gunderson, L. L., and Sosier, H.: Areas of failure at reoperation following "curative" surgery for adenocarcinoma of the rectum, Cancer 34:1278, 1974.
12. Whitley, H. W., Jr., and Stearns, M. W., Jr., et al.: Palliative radiation therapy in patients with cancer of the colon and rectum, Cancer 25:343, 1970.
13. Moertel, C. G., et al.: Combined 5-fluorouracil and supervoltage radiation therapy of locally irreversible gastrointestinal cancer, Lancet 2:865, 1969.
14. Moertel, C. G., et al.: Therapy of advanced colorectal cancer with combination of 5-FU, methyl-CCNU and vincristine, J. Natl. Cancer Inst. 54:69, 1975.
15. Higgins, G. A., et al.: Adjuvant chemotherapy in the surgical treatment of large bowel cancer, Cancer 38:1461, 1976.
16. Mathe, G., et al.: Active immunotherapy for acute lymphoblastic leukemia, Lancet 1:697, 1969.
17. Mauligit, G. M., et al.: Prolongation of postoperative disease free interval and survival in human colorectal cancer by BCG plus 5-fluorouracil, Lancet 1:871, 1976.
18. Jaffe, N., Frei, E., et al.: Adjuvant methotrexate and citrovorum factor treatment of osteogenic sarcoma, N. Engl. J. Med. 291:994, 1974.
19. Cortes, E. P., et al.: Amputation and Adriamycin in primary osteogenic sarcoma (CALGB-7181), Cancer Treatment Reports, 1976. In press.
20. Mountain, C. F.: Keynote address on surgery in the therapy for lung cancer, Cancer Chemother. Rep. 4:19, 1973.
21. Hansen, J. J., and Muggia, F. N.: Staging of inoperable patients with bronchogenic carcinoma, Cancer 30:1395, 1972.
22. Walker, M. D.: Chemotherapy adjuvant to surgery and radiation therapy, Semin. Oncol. 2:69, 1975.
23. Staubitz, W. J., et al.: Surgical management of testes tumor, J. Urol. 111:205, 1974.

24. Samuels, M. L., *et al.*: Bleomycin and combination chemotherapy in the management of testicular neoplasia, Cancer 36:318, 1975.
25. MacKenzie, A. R.: Chemotherapy of metastatic testis cancer: results in 154 patients, Cancer 19:1369, 1965.
26. Skinner, D. G.: Non-seminomatous testis tumors: A plan of management based on 96 patients to improve survival in all stages by combined therapeutic modalities, J. Urol. 115:65, 1976.
27. Schabel, F. M.: Concepts for systemic treatment of micrometastases, Cancer 35:15, 1975.
28. Fisher, B., *et al.*: Ten year follow-up results of patients with carcinoma of the breast in a co-operative clinical trial evaluating surgical adjuvant chemotherapy, Surg. Gynecol. Obstet. 140:528, 1975.
29. Bonadonna, G., *et al.*: Combination chemotherapy as an adjuvant treatment in operable breast cancer, N. Engl. J. Med. 294:405, 1976.
30. McDonald, A. M., *et al.*: Treatment of early cancer of the breast: Histological staging and role of radiotherapy, Lancet 1:1098, 1976.

Name Index

(Numbers in italics indicate original contributions to this volume.)

A

Aarseth, P., 213, 224
Abbott, W. M., 2, 62, 63, 64, 68
Abbruzzese, A., 266
Abel, R. M., 28, 62, 63, 64, 68
Abrams, J. S., 215, 223
Accurso, J., 211
Acland, R. D., 293, 331, 332
Adams, J. E., 338
Adkins, P. C., 215
Adson, M.A., 96
Agee, R. N., 224
Aguirre, A., 63, 65
Aiken, B., 210
Aldrete, J. A., 212, 221
Alexander, C. S., 167
Alexander, J. I., 219
Alexander, J. K., 217
Alexander, R. S., 216
Alexander-Williams, J., 98
Alfrey, C., 217
Ali, J., 215, 219
Alldred, A., 372
Allen, C. V., 383
Allen, C. V., 383
Allison, J. B., 67
Alpert, L. I., 97
Altschule, M. D., 220
Altug, K., 210
Ames, A., 66
Anderson, A. F., 96
Anderson, G. H., 63, 65
Anderson, J. T., 333
Anderson, M. W., 221
Anderson, R., 95, 96
Anderson, R. W., 180, 208, 214, 222
Anderson, W. R., 280, 281, 283
Anderson, W. T., 124 ·

Anscombe, A. R., 219
Aoki, T. T., 63
Aoyagi, F., 332
Arers, J. F., 126
Arima, E., 212, 220
Artz, C. P., 216
Asch, M. J., 64
Ashbaugh, D. G., 120, 123, 212
Ashbell, T. S., 167
Asher, W. M., 243, 263, 264, 265
Asuncion, Z., 208
Atkinson, A. J., Jr., 168
Attik, A., 67
Aubaniac, 2
Ault, G. W., 96
Ausinsch, M., 168
Austen, W. G., 62
Avello, F., 211
Avioli, L. V., 222
Axelrod, M. A., 217
Aylett, S. O., 72, 96

B

Babcock, J. B., 211
Babington, P. C., 211
Badger, F. C., 372
Baek, S. M., 123
Bakamjian, V. Y., 314, 332
Baker, A. B., 211
Baker, D. W., 266
Baker, J., 210
Baker, L. H., 168
Baker, W. N. W., 96
Baldessarini, R. J., 33, 63, 64
Balis, J. V., 209
Ballantine, T. V., 208
Ballard, B. E., 166
Banas, J. S., 217

385

Hepatotoxic drugs, 140–142
Hepatotoxicity: postoperative drug-
  induced, diagnosis of, 143–145
Hepatotoxins
  allergy and, 142
  cholestatic, indirect, 141–142
  cytotoxic, indirect, 140–141
  direct, 140
  hypersensitivity and, 142
Hollister ileostomy bag, 76
Hormones: and parenteral nutrition,
  9–10
Hyperalimentation, 1–69
  (See also Parenteral nutrition)
  at home, 55–56
  outpatient, 55–56
Hyperglycemia: common causes of, 53
Hypersensitivity: and hepatotoxins, 142
Hypertrophy: prostatic, ultrasonography
  of, 244
Hypokalemia: and parenteral nutrition,
  50–51
Hypomagnesemia: and parenteral
  nutrition, 51
Hyponatremia: and parenteral nutrition,
  50
Hypophosphatemia: and parenteral
  nutrition, 51

I

Ileorectal anastomosis
  recurrence of Crohn's disease after, 93
  in ulcerative colitis, 71–73
Ileosigmoid anastomosis: recurrence of
  Crohn's disease after, 93
Ileostomy
  bag
    Coloplast, 77
    Hollister, 76
  complications of, 77–78
  reservoir, 79–83
    construction of, 80
  stomal care, 76–77
  technique, 74–76
  trephine wounds for, 74
  in ulcerative colitis, 73–83
Ileum: narrowing of, in Crohn's disease,
  92
Ileus: prolonged, and parenteral
  nutrition, 30
Iliofemoral flap by microsurgery,
  312–313
  flap design, 313

Immunostimulants: as adjuvant in
  colonic cancer, 378–379
Inguinal mass: ultrasonography of, 260
Instruments, microinstruments, 290–291
  for microneural techniques, 302–303
Intestine
  large, Crohn's disease of, 87–96
  monitoring of, 121–122
Intracranial tumors: microsurgery of,
  325–326
Intralipid, 16
Intrauterine contraceptive device:
  ultrasonography of, 245

J

Joints
  carpometacarpal (see Carpometacarpal
    joints)
  metacarpal (see Metacarpal joints)
  metacarpophalangeal (see
    Metacarpophalangeal joints)
Jugular vein in parenteral nutrition, 40

K

Kidney
  artery embolism, 276
  bench surgery, in microsurgery, 331
  failure
    causes of, 113
    management, 21–23
    parenteral nutrition in, 20–23
    types of, 114
  function
    drug excretion and, 133–136
    monitoring of, 112–120
    monitoring of, tests for, 115
    tests of, 113
  mass lesions, ultrasonography of, 254
  polycystic, ultrasonography of, 253
  transplants, ultrasonography of,
    247–248
  ultrasonography of, 252–256

L

Lens: objective, for microsurgery, 288
Lidocaine infusion, 155–159
  nomogram to determine rate of, 158
Limb (see Extremities)
Lipid: intralipid, 16

edema, 240
masses, 242
normal, 239
pseudocyst, 241
of pelvis, 243–248
masses, 246
of prostate, 243–245
hypertrophy, 244
radiotherapy planning and, 258–259
of retroperitoneum, 248–257
of spleen, 242–243
abscess, 256–257
tomography and, computerized,
261–263
of uterus, 245–247
myoma, 245
of vena cava, 250–251
venacavography and, 251
Ultrasound (see Ultrasonography)
Urology (see Microsurgery, in urology)
Uterus
myoma, ultrasonography of, 245
ultrasonography of, 245–247

V

Vasoactive materials: in respiratory
distress syndrome, 193–195

Vasovasotomy: by microsurgery,
329–331
Veins
anastomosis, by microsurgery, 296
central (see Central venous)
jugular, in parenteral nutrition, 40
shunts, lymphnodocapsular, by
microsurgery, 300–301
subclavian, in parenteral nutrition, 39
Vena cava: ultrasonography of, 250–251
Venacavography: ultrasonic, 251
Ventilatory treatment: assessment of
adequacy of, 118–119
Vessels
changes, effect on oxygen delivery and
uptake, 149–151
diameter discrepancies, in
microsurgery, 296
disease, microsurgery of, 326–328
microvascular techniques in
microsurgery, 292–297
Vitamins
dosage during severe illness, 11
requirements in disease, 10

Z

Zinc deficiency: and parenteral nutrition,
51